CRASH COURSE
Gastroenterology
SECOND EDITION

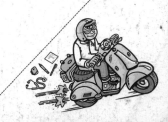

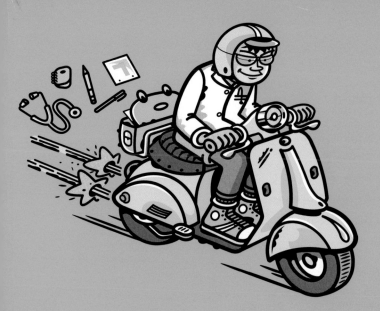

Series editor
Daniel Horton-Szar
BSc (Hons) MBBS (Hons)
GP Registrar
Northgate Medical Practice
Canterbury
Kent

Gastroenterology

SECOND EDITION

Christopher Fox
MBCh B (Hons) MRCP (Lond)
Specialist Registrar, Nottingham City Hospital, Nottingham

Martin Lombard
MD MSc FRCPi FRCP (Lond)
Consultant Physician and Gastroenterologist, Royal Liverpool University Hospital, and Senior
Lecturer in Medicine, University of Liverpool, Liverpool

First edition authors
Emma Lam, Martin Lombard

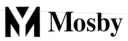 Mosby

Edinburgh • London • New York • Oxford • Philadelphia • St Louis • Sydney • Toronto 2004

MOSBY
An imprint of Elsevier Science Limited

Commissioning Editor: **Alex Stibbe, Fiona Conn**
Project Development Manager: **Fiona Conn**
Project Manager: **Frances Affleck**
Designer: **Andy Chapman**
Illustration Management: **Bruce Hogarth**

First edition 1999

Second edition 2004

ISBN 072343333X

British Library Cataloguing in Publication Data
A catalogue record for this book is available from the British Library

Library of Congress Cataloging in Publication Data
A catalog record for this book is available from the Library of Congress

Notice
Medical knowledge is constantly changing. Standard safety precautions must be followed, but as new research and clinical experience broaden our knowledge, changes in treatment and drug therapy may become necessary or appropriate. Readers are advised to check the most current product information provided by the manufacturer of each drug to be administered to verify the recommended dose, the method and duration of administration, and contraindications. It is the responsibility of the practitioner, relying on experience and knowledge of the patient, to determine dosages and the best treatment for each individual patient. Neither the publisher nor the authors assume any liability for any injury and/or damage to persons or property arising from this publication.
The Publisher

 ELSEVIER SCIENCE your source for books, journals and multimedia in the health sciences

www.elsevierhealth.com

The Publisher's policy is to use **paper manufactured from sustainable forests**

Typeset by SNP Best-set Typesetter Ltd, Hong Kong
Printed in Spain

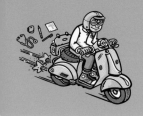

Preface

Having recently negotiated the daunting hurdles of medical finals and MRCP, I can certainly appreciate the value of a book such as this. The logical structure and friendly format provides enough detail for a distinction student, whilst simultaneously serving as a concise revision text.

I hope that, in addition to facilitating success with your undergraduate exams, it will also aid the transition to pre-registration house officer, and assist with the various gastrointestinal problems that you will undoubtedly face.

There is light at the end of the tunnel. This book will help prevent you becoming lost along the way!

Christopher Fox

Dispite their best intentions and notice of timetables, all students find that exams come too soon. *Crash Course* is written by people who've been there for people who are getting there! The clinical series is largely written by young doctors in training who have recently passed their exams and who know what you need to know to pass and excel in your exam. This book on gastroenterology tells you that, but I hope is comprehensive enough to give you even more—a good grounding in gastroenterology. It may therefore prove useful as a brief reference for forgotten facts even for those not doing exams. It doesn't pretend to give all of the detail required to practice gastroenterology, but should be used as a primer for those starting out in a career in gastroenterology and as a crash course for those coming up to examinations. The illustrations in this book pack in thousands more words than we could in the text and I hope you will enjoy learning from them.

Martin Lombard

Over the last six years since the first editions were published, there have been many changes in medicine, and in the way it is taught. These second editions have been largely rewritten to take these changes into account, and keep *Crash Course* up to date for the twenty-first century. New material has been added to include recent research and all pharmacological and disease management information has been updated in line with current best practice. We've listened to feedback from hundreds of medical students who have been using *Crash Course* and have improved the structure and layout of the books accordingly: pathology and disease management material has been moved closer to the diagnostic skills chapters; there are more MCQs and now we have Extended Matching Questions as well, with explanations of each answer. We have also included 'Further Reading' sections where appropriate to highlight important papers and studies that you should be aware of, and the clarity of text and figures is better than ever.

The principles on which we developed the series remain the same, however. Clinical medicine is a huge subject, and teaching on the wards can sometimes be sporadic because of the competing demands of patient care. The last thing a student needs when finals are approaching is to waste time assembling information from different sources, or wading through pages of irrelevant detail. As before, *Crash Course* brings you all the information you need in compact, manageable volumes that integrate an approach to common patient presentations with clinical skills, pathology and management of the relevant diseases. We still tread the fine line between producing clear, concise text and providing enough detail for those aiming at distinction. The series is still written by junior doctors with recent exam experience, in partnership with senior faculty members from across the UK.

I wish you the best of luck in your future careers!

Dr Dan Horton-Szar
Series Editor

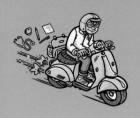

Acknowledgements

Grateful thanks to the following at Royal Liverpool University hospital for their helpful contributions and comments to this book: Dr Conall Garvey, Consultant Radiologist for all of the radiology pictures; Dr Fiona Campbell, Consultant Pathologist for all of the histology photomicrographs, and Tracy Norris for the graphs of oesophageal manometry and pH. We would also like to thank our mentors and students respectively for all that they have taught us and Emma Lam, the author of the first edition of Crash Course Gastroenterology.

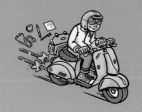

Dedication

For our families

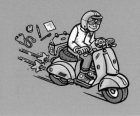

Contents

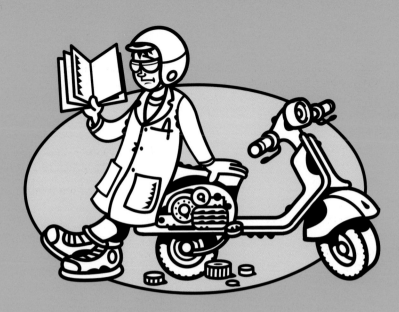

THE PATIENT PRESENTS WITH...

1. Indigestion

'Indigestion' encompasses a vast number of symptoms representing upper digestive tract problems with which a patient may present. These include:

- Heartburn.
- Fullness.
- Early satiety.
- Upper abdominal pain or ache.
- Flatulence.
- Hiccups.
- Belching.

The generic term that is useful to describe this constellation of symptoms is dyspepsia.
   Dyspepsia:
- Is very common and occurs in up to 10% of the adult population. At least half of these 10% seek advice from their family doctor.
- Accounts for 40% of referrals to gastroenterology clinics.

Dysphagia, or difficulty in swallowing, is dealt with separately.

History of the patient with indigestion

When taking a history from a patient with dyspepsia, it is useful to classify the problem according to the group of symptoms present, although this does not always correlate with the pathology. Dyspepsia is characterized as:

- 'Reflux-like', if heartburn or chest pain predominate.
- 'Ulcer-like', if the characteristics convey the impression of peptic ulcer disease. This can be confirmed by the presence of *Helicobacter pylori* in the gastric antrum (see Chapter 19).

'Non-ulcer dyspepsia' describes similar symptoms in the absence of *H. pylori*.

History of heartburn
Heartburn is the key to differentiating reflux-like dyspepsia from other forms. It is described as a

burning sensation which the patient locates retrosternally (behind the sternum). It is a diffuse and poorly localized sensation, typically worse on lying and leaning forward.

Excess saliva
'Waterbrash' is a specific phenomenon which the patient will describe as a flood of saliva in the mouth. Excess saliva is produced in the mouth and pharynx as a reflex response to acid in the lower oesophagus.

Chest pain
This is a common feature of gastro-oesophageal reflux.
   Pain due to heartburn often radiates between the shoulder blades. Oesophageal spasm more commonly causes chest pain, which occurs after a meal but can arise spontaneously. The pain is:

- Typically felt behind the sternum.
- Often severe.
- Sometimes described as 'something squeezing my inside'.

Unlike cardiac pain, oesophageal spasm tends not to be provoked by exertion. However, radiation of the pain to the jaw and left shoulder/arm can occur in severe cases. Exacerbation of the pain by changes in body position can be a helpful clue, since reflux symptoms are worse when lying flat or stooping forward and are often relieved by adopting an upright posture. Nausea and vomiting are uncommon with reflux, but can accompany myocardial infarction.

This pain is often confused with cardiac chest pain and, rather misleadingly, nitrates will relieve both spasm and angina, making it a diagnostic conundrum.

Other common causes of oesophageal spasm are:
• Underlying acid reflux.
• Achalasia.

A history of either condition should raise suspicion in someone presenting with atypical chest pain.

Other causes of chest pain are usually easy to differentiate. Pain due to pulmonary disease (pleural inflammation) is more often sharp or stabbing 'like a knife-cut', and is referred to as pleuritic. It is exacerbated by deep breaths and coughing, which does not affect pain of oesophageal origin.

Nocturnal cough/asthma

Some patients with severe acid reflux do not complain of heartburn or chest pain, but develop cough or wheeze during the night when they are lying flat. They often lack symptoms during the daytime. Characteristically, they will demonstrate a 'morning dip' in their peak-flow recordings (Fig. 1.1). The bronchospasm is thought to be due to microaspiration of acid, but a vagal reflex may also be involved because, experimentally, oesophageal acid-induced bronchospasm is ablated by vagotomy.

Asthmatics have a higher than average prevalence of heartburn. Increased intra-abdominal pressure may play a role, but some drugs such as theophylline reduce the lower oesophageal sphincter tone.

Aggravating and risk factors for reflux

The most important risk factor is increased intra-abdominal pressure (Fig. 1.2) which can 'squeeze' the stomach contents upwards and, ultimately, squeeze the stomach itself through the hiatus in the diaphragm (hiatus hernia).

Ask about lifestyle habits and medication as:
• Stooping and bending (occupation or sport) aggravate the problem.
• Spicy foods, or those with a high fat content, often aggravate the problem.
• Alcohol ingestion can result in increased acid secretion, delayed gastric emptying, and gastritis.
• Cigarettes often make reflux symptoms worse: nicotine causes smooth muscle relaxation in the lower oesophageal sphincter.
• Non-steroidal anti-inflammatory drug (NSAID) ingestion can interfere with prostaglandin cytoprotection.

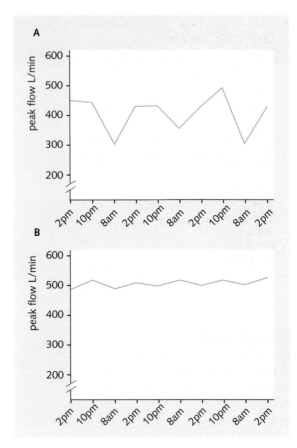

Fig. 1.1 (A) Peak flow measurement in an asthmatic demonstrating 'morning dip' due to acid reflux. (B) This was ablated when the patient took antisecretory medication before going to bed.

Risk factors for gastro-oesophageal reflux
increased intra-abdominal pressures
• sport e.g. weight lifting
• occupation e.g. stooping
• asthma
• obesity
• pregnancy
drugs
• alcohol
• cigarette smoking
• caffeine
• anti-cholinergics

Fig. 1.2 Risk factors for gastro-oesophageal reflux.

- Caffeine and theophylline cause relaxation of the lower oesophageal sphincter.
- Those drugs with an anticholinergic action can also lower oesophageal tone (e.g. neuroleptics).

For most patients, antacids will provide some form of relief and are readily available as an over-the-counter medication.

All of these dyspeptic symptoms constitute 'gastro-oesophageal reflux disease' (GORD).

A long history of heartburn followed by difficulty in swallowing (dysphagia), but improvement in the heartburn, may herald a fibrotic stricture in the lower oesophagus.

Epigastric pain

Epigastric pain is not a feature of GORD, but characterizes dyspepsia as 'ulcer-like'. It is a very common presenting complaint, but:

- The history is often vague.
- Sometimes patients have difficulty ascribing the term 'pain' to what they feel. The pain is often described as 'gnawing' or a persistent dull ache.

Pain due to:

- Peptic ulcer disease is occasionally more easily localized. The patient may point to a spot with one finger, although this is not a reliable sign.
- A gastric ulcer is often worse immediately after eating.

Peptic ulcers associated with NSAID use are usually painless and often present with occult bleeding.

Duodenal ulcer pain is:

- Commonly relieved by antacids.
- Worse at night, or in the fasted state, so the patient will often eat or drink milk before going to bed at night.

A family history is common. Find out about lifestyle habits such as smoking and alcohol consumption; these are important because they may contribute to

gastritis. Medication such as NSAIDs can also cause gastritis, erosions, and ulcers.

Epigastric pain presenting with weight loss may indicate gastric carcinoma and warrants urgent investigation.

Flatulence, belching, bloating, and early satiety

These symptoms are characteristically more vague. The term 'non-ulcer dyspepsia' is used to account for symptoms that occur in the absence of demonstrable acid reflux or *Helicobacter*-related disease (duodenal and gastric ulcer; duodenitis and gastritis).

Non-ulcer dyspepsia and peptic ulcer pain can be difficult to differentiate from other causes of acute and chronic abdominal pain (see Chapters 3 and 4). Some non-ulcer dyspepsia is thought to be due to abnormal motility or abnormal sensitivity of the upper gastrointestinal (GI) structures to distension.

Examining the patient with indigestion

Physical examination is usually unrevealing in the patient with reflux disease or oesophageal spasm.

Check for:

- Obesity or pregnancy—these may support a diagnosis of GORD.
- Chronic GI blood loss and signs of iron deficiency—these may be caused by ulceration of the oesophageal mucosa and may indicate chronic severe acid reflux, or alternative GI pathology.
- Tooth erosion by acid—this may be a sign of very severe reflux.

Cardiac pain can sometimes be very difficult to differentiate from the pain of GORD and associated spasm. Features that may predispose to ischaemic heart disease should be looked for, such as:

- Tar staining on the fingers.
- Obesity.
- Stigmata of hypercholesterolaemia, such as xanthomas.

Tenderness on deep palpation may indicate that the patient has 'ulcer-like' dyspepsia due to gastritis or ulcer disease. Careful examination is important to exclude other causes of abdominal pain.

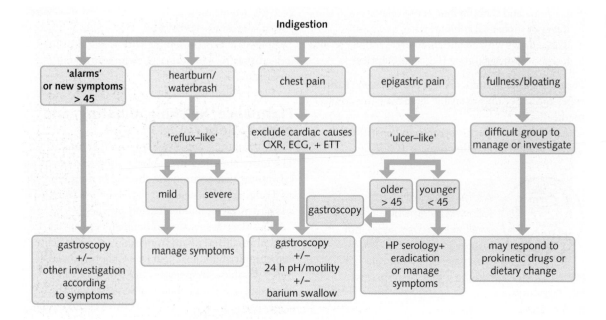

Fig. 1.3 Algorithm for the investigation of patients with dyspepsia. (CXR, chest X-ray; ECG, electrocardiography; ETT, exercise tolerance test; HP, *Helicobacter pylori*.)

Investigating indigestion

An algorithm for the investigation of the patient with indigestion is shown in Fig. 1.3.

In the majority of cases of reflux, the symptoms are mild and the diagnosis can often be made clinically and appropriate treatment commenced. More symptomatic cases may require investigation to exclude or confirm underlying oesophagitis. Any 'ALARMS' symptoms are an indication for urgent referral and investigation.

ALARMS symptoms in dyspepsia:
- Anaemia
- Loss of weight
- Anorexia
- Refractory to anti-secretory medication
- Melaena
- Swallowing problems
- Persistent continuous vomiting

Upper GI malignancy can also present with these symptoms, and therefore patients over 45 years of age with recent onset, persisting, dyspeptic symptoms should usually undergo prompt endoscopy (upper GI cancer is exceptionally rare under the age of 45 years except in familial cancer syndromes).

Many practitioners now use *Helicobacter* serology in association with the symptom of dyspepsia to identify those patients that may benefit from empiric eradication treatment for *Helicobacter* (see below).

Investigations to consider are discussed below.

Full blood count

A full blood count may be performed to exclude underlying anaemia. Microcytic anaemia is common with severe oesophagitis but rare in peptic ulcer disease. Plummer–Vinson syndrome comprises iron deficiency anaemia associated with an oesophageal web. A high platelet count can indicate chronic GI bleeding.

Electrocardiography

Electrocardiography is particularly useful for patients with atypical sounding pain that may be due to

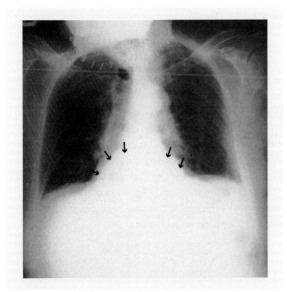

Fig. 1.4 Chest X-ray showing a hiatus hernia behind the cardiac shadow. (Incidentally shown on this X-ray are surgical staples around the neck following operative dissection.)

oesophageal spasm or angina pectoris. However, non-specific T-wave changes can occur with reflux. An exercise tolerance test may be necessary to differentiate between oesophageal and cardiac pain.

Occasionally, other investigations such as a thallium scan and coronary angiography are necessary to discriminate between cardiac and oesophageal symptoms.

Chest X-ray
A chest X-ray may demonstrate a hiatus hernia behind the cardiac shadow (Fig. 1.4).

Barium swallow
Barium swallow or scintigraphy is useful in demonstrating reflux. It can give rise to a 'corkscrew' appearance during an attack of spasm, and this is usually diagnostic (Fig. 1.5).

Oesophageal motility studies
These may be required to demonstrate the diffuse contraction and reduced peristalsis during a provoked attack. Pressures in the oesophagus can be exceedingly high, and the term 'nutcracker oesophagus' has been coined for these cases.

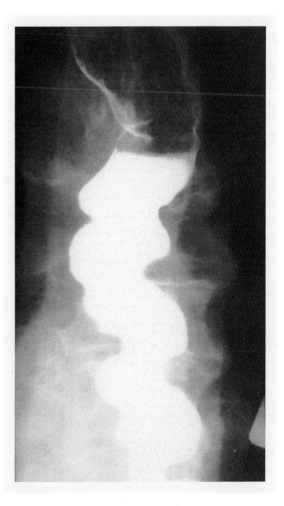

Fig. 1.5 Barium swallow demonstration of 'corkscrew' oesophagus caused by oesophageal spasm.

pH monitoring
pH monitoring is usually reserved for patients whose symptoms are more marked than expected from the endoscopic findings.

Breath tests
Breath tests have been devised to detect the presence of *H. pylori* without the requirement of endoscopy and biopsy (see Chapter 24).

Serology
Serology may be used to identify past infection with *H. pylori*. However, the immunoglobulin G antibody test gives no indication of current state of

infection and is not useful for assessing response to treatment.

Endoscopy

Endoscopy is useful for the assessment of the presence, extent and severity of oesophagitis. It may also be used to identify:

- Hiatus hernia—this may be noted on endoscopy but itself is not diagnostic of acid reflux because it is often an incidental finding, especially in elderly people.
- Ulcer disease and gastritis—biopsies can be taken to differentiate each type, exclude malignancy and also to look for the presence of *H. pylori*.

Barium meal

This is an alternative for patients for whom endoscopy may be difficult. It may demonstrate ulcer disease or malignancy. Oesophageal spasm tends not to be exercise-related. However, radiation of the pain to the jaw and left shoulder/arm can occur in severe cases, similar to cardiac pain. Change in severity of the pain in relation to body position is a helpful clue, since reflux symptoms will worsen when lying flat (e.g. in bed) or stooping forward (i.e. to pick something off the floor), and can be relieved when the patient sits or stands upright. Nausea or vomiting is unusual with reflux, but not uncommon with myocardial infarction.

Differential diagnosis

The patient will usually complain of difficulty swallowing or the sensation of food sticking as it goes down (dysphagia). Difficulty with the passage of food typically begins with solids like bread or meat, followed by liquids if the condition is progressive. The condition is usually painless and is due to a narrowing of the oesophageal lumen.

The differential diagnosis therefore includes, in order of importance:

- Oesophageal carcinoma.
- Achalasia.
- Benign oesophageal stricture.
- Oesophagitis.
- Oesophageal spasm.
- Failure of peristalsis due to other reasons (e.g. scleroderma).
- Oesophageal pouch or diverticulum.
- Oesophageal web.
- Incarcerated hiatus hernia.
- Foreign body obstruction.

Dysphagia is often unnoticed or even denied by patients until it becomes troublesome. They may also relieve their distress by changing posture, belching, regurgitating food, or by taking a drink.

History of the patient with swallowing problems

Taking a careful history of the presenting complaint is the key to sorting out the differential diagnosis. Important features to ask about are discussed below.

Duration of symptoms

A long or intermittent history, usually accompanied by manoeuvres to relieve the symptoms, often indicates anatomical or mechanical obstruction due to:

- Pouch.
- Diverticulum.
- Webs.
- Incarcerated hernia.

The first three are more common in younger adults; the last in elderly people.

Level at which dysphagia occurs

Attempt to determine the level at which dysphagia is experienced, as:

- High-level dysphagia can be due to cricopharyngeal spasm, a contraction of the cricopharyneus muscle and inferior constrictors, which is closely associated with pharyngeal pouch.
- Low-level dysphagia is more common with peptic strictures.
- Carcinoma occurs at all levels (Fig. 2.1).

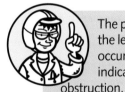

The patient's perception of the level at which dysphagia occurs is not a reliable indication of the level of obstruction.

Weight loss

Minor weight loss is common because patients may have modified their diet to cope with dysphagia. Significant weight loss is an ominous sign and almost always indicates carcinoma.

History of heartburn

A history of heartburn preceding the dysphagia is highly suggestive of benign oesophageal stricture, which often prevents further reflux.

Reflux

Reflux and dysphagia occurring together suggest achalasia, a condition in which there is uncoordinated

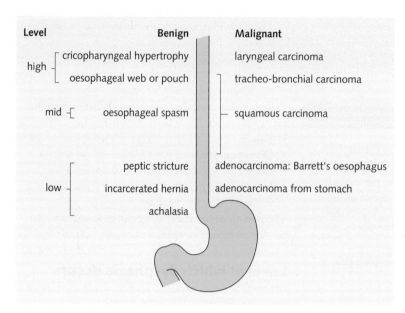

Fig. 2.1 Sites at which oesophageal lesions cause dysphagia. The patient will often describe the level of obstruction as high, mid-chest, or lower chest but this does not reliably correlate with site or nature of pathology.

oesophageal peristalsis and failure to relax the lower oesophageal sphincter. This tends to present in early adulthood with chest pain, occurring due to oesophageal spasm, which can be mistaken for cardiac pain.

Regurgitation of food

This is common if pouches are present. It differs from vomiting in that:
- There is an absence of nausea.
- Only small boluses are regurgitated back into the mouth and are often swallowed immediately.

Fluids are often more problematic than solids. Occasionally, dysphagia may be present because of obstruction by the pouch itself, but this is usually intermittent.

Regurgitation is not a feature of oesophageal carcinoma or benign strictures.

Recurrent pulmonary infections

Recurrent pulmonary infections resulting from aspiration can be due to:

- Achalasia.
- Pouches.
- Diverticula.

Progression of dysphagia

Progressive dysphagia is manifest by the patient finding increasing difficulty with soft foods or liquids, following difficulty with solids. This may occur over a relatively short duration (weeks or months) and is an ominous development, most often signifying an oesophageal carcinoma.

Pain with dysphagia

Pain on swallowing is termed odynophagia and may or may not be accompanied by dysphagia. Odynophagia may be caused by:

- Infection with *Candida*—this is the most common cause, and may result from underlying immunosuppression (e.g. corticosteroids or other immunosuppressive treatments, diabetes, malignancy, or immunodeficiency). Herpes and cytomegalovirus (CMV) infection of the oesophagus are more likely to be found in people infected with the human immunodeficiency virus (HIV).
- Impaction of a foreign body—this may cause dysphagia and will usually have an obvious history (e.g. fish bones represent the most common cause).

Oesophageal candidiasis should always prompt the clinician to look for underlying immunosuppression.

Pain between the shoulder blades in association with heartburn usually signifies oesophagitis.

A 'lump' in the throat can be due to pharyngitis, but is also a presentation of globus hystericus. Globus is a functional disorder that usually affects young females. True dysphagia of solids followed by difficulty with liquids is absent. A history suggestive of depression and/or anxiety can often be elicited, and it is important to establish the root of the patient's concern in order to allay unfounded fears (e.g. 'My father died of throat cancer, etc.').

 The diagnosis of globus should not be accepted without investigation and exclusion of more common or more sinister causes of dysphagia.

Important past medical history

Find out about the patient's past medical history, particularly:

- Risk factors for carcinoma—these include Barrett's oesophagitis, tylosis, and smoking.
- Chronic systemic diseases —neuromuscular disorders such as motor neuron disease, myasthenia gravis, and mytonia dystrophica are associated with disordered peristalsis.
- Collagen vascular disease, for example, scleroderma, which can interfere with the elasticity of the oesophagus and impair peristalsis.

Examining the patient with swallowing problems

Look out for:

- Weight loss—if marked, should give cause for concern; patients with carcinoma are often cachectic. A healthy, well-nourished patient with

a history of dysphagia usually indicates a benign aetiology, but not exclusively so.

- Anaemia—sometimes clinically evident, can occur with oesophagitis and classically has been a feature associated with oesophageal web (Plummer–Vinson or Paterson–Kelly syndrome). It is more common with malignant disease.
- Systemic features such as clubbing, tylosis (thickening of the palms of the hand and soles of the feet), supraclavicular lymph nodes, and hepatomegaly are suggestive of malignant disease in the context of dysphagia.
- An epigastric mass—may be palpable if the tumour extends into the cardia and certainly signifies extensive disease. However, there are no clinical signs that are specific for oesophageal carcinoma.

Investigating swallowing problems

It is imperative to investigate any patient who presents with dysphagia. A summary algorithm is shown in Fig. 2.2.

Full blood count and biochemistry

Full blood count and biochemistry should be performed to assess anaemia and, in severe cases, dehydration. Blood tests such as serum glucose and thyroid function test will exclude other causes of weight loss such as diabetes and thyrotoxicosis. Occasionally, a retrosternal goitre may cause dysphagia. Liver biochemistry and calcium levels may be deranged in advanced malignancy.

Endoscopy

Endoscopy is the investigation of choice for most patients with a history of dysphagia because, in addition to directly visualizing the oesophageal mucosa, biopsies can be undertaken to allow histological differentiation of benign and malignant lesions.

Laryngoscopy

This procedure may be necessary to investigate high causes of dysphagia.

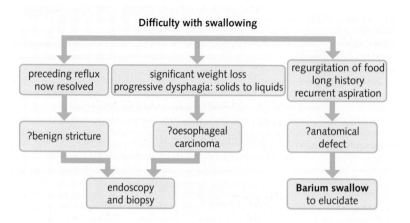

Difficulty with swallowing

preceding reflux
now resolved

significant weight loss
progressive dysphagia: solids to liquids

regurgitation of food
long history
recurrent aspiration

?benign stricture

?oesophageal
carcinoma

?anatomical
defect

endoscopy
and biopsy

Barium swallow
to elucidate

Fig. 2.2 Algorithm for the investigation of a patient with difficulty in swallowing.

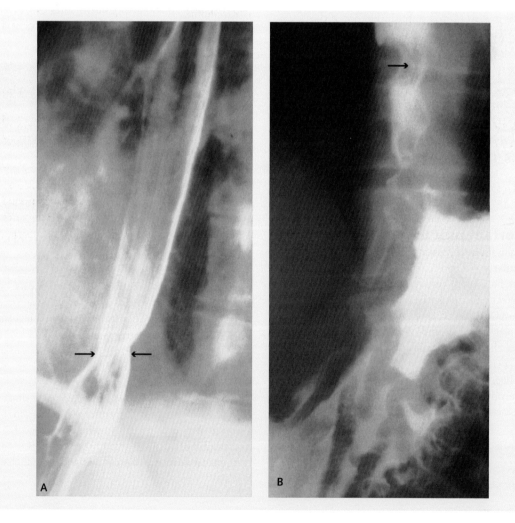

A

B

Fig. 2.3 (A) Barium swallow showing smooth tapering stricture of benign oesophageal type (arrows), and (B) the 'shouldered' appearance of malignant stricture (arrow) due to infiltration of the oesophagus from adenocarcinoma of the stomach cardia.

When endoscopy is unrevealing and dysphagia persists or is high level, a barium swallow should always be done as well.

Barium swallow

Barium swallow can be undertaken for patients who are unable to tolerate endoscopy, but appearances between benign and malignant strictures can be difficult to interpret. Generally:
- Benign strictures are smooth and tapering.
- Malignant strictures are irregular and 'shouldered' (Fig. 2.3).

Barium swallow is very useful in demonstrating anatomical anomalies such as:
- Pouches, usually high in the midline, caused by a defect in the overlapping muscle layers.
- Diverticula—usually small and associated with disordered peristalsis.
- Webs can be high at the cricopharyngeus or lower down the oesophagus.
- A Schatzki ring is a fibromuscular attachment originating from the diaphragm usually associated with a small hiatus hernia.

Barium swallow can be diagnostic of achalasia with the typical appearance of:
- A dilated oesophagus with no peristalsis.

- A narrowed lower oesophagus (bird's beak appearance) due to the failure of the lower oesophageal sphincter to relax (see Fig 14.6).

Achalasia is often missed at endoscopy.

Oesophageal motility studies

These are useful to confirm spasm or achalasia. Twenty-four hour oesophageal pH monitoring is useful to confirm acid reflux (see Figs 24.9 and 24.10).

Chest X-ray

A chest X-ray, often forgotten, provides useful information about patients with swallowing problems, especially those who present with pneumonia. A dilated oesophagus can be seen as a double cardiac shadow with a fluid level behind the heart.

Other investigations

Occasionally, the cause of dysphagia may be difficult to find.

Bronchoscopy or a computed tomography (CT) scan may be required if tracheobronchial carcinoma is suspected.

Patients found to have a malignant stricture will need to be assessed for surgical resection. Gross metastatic spread can be identified by ultrasound of the liver or CT scan of the thorax. For loco-regional spread, endoscopic ultrasound is the best single staging test.

3. Acute Abdominal Pain

Acute abdominal pain is a common presentation in clinical medicine and often the most difficult to deal with. It usually refers to pain of sudden onset and a duration of less than 48 hours.

It is important to organize management (e.g. intravenous access, analgesia, etc.) at the same time as attempting to make a diagnosis.

The differential diagnosis of acute abdominal pain includes:
- Acute peptic ulceration.
- Biliary colic.
- Acute cholecystitis.
- Acute pancreatitis.
- Acute appendicitis.
- Acute diverticulitis.
- Perforation of abdominal viscus.
- Bowel obstruction.
- Acute renal colic, pyelonephritis or acute urinary retention.
- Acute infarction of bowel, spleen, or kidney.
- Myocardial infarction occasionally presents with acute upper abdominal pain (particularly in the elderly).
- Acute hepatic vein thrombosis (Budd–Chiari syndrome).
- Lower lobe pneumonia can present with referred abdominal pain.
- Rupture of an abdominal aortic aneurysm.
- Metabolic causes: diabetic ketoacidosis, Addison's disease, acute intermittent porphyria.
- Gynaecological causes: ectopic pregnancy, acute salpingitis, ovarian cyst rupture.

History of the patient with acute abdominal pain

A carefully elicited history is vital in helping to discern the cause of acute abdominal pain. The following points should be considered.

Site of pain
The site of pain gives the most important clue to its cause (see Fig. 21.1). Acute epigastric pain is suggestive of:
- Peptic ulcer disease.
- Acute pancreatitis.
- Biliary colic.

By contrast, acute lower abdominal pain is suggestive of:
- Gynaecological problems (e.g. acute salpingitis).
- Acute appendicitis.
- Acute diverticulitis.
- Acute urinary retention.

Particular sites of pain tend to be associated with specific conditions, for example:
- Pain in the right iliac fossa due to appendicitis.
- Pain in the right upper quadrant due to acute cholecystitis.
- Pain in the left iliac fossa due to acute diverticulitis.
- Pain in the loin due to renal colic.

Generalized pain is more likely to be due to a metabolic cause or peritonitis from perforation or infarction.

Radiation of pain
Pain due to certain conditions characteristically radiates to particular sites. For example:
- Pancreatic pain radiates 'through' to the middle of the back.
- Gall bladder pain commonly radiates around the right side to the back.

- Myocardial pain, when caused by ischaemia in the diaphragmatic surface, radiates to the epigastrium.
- Renal pain starts in the loin but radiates to the groin.

Character of the pain

The character may be difficult to ascertain and is not always reliable, but the following may be useful:
- 'Colicky' describes pain that builds to a crescendo and subsides. It is characteristic of hollow organ pain (e.g. distension of the bowel, bile duct, or ureter wall in obstruction). It implies spasm of the smooth muscle wall of the viscus, often due to obstruction (e.g. ureteric calculus).
- A sharp stabbing pain worsened by movement or respiration suggests pleural or peritoneal irritation (e.g. peritonitis from acute appendicitis or cholecystitis).

Generalized peritonitis has a similar characteristic, but is less well localized and is seen with perforation or ruptured aortic aneurysm.

Relieving and exacerbating factors

These are not often helpful in the acute situation. With any painful condition, the patient will usually adopt the most comfortable posture:
- Peptic ulcer disease may reveal a history of pain exacerbated or relieved by food.
- Acute pancreatitis is classically relieved by sitting forward while holding the abdomen.
- Vomiting may relieve the pain of bowel obstruction.

Past medical history

Past history and risk factors are important, for example:
- In an elderly patient with known abdominal aortic aneurysm, a sudden onset of abdominal pain may be due to rupture.
- A patient with a history of constipation may present with acute obstruction.

Risk factors for acute pancreatitis include:
- Gallstones.
- Alcohol.

- Recent endoscopic retrograde cholangiopancreatography (ERCP).

A menstrual history accompanied by a urinary human chorionic gonadotrophin test is essential to exclude the possibility of a ruptured ectopic pregnancy.

Family history

This may be relevant (e.g. porphyria is a hereditary condition that commonly presents with acute abdominal pain).

Examining the patient with acute abdominal pain

A general inspection can reveal a lot about your patient while you are taking the history and instigating management. Decide whether the patient looks 'ill'. This is a good indicator of serious underlying pathology. Other pointers are:
- Is the patient lying still with shallow breathing (generalized peritonitis)?
- Is the patient agitated and restless (colicky pain) or holding a particular part of the abdomen (localized peritonitis)?
- Is the patient tachycardic, peripherally cool and/or hypotensive, suggesting hypovolaemic shock (ruptured abdominal aneurysm, ectopic pregnancy)?
- Is there any external bruising (acute pancreatitis)?
- Is the patient tachypnoeic (a sign of significant metabolic acidosis)?
- Is there a fever indicative of an infective or inflammatory process?

Guarding and rebound tenderness

If the patient tends to hold the abdominal muscle rigid (guarding), this may suggest peritonitis is present. The abdomen will be tender but the patient will allow gradual gentle pressure. Sudden removal of the palpating hand produces rebound tenderness—this is an important sign of peritonitis which can also be elicited by the patient being reluctant to 'blow out' the abdomen to touch your hand positioned at about 5 cm above the resting abdomen.

Site of tenderness

If tenderness is more localized, think of the underlying structure, for example:

- Appendix in the right iliac fossa.
- Descending colon in the left iliac fossa.
- Ovaries in lower abdomen.
- Stomach or pancreas in the upper abdomen.

Beware of a ruptured abdominal aortic aneurysm masquerading as a history of renal colic, particularly in older patients with arterial disease.

Pulsation

A pulsating or expansile mass may suggest an aortic aneurysm but, in some cases of rupture, the pulsation may be absent. Peripheral pulses should be palpated.

Distension

Acute obstruction of small or large bowel can cause painful abdominal distension with a resonant percussion note. In the presence of chronic liver disease, ascites may be present and can become infected (spontaneous bacterial peritonitis, SBP). Acute onset of painful ascites is sometimes seen in hepatic vein thrombosis (Budd–Chiari syndrome).

Hernial orifices and male genitalia

Examination of the hernial orifices (inguinal and femoral) is important to exclude the possibility of an incarcerated hernia giving rise to small bowel obstruction. Testicular torsion can also manifest as lower abdominal pain.

Internal examination

Rectal examination is essential to exclude melaena from acute upper gastrointestinal ulceration. Constipation may give a clue about obstruction or a

tender rectal examination may be due to a locally inflamed retrocaecal appendix.

Vaginal examination may be indicated in certain circumstances (e.g. a tender fornix may suggest torsion or rupture of an ovarian cyst).

Investigating acute abdominal pain

Investigations are usually important to confirm your diagnosis or to determine the severity of the illness.

Full blood count

A full blood count may aid diagnosis:

- A raised white cell count may support a diagnosis of underlying sepsis or peritonitis, but is relatively non-specific. There may be haemoconcentration due to dehydration, manifest by a high/normal haemoglobin and supported by an elevated urea.
- Platelets will be high in inflammatory disease or chronic gastrointestinal blood loss.
- A low haemoglobin should raise suspicion of bleeding in association with the acute abdominal pain.

Biochemistry

Specific biochemical tests and their correct interpretation in the context of acute abdominal pain can be very helpful:

- A raised amylase is important to support a diagnosis of acute pancreatitis, but it can be slightly raised in cholecystitis, biliary colic, ectopic pregnancy, perforated peptic ulcer and other intra-abdominal catastrophes.
- Urea and electrolytes may be disturbed if the patient is ill or dehydrated. The combination of hyperkalaemia with hyponatraemia should suggest the possibility of Addison's disease.
- A high sugar with acidosis in a patient with acute abdominal pain may be due to diabetic ketoacidosis.
- Raised liver enzymes may point to a diagnosis of obstructive jaundice due to gallstones or acute cholestasis associated with Budd–Chiari syndrome.
- Hypercalcaemia can cause constipation and abdominal pain.

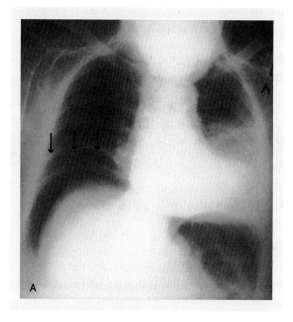

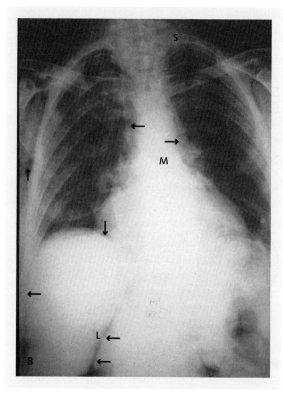

Fig. 3.1 Chest X-rays. (A) A patient with acute abdominal pain due to visceral perforation. Air under the diaphragm is more obvious on the right side above the liver (arrows). (B) A patient with retroperitoneal perforation: arrows show where air tracks up around the liver (L), into the mediastinum (M), and subcutaneously (S) (felt as crackling under the skin).

- Urine analysis may reveal haematuria suggestive of renal colic, or nitrites and leucocytes indicative of a urinary tract infection.
- Urinary porphyrin estimation has been superseded by measurement of specific enzyme activity in the blood.
- A pregnancy test is mandatory in women of a child-bearing age.
- C-reactive protein is a sensitive acute phase protein indicative of ongoing infection or inflammation and it would be unusual for this to be normal in any significant cause of acute abdominal pain.

A low venous bicarbonate or arterial blood gas analysis consistent with metabolic acidosis is suggestive of acute intraabdominal pathology (e.g. bowel infarction, pancreatitis or peritonitis).

Radiology

An erect chest radiograph is essential to exclude air under the diaphragm, indicative of a perforated intraabdominal viscus (Fig. 3.1).

A plain abdominal X-ray may reveal:
- Dilated bowel loops indicative of obstruction (Fig. 3.2).
- Faecal loading associated with constipation or obstruction.
- Calcification in gallstones, ureteric stones (commonly radio-opaque), or aortic aneurysm.

Ultrasound is not routinely performed as an emergency, but may be helpful in confirming:
- Dilated bile ducts due to stones.
- Stones in gallbladder.
- Congested liver (Budd–Chiari).
- Ovarian cysts.

A computed tomography scan similarly is rarely needed in the emergency situation, but can be useful when the diagnosis is not apparent (e.g. ruptured

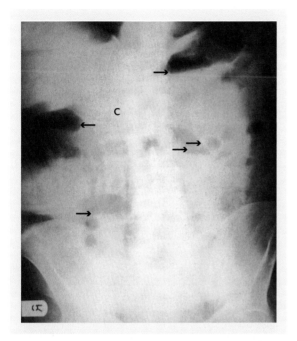

Fig. 3.2 Abdominal X-ray from a patient with intestinal obstruction, showing fluid levels in the bowel (arrows), a grossly distended caecum (C), and a collapsed colon.

liver or renal cysts), or if a ruptured aortic aneurysm is suspected.

Electrocardiography

All patients who present with chest or abdominal pain should have an electrocardiogram to exclude myocardial infarction (Fig. 3.3). Some T-wave changes are non-specific and can be seen in many causes of acute abdominal pain, although ultimately cardiac enzyme levels may need to be measured to exclude myocardial injury.

Endoscopy

Gastroscopy may be indicated if peptic ulcer disease is suspected but would be contraindicated in many causes of acute abdominal pain (e.g. perforation).

Urgent ERCP may be indicated for suspected gallstone pancreatitis or acute cholangitis. This would usually follow ultrasound examination.

In both conditions, emergency sphincterotomy has been shown to be effective.

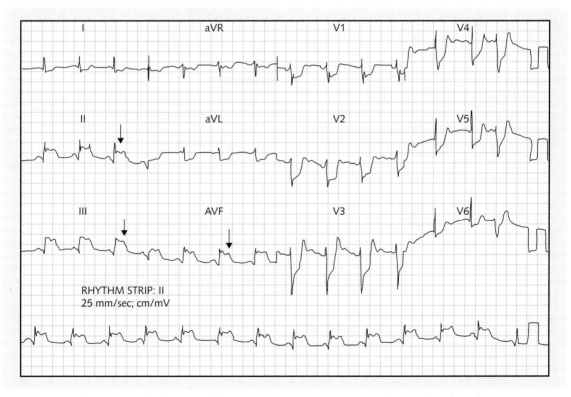

Fig. 3.3 Electrocardiogram from a patient presenting with acute abdominal pain. ST segment elevation in leads II, III, and AVF (arrows) supports a diagnosis of inferior myocardial infarction.

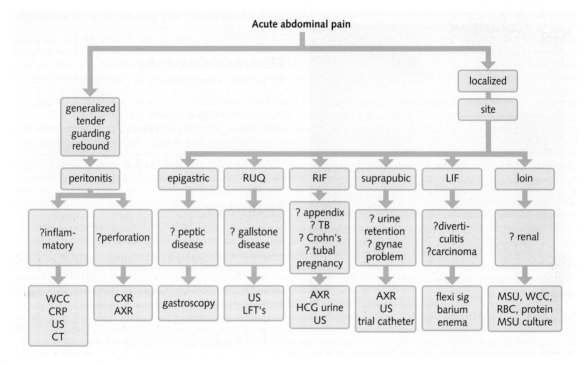

Fig. 3.4 Algorithm for the investigation of acute abdominal pain. (WCC, white cell count; CRP, C-reactive protein; US, ultrasound; CT, computed tomography; CXR, chest X-ray; AXR, abdominal X-ray; LFTs, liver function tests; HCG, human chorionic gonadotrophin (pregnancy test); RUQ, right upper quadrant; LIF, left iliac fossa; RIF, right iliac fossa; MSU, midstream urine; RBC, red blood cells.)

Surgery

Many of the causes of acute abdominal pain are surgical emergencies. Occasionally, no cause is apparent and diagnostic laparotomy or laparoscopy can be useful in these situations (e.g. peritonitis of uncertain cause).

Summary

An algorithm summarizing the investigation of acute abdominal pain is shown in Fig. 3.4.

4. Chronic Abdominal Pain

Chronic abdominal pain is a common complaint that accounts for about 40% of referral to gastroenterology outpatient clinics. The symptoms are often of an intermittent nature, with pain-free periods in between. The list of differential diagnoses is vast, and only those commonly seen in clinical practice are discussed here. There is considerable overlap between some of these symptoms and 'indigestion' discussed in Chapter 1, but pain is not really a prominent symptom in dyspepsia and is discussed in more detail here.

The common differential diagnoses for chronic abdominal pain include:
- Peptic ulcer disease.
- Chronic pancreatitis.
- Chronic cholecystitis.
- Chronic appendicitis.
- Irritable bowel syndrome.
- Constipation.
- Subacute bowel obstruction.
- Crohn's disease.
- Intestinal malignancy.
- Mesenteric ischaemia.
- Gynaecological causes (e.g. endometriosis, pelvic inflammatory disease).

History of the patient with chronic abdominal pain

As with acute abdominal pain, a detailed history is essential to focus the differential diagnosis. Several important features need to be discovered, and these are discussed below.

Site and radiation of the pain
The most obvious clue to the aetiology is the site of the pain and its radiation.

Chronic pain in the upper abdomen is suggestive of:
- Peptic ulcer disease.
- Chronic cholecystitis.
- Chronic pancreatitis.

Pain at particular sites may be even more specific:
- Pain in the right upper quadrant is commonly of liver or biliary origin.
- Pain in the right iliac fossa may suggest Crohn's disease (terminal ileal disease).
- Pain in the loin may be due to chronic pyelonephritis.
- Pain in the lower abdomen is usually due to colonic or gynaecological problems.

Character
The character of chronic pain is often vague, but certain features are helpful:
- Most chronic abdominal pain is described as a dull ache which is suggestive of visceral peritoneal involvement (e.g. chronic pancreatitis, intestinal malignancy, gynaecological causes).
- Sharp, stabbing, or colicky pain may be associated with distension of a viscus (e.g. biliary colic, constipation, or irritable bowel syndrome).

Take a history of each episode of pain. Has hospital admission been necessary? Evaluation of old medical notes can be very revealing.

Exacerbating and relieving factors
These are sometimes helpful. The patient may have had the pain for some time and may have experimented with ways to relieve or exacerbate the pain, such as with food or alcohol.

Food can have the following effects:
- It may aggravate biliary causes, characteristically occurring 20–30 minutes after a meal, and there may be fat intolerance, although this is not specific for a particular diagnosis.
- With mesenteric ischaemia ('abdominal angina'), the patients may notice that pain occurs 1–2 hours after food and this results in a reluctance to eat, for fear of pain.
- It can relieve the pain of a duodenal ulcer, particularly if the patient drinks milk at bedtime.

Alcohol:
- Worsens chronic pancreatitis and gastritis, but the patient does not always modify his or her behaviour.

Defaecation or passage of flatus:
- Relieves lower abdominal pain due to constipation or irritable bowel.
- May exacerbate pain due to local inflammatory conditions of the anus or rectum, or in obstruction.

Menstruation:
- Painful periods should be obvious but ectopic areas of endometriosis may also induce pain at time of menstruation.
- Pain in mid-cycle can occur with ovulation ('mittelschmerz') or occasionally with ovarian cysts.

Associated features

Patients may not notice other symptoms or realize their significance in relation to the pain. It is therefore important to ask specifically about:
- Distension or bloating—if intermittent, this is suggestive of irritable bowel syndrome or subacute obstruction; if progressive, it may indicate development of a mass or ascites.
- Weight loss—think of underlying malignancy (i.e. pancreatic or intestinal), especially in elderly patients. In younger patients, think of Crohn's disease or lymphoma. Weight loss may also result from avoidance of food.
- Change in bowel habit—alternating constipation or diarrhoea may be due to a change in diet but intestinal malignancy must be excluded in patients aged over 45 years.
- Rectal bleeding—may signify an underlying inflammatory or malignant process (see Chapter 10).
- Vaginal discharge—pelvic inflammatory disease is something the patient may be embarrassed to volunteer information about.

Many patients will be reluctant to reveal their level of alcohol consumption. Careful questioning is often required! Try to ascertain their habit from several angles.

Examining the patient with chronic abdominal pain

On general inspection, important features to note include:
- Obvious signs of weight loss.
- Pigmentation, pallor or jaundice.
- Signs of dehydration.

In the neck, look for:
- Lymphadenopathy, particularly in the supraclavicular regions.
- Goitre.

Abdominal inspection and palpation may reveal:
- Scars from previous surgery—patients occasionally omit information about previous operations.
- Distension—is it uniform due to ascites or asymmetrical due to a mass?
- Peristalsis may be obvious in thin people with intestinal obstruction.
- A mass may be present, and its anatomical location usually indicates the aetiology (e.g. epigastric in gastric malignancy, right iliac fossa in Crohn's disease, or an appendix mass).
- Stigmata of chronic alcohol misuse may be present (spider naevi, umbilical varices and other signs of chronic liver disease).

Other features to note are:
- Signs of peripheral vascular disease which may accompany mesenteric ischaemia.
- Tenderness in the fornix or vaginal discharge, suggesting pelvic inflammatory disease.
- Rectal examination should always be performed for patients with lower abdominal pain.

Investigating chronic abdominal pain

Full blood count

Anaemia may be due to blood loss giving rise to a microcytic hypochromic picture of iron deficiency. In malignant or inflammatory disease, a normocytic anaemia may also occur. Raised white cell count is indicative of underlying infection or inflammation. Platelets can be raised in chronic inflammatory disease or chronic gastrointestinal blood loss.

Iron deficiency anaemia in the context of chronic abdominal pain should always prompt endosopic examination of either the upper or lower gastrointestinal tract (or both—in context with the clinical findings).

Biochemistry

Often a range of biochemistry tests is undertaken as a routine, but is essential to interpret these in the clinical context. The following may be helpful:

- Electrolytes can be disturbed if diarrhoea or vomiting have occurred (e.g. low potassium).
- Calcium can be raised in malignant disease, but hypercalcaemia for other reasons (e.g. hyperparathyroidism) may also cause chronic abdominal pain.
- Amylase can be raised slightly and non-specifically with many causes of abdominal pain. It is usually normal in chronic pancreatitis, in contradistinction to acute pancreatitis.
- Liver enzyme abnormalities are common with cholangitis or gallstone problems.
- Urea may be raised if dehydration is present, or low if the patient has been anorectic, has malabsorption or has liver disease.
- A thyroid function test should be performed because hypothyroidism is an occasional cause of abdominal pain.
- Tumour markers such as CEA or CA19.9 may be useful, but need to be interpreted in context.

Radiology

Although often unrevealing, a plain abdominal radiograph may reveal:

- Calcification indicative of chronic pancreatitis, gallstones, or aortic aneurysm (Fig. 4.1).
- Faecal loading suggestive of chronic constipation.
- Dilated bowel indicative of subacute obstruction.

Abdominal ultrasound is useful to identify:

- Gallstones causing chronic cholecystitis or bile duct obstruction.

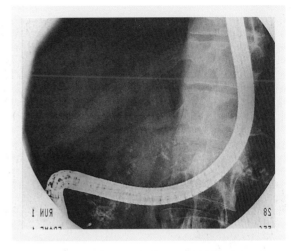

Fig. 4.1 Abdominal calcification is seen across the pancreatic area in a pre-injection endoscopic retrograde cholangiopancreatogram.

- Liver metastases which commonly arise from colon or breast (Fig. 4.2).
- Chronic pancreatitis or carcinoma of the body of pancreas.

Intra-abdominal lympadenopathy—suggesting lymphoma or metastatic disease
Contrast studies can be helpful:

- Small bowel barium enema can be used to identify stricture in the terminal ileum due to Crohn's disease.
- Large bowel barium enema is used to confirm diverticular disease or exclude colonic carcinoma.

Computed tomography of the abdomen may be required to visualize chronic pancreatitis or pancreatic carcinoma and to search for, or stage, lymphoma.

Endoscopy

Gastroscopy is useful to investigate dyspepsia (see Chapter 1) and to exclude gastric carcinoma. Colonoscopy may be required to confirm diverticular disease or to exclude colonic carcinoma.

Surgery

Despite extensive (and sometimes expensive!) investigation, no cause for chronic abdominal pain

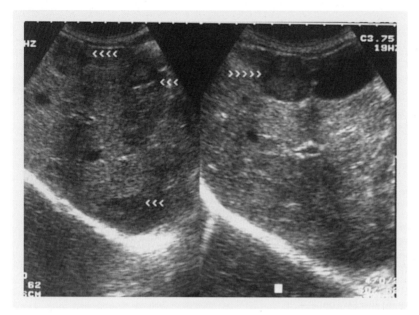

Fig. 4.2 Ultrasound scan showing multiple areas of different echogenicity and size in the liver suggestive of metastases.

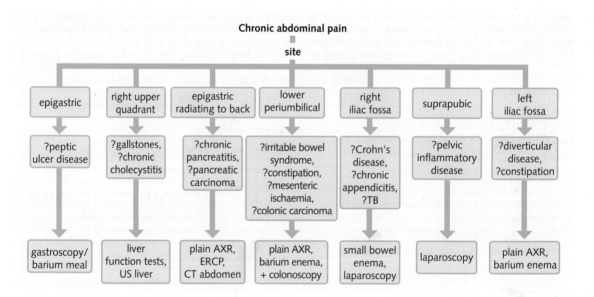

Fig. 4.3 Algorithm for the investigation of chronic abdominal pain. (AXR, abdominal X-ray; CT, computed tomography; ERCP, endoscopic retrograde cholangiopancreatography; US, ultrasound.)

may be found. In this situation, and after careful consideration, a diagnostic laparoscopy can be useful (e.g. to identify endometriosis).

Summary

An algorithm summarizing the investigation of chronic abdominal pain is shown in Fig. 4.3.

5. Abdominal Distension

Swelling of the abdomen rarely presents in isolation: it usually accompanies other symptoms such as abdominal pain, diarrhoea, jaundice or weight loss.

History of the patient with abdominal distension

Patients may complain that their abdomen is abnormally distended. They may have noticed that their clothes are fitting too tightly. Others may have commented that they have put on weight or look pregnant.

Occasionally, patients do not realize they have abdominal distension until it is detected on physical examination. Several specific features in the history can give important clues to the aetiology or pathogenesis.

Traditionally, all medical students are taught abdominal distension is caused by Fat, Faeces, Flatus, Fluid, or Foetus (the five Fs) and, although this is not strictly accurate, it is worth remembering, especially when one comes across a difficult examiner!

Onset of symptoms
The onset may give a clue about its cause:
- Distension caused by ascites often takes several days or weeks to develop and progresses with time (Fig. 5.1).
- Acute abdominal distension accompanied by pain suggests the diagnosis of Budd–Chiari syndrome (i.e. hepatic vein thrombosis).
- Distension due to acute bowel obstruction may only have a relatively short period of onset (i.e. 12–24 hours) and will have associated features such as vomiting, abdominal pain and absolute constipation.

- Menstrual history is important in women of child-bearing age: unexpected pregnancies occur and have occasionally gone unnoticed or been denied, even up to full term.
- Intermittent distension is suggestive of subacute obstruction or, more commonly, irritable bowel syndrome, in which patients obtain relief from opening their bowels.

Bowel habit
Abdominal distension due to gastrointestinal disease will usually be associated with a disturbance of gastrointestinal function.

A long history of constipation may suggest that the distension is due to faeces. In severe cases, subacute or acute obstruction occurs and the distension is further aggravated by flatus. Abdominal pain and vomiting may also be a prominent feature.

Alternating diarrhoea and constipation associated with intermittent distension and borborygmi are highly suggestive of irritable bowel syndrome.

Past history
As always, the patient's past medical history can give helpful clues:
- A history of liver disease may suggest ascites.
- Pericardial disease due to rheumatic fever in the past, or even tuberculosis, can produce constrictive pericarditis, and is often forgotten as a cause of ascites.
- Cardiac failure can also cause ascites.
- Nephrotic syndrome can result in hypoalbuminaemic ascites.

A family history may be important (e.g. polycystic kidney or polycystic liver disease, which can produce distension if cysts are large). The condition is autosomal dominant.

Examining the patient with abdominal distension

On general examination, several features can be helpful:

Causes of ascites	
High protein (exudative)	**Low protein (transudative) >10 g⁻ less than serum albumin**
• intra-abdominal malignancy (primary or secondary) • infection (especially TB) • pancreatitis • Budd–Chiari syndrome	• hypoalbuminaemia (from any cause e.g. nephrotic syndrome) • cirrhosis • cardiac failure or constrictive pericarditis

Fig. 5.1 Causes of ascites—differentiated by protein concentration of ascitic fluid. Protein level should be compared to serum albumin concentration, and correlated with cell count, culture, cytology and amylase level in fluid.

- Presence of jaundice, parotitis, or encephalopathy suggests the possibility of liver-related ascites.
- The patient may not be able to lie down flat for the examination due to pulmonary oedema, secondary to congestive cardiac failure.

- Truncal obesity together with abdominal striae may alert one to the diagnosis of Cushing's disease.
- A paradoxical rise in the jugular venous pulse on inspiration may suggest constrictive pericarditis, and the heart sounds may be diminished.

On examination of the abdomen:

- Look for any asymmetry present—is the lower abdomen more distended? This may be the case in pregnancy, urinary retention, ovarian tumour or fibroids protruding from the pelvic cavity (Fig. 5.2).
- Look for scars that may be present—has the patient had previous surgery for malignancy or obstruction?
- Faecal loading is often palpable over the descending colon and can be indented, unlike a malignant mass.
- Hepatosplenomegaly may be evident if underlying cirrhosis or right ventricular failure is present.
- A rectal examination is mandatory for masses arising from the pelvis.
- Supplemental vaginal examination may be required if an ovarian or uterine origin is suspected.

		Possible diagnoses
Abdominal distension arising out of pelvis	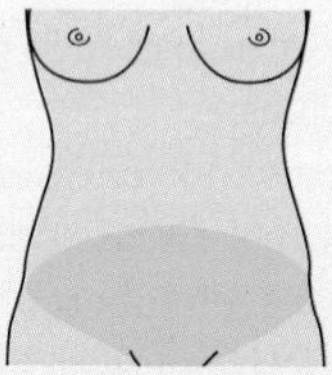	urinary retention pregnancy ovarian cysts
Abdominal distension in the flanks	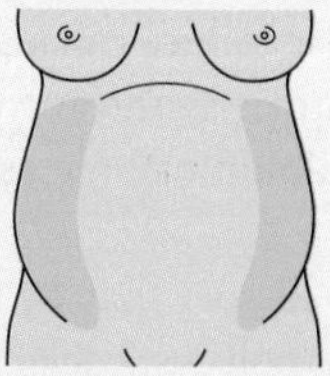	obesity ascites
Asymmetrical abdominal distension	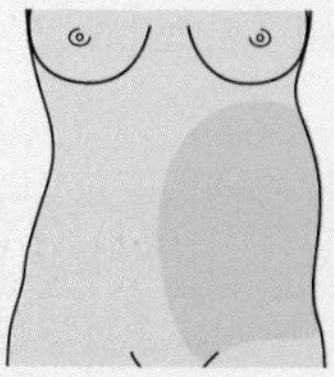	pregnancy cystic masses infiltrating cancers organs, e.g. kidney, liver, colon

Don't forget that hepatomegaly and splenomegaly are also asymmetric masses!

Fig. 5.2 Illustration of patterns of abdominal distension.

Percussion of the abdomen is most helpful in differentiating types of distension:

- A tympanitic note is produced by gaseous distension.
- A dull note is produced by a solid mass.
- 'Shifting dullness' is demonstrable when a dull note in the flank becomes resonant following the patient rolling onto the opposite side. This suggests gravity-dependent free fluid in the abdomen (i.e. ascites).

Auscultation can be useful in complete obstruction, when bowel sounds may be hyperactive (often described as tympanic or tinkling) or absent.

Investigating abdominal distension

Investigation is largely influenced by the clinical scenario, but radiological investigation has a key role in differentiating between causes of abdominal distension.

Radiology

Different imaging modalities may be used for diagnosis:

- Chest X-ray is useful to demonstrate an enlarged heart or signs of cardiac failure. The heart size may be normal in constrictive pericarditis.

- Plain abdominal X-ray is indicated if the patient is suspected clinically of having bowel obstruction, when fluid levels in the bowel will be obvious. Occasionally, a calcified mass may be seen in the pelvis due to fibroids or dermoid cysts of the ovaries. Faecal loading may also be shown in the colon.
- Abdominal ultrasound is the diagnostic modality of choice to identify ascites. It is also helpful to differentiate pelvic from intra-abdominal masses.

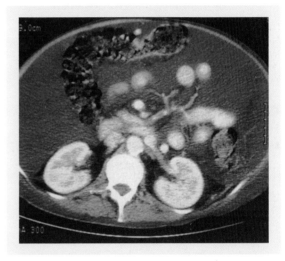

Fig. 5.3 Distension caused by ascites (ground glass appearance). Small bowel is floating in the fluid.

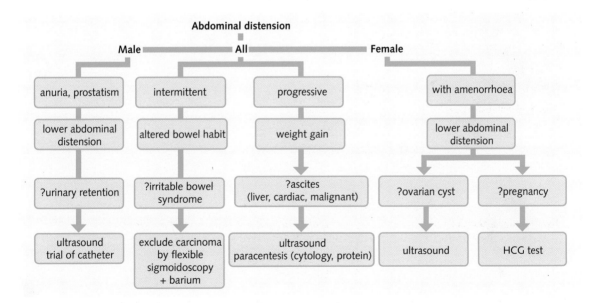

Fig. 5.4 Algorithm for the investigation of abdominal distension. (HCG, human chorionic gonadotrophin.)

- A computed tomography or magnetic resonance imaging scan of the abdomen may be indicated for some patients when ultrasound is equivocal (Fig. 5.3) or for a diagnosis of underlying malignancy.

A pregnancy test is essential if the cause of abdominal distension is not obvious for other reasons in women of child-bearing age. This is achieved by measuring the level of human chorionic gonadotrophin in the urine. Protein in the urine should alert one to the possibility of nephrotic syndrome.

Cardiac investigation

Further tests may be necessary if cardiac failure or constrictive pericarditis is considered likely.

Electrocardiogram may show:
- Elevated ST segment.
- T-wave changes.
- Low voltage QRS complexes (if a pericardial effusion is present).

Echocardiography is useful to demonstrate:
- Valvular stenosis or regurgitation.
- Pericardial effusion.
- Pericardial thickening.
- Poor ventricular myocardial function.

Summary

An algorithm summarizing the investigation of abdominal distension is shown in Fig. 5.4.

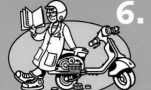

6. Weight Loss and Anorexia

Weight loss can be a very subjective assessment and, for a comprehensive investigation, it is important to try to attain objective evidence so that the rate and quantity of weight loss can be ascertained. Anorexia is loss of appetite which commonly accompanies weight loss, and it is appropriate to consider these entities together. The causes are myriad and include:

- Malignancy of any variety due to hypermetabolic effects; gastrointestinal (GI) malignancy clearly can also cause weight loss by interfering with the digestive process.
- Endocrine causes (e.g. diabetes mellitus, hyperthyroidism, adrenal insufficiency).
- Malabsorption (e.g. coeliac disease, Crohn's disease, bacterial overgrowth, intestinal parasitosis, chronic pancreatitis).
- Infection (e.g. underlying abscess, tuberculosis).
- Psychiatric cause (e.g. anorexia nervosa or bulimia, depression).
- Neurological cause (e.g. bulbar palsy, myasthenia causing difficulty in swallowing).

> Documentation of weight over a period of time is often extremely useful (e.g. clinic notes, general practitioner records). For reasons of posterity, it is important to document weight at every opportunity when you clerk a patient.

History of the patient with weight loss

An inquisitive history is required to assess weight loss objectively. Important aspects to enquire about include:

- How much weight loss and over what period of time? Weight loss of 10kg over 2 months is clearly more significant than over 1 year.
- Do their clothes fit them more loosely? How much tighter do belts have to be?
- Do they have any recent photographs to compare weight over a period of time?

Anorexia

It is very important to assess appetite when considering weight loss. The following should be considered:

- Are there any features of psychiatric illness such as distorted body image, early wakening, depression, behavioural changes?
- Is appetite out of step with weight loss? Hyperthyroidism causes increased appetite with weight loss. Brain tumours occasionally present with 'omniphagia'.

Associated features

These may give a clue to underlying disease, especially those resulting in malabsorption. Look for any GI symptoms such as:

- Diarrhoea or steatorrhoea (malabsorption, inflammatory bowel disease, hyperthyroidism).
- Vomiting.
- Change in bowel habit (possible malignancy).
- Increased activity due to change of lifestyle.
- Has there been excessive thirst (polydipsia) or excessive passage of urine (polyuria) suggestive of diabetes mellitus?
- Has there been fever, heat intolerance or night sweats, suggesting underlying infection or malignancy?

Past medical history

A history of previous GI surgery, particularly partial gastrectomy or small bowel resection, is important, because this may interfere with normal digestion. Patients who have had a stroke or neuromuscular problem such as myasthenia may find chewing or swallowing difficult.

Examining the patient with weight loss

There may be obvious cachexia or weight loss when looking at the patient. Look out for additional signs such as:

- Pallor indicative of anaemia, which may accompany malabsorption, malignancy or chronic infection/inflammation.
- Lymphadenopathy, suggestive of malignancy or lymphoma.
- Tremor with exophthalmos and a goitre, suggestive of thyrotoxicosis.
- Pigmentation of the skin and buccal membrane with postural hypotension, suggesting adrenal insufficiency.
- Hepatomegaly, ascites, or jaundice, suggesting possible malignancy or liver abscess.
- Lack of eye contact, withdrawn demeanour, or unkempt appearance, suggestive of depression or self-neglect.

Although amenorrhoea is characteristic of anorexia nervosa, it will occur with any condition causing profound weight loss. It should also be differentiated from primary amenorrhoea or pituitary failure.

Abdominal and particularly rectal examination must not be omitted when considering weight loss.

In a young female who is very thin, the following features ought to arouse suspicion of anorexia nervosa or bulimia:
- A history of excessive dieting or of binge eating.
- Delayed sexual maturation or amenorrhoea.
- Tooth erosion (due to acidic vomiting).
- Wearing loose clothes to disguise a perceived distorted body image.
- Lanugo hair on the arms and trunk.
- Callosities on dorsum of fingers from repeated self-induction of gag-reflex vomiting.

Investigating weight loss

A broad spectrum of investigations may be necessary to establish the aetiology of weight loss. The following investigations are confined to weight loss of GI causes and those that may present to a gastroenterologist.

Blood tests

The following blood tests may aid diagnosis:
- A full blood count is important to look for anaemia. A pancytopaenia may be indicative of marrow failure (e.g. malignant infiltration) or malabsorption of vitamin B_{12} or folate, resulting in megaloblastic change.
- Erythrocyte sedimentation rate is a useful test in this context because it is almost always raised if significant malignant or infectious pathology is present. C-reactive protein is a more sensitive marker of inflammatory disease.
- A coagulopathy and low blood urea is indicative of profound malabsorption or malnutrition.
- Measurement of blood sugar is essential to exclude diabetes mellitus.
- Hyperkalaemia with hyponatraemia should arouse suspicion of adrenal insufficiency. A Synacthen test may be indicated.
- Raised liver enzymes in the absence of discernible liver problems should arouse suspicion of malignant disease.
- Thyroid function tests are essential to exclude hyperthyroidism.
- Gonadal function tests may be useful to differentiate primary and secondary causes of amenorrhoea.
- Tumour markers can occasionally be helpful if other investigations prove unrevealing, but need to be interpreted with caution.

A careful drug history is important to enquire about laxative abuse and recreational drugs such as amphetamines—both of which can lead to weight loss.

Radiology

The tests that will be most helpful depend on the clinical context:
- Chest radiograph is important to exclude occult lung tumour, lymphadenopathy (lymphoma), or tuberculosis.
- Ultrasound of the abdomen and pelvis is useful to look for underlying malignancy.
- Barium enema should be performed in older age groups to exclude colonic malignancy. In younger

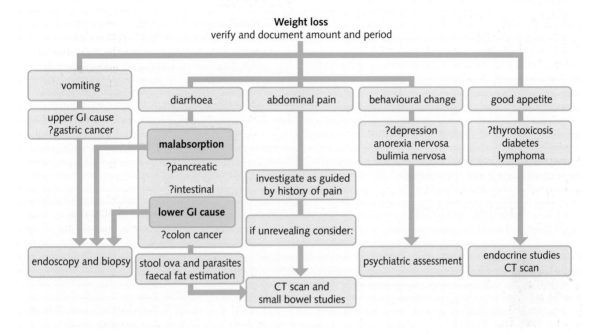

Fig. 6.1 Algorithm for the investigation of weight loss. (CT, computed tomography.)

patients, a small bowel enema may be indicated to look for evidence of Crohn's disease.

- Computed tomography of the abdomen is the best modality to look for occult malignancy such as pancreatic tumours and intra-abdominal lymphadenopathy.

Endoscopy

Gastroscopy:

- May be important to exclude occult gastric carcinoma in elderly patients.

- Is a useful investigation in younger patients allowing a small bowel biopsy to be taken to exclude coeliac disease.

Colonoscopy may be necessary to evaluate further any lesion in the colon found on barium enema.

Summary

An algorithm summarizing the investigation of weight loss is shown in Fig. 6.1.

7. Vomiting

Vomiting is the forceful ejection of gastric contents through the mouth. It is most often mediated through a vagal reflex involving chemoreceptor trigger zones in the medulla of the brain. It can be differentiated from regurgitation of oesophageal contents due to obstruction or pouch because of its greater force and volume. It is frequently preceded by nausea or abdominal pain. Vomiting can also occur because of intracranial phenomena or direct toxic effects on the trigger zone by drugs.

The common causes of vomiting include:
- Raised intracranial pressure or inflammation of the brain lining: meningitis or encephalitis.
- Migraine.
- Vestibular disturbances.
- Gastric causes such as gastritis, consequent upon alcohol excess, noxious substances, viral infection, bile, non-steroidal anti-inflammatory drugs.
- Gastrointestinal (GI) obstruction due to malignancy/pyloric stenosis/herniae/adhesions/volvulus/stricture.
- Liver disease such as acute hepatitis or hepatic failure.
- Gastroparesis secondary to autonomic dysfunction (e.g. diabetes mellitus).
- Metabolic derangement (e.g. adrenal insufficiency, uraemia, hypercalcaemia, porphyria, diabetic ketoacidosis).
- Drug toxicity.
- Pregnancy.
- Psychogenic vomiting.

History and differential diagnosis of vomiting

A detailed history is important to differentiate GI from central nervous systems (CNS) causes. Psychogenic or metabolic causes can be very difficult to discern, but are often more chronic or recurrent than is the case with GI causes. Features to consider are discussed below.

Onset and duration
Onset is an important feature: a short history is more likely to be due to an acute cause similar to those

seen in acute abdominal pain (e.g. infection or acute intestinal obstruction).

Ensure that you establish whether abdominal pain preceded or followed the vomiting. If the pain is precedent, then an intra-abdominal aetiology is likely.

Drugs and alcohol
A drug history is essential: probably the most common cause of nausea and vomiting.

The list of drugs causing nausea or vomiting is exhaustive but particular ones to note are:
- Opiates, from codeine to diamorphine.
- Cytotoxic drugs.
- Antibiotics (e.g. Erythromycin).
- Digoxin toxicity.

Alcohol excess results in gastritis, and vomiting commonly occurs the morning after excessive alcohol intake.

Infections and toxins
Recent contact with people with similar symptoms should alert you to viral gastritis or food poisoning.

Food poisoning is caused by ingestion of bacteria or their toxins in contaminated food. The time course of symptoms in relation to a meal is important:
- Symptoms occurring 1–4 hours after a meal is indicative of toxin such as heat-stable enterotoxin from *Staphylococcus aureus*.
- Symptoms occurring 12–48 hours after a meal are more often due to direct bacterial effects, although with some (e.g. *Shigella*), toxins also play a role. Most will also cause diarrhoea. *Salmonella* spp. is possibly the most common bacterial contaminant causing vomiting.

Past history

In addition to medication the patient may be taking for an unrelated condition, the following may also be of significance:

- Previous gastric surgery may give rise to biliary gastritis causing vomiting.
- Chronic duodenal ulceration can cause pyloric stenosis with gastric outlet obstruction.
- Chronic liver disease progressing to hepatic failure can also cause vomiting.
- Long-standing diabetes can result in gastroparesis and obstruction due to autonomic neuropathy.

Associated features

These can often give a clue to the underlying abnormality:

- Diarrhoea is common with vomiting induced by food poisoning.
- Weight loss may be prominent if underlying malignancy is present.
- Postural hypotension may be apparent if adrenal insufficiency is the cause.
- Headache is usually prominent with any CNS cause.
- Psychological factors, particularly in young females, may have a role in recurrent vomiting without anorexia nervosa.

Pregnancy is a very common cause of early morning sickness and vomiting in young women. Do not forget to take a menstrual history, but you cannot always rely on it—if in doubt do a pregnancy test!

Examining the patient with vomiting problems

General examination is important to ascertain whether a systemic condition is responsible for the vomiting. Important points to consider are:

- Altered level of consciousness, suggestive of drug toxicity or intracranial pathology.
- Neck stiffness or photophobia indicative of meningitis.

- Cachexia may suggest underlying malignancy.
- Pallor or pigmentation indicating anaemia, hypoadrenalism, or renal failure.
- Dehydration may indicate that vomiting has been severe and prolonged.
- Pyrexia or tachycardia possibly indicative of sepsis.

Abdominal examination is necessary to establish whether there is any evidence of intestinal obstruction and to identify any masses that may be responsible.

A succussion splash may be present with gastric outlet obstruction.

Investigating vomiting problems

Investigation may be necessary both to identify the cause of vomiting and to monitor its metabolic effects.

Blood tests

Consider the following blood tests:

- Full blood count may support an impression of dehydration if haematocrit is high. Raised white cell count can indicate infection.
- Blood urea is mildly raised in dehydration, but higher levels may be indicative of renal failure or upper GI bleeding which can both cause vomiting.
- Blood glucose is high in diabetic ketoacidosis.
- Hyperkalaemia with hyponatraemia may suggest adrenal insufficiency. Persistent vomiting will also cause hypokalaemic alkalosis (low potassium with elevated bicarbonate).
- Hypercalcaemia from any cause can present with vomiting.
- Liver enzymes may reveal a pattern of acute hepatitis which sometimes presents with vomiting.

Microbiological tests

Blood cultures and cerebrospinal fluid tap may be indicated if the patient is very ill or if meningitis is suspected.

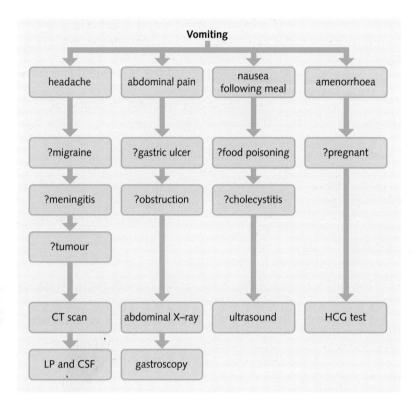

Fig. 7.1 Algorithm for the investigation of vomiting. (LP, lumbar puncture; CSF, cerebrospinal fluid; CT, computed tomography; HCG, human chorionic gonadotrophin or pregnancy test.)

Radiology

Plain abdominal X-ray is useful to exclude obstruction (e.g. due to pyloric stenosis).

A computed tomography scan of the head may be indicated by the clinical picture.

Summary

An algorithm summarizing the investigation of vomiting is shown in Fig. 7.1.

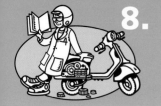

8. Haematemesis and Melaena

Haematemesis refers to the vomiting of blood. Melaena is the passage of black tarry and foul-smelling stools, resulting from the effect of the digestive process on fresh blood. Haematemesis and melaena are usually caused by upper gastrointestinal (GI) bleeding.

Common causes include:
- Reflux oesophagitis.
- Mallory–Weiss tear.
- Oesophageal varices.
- Gastric ulcers or erosions.
- Gastric carcinoma.
- Duodenal ulceration.
- Hereditary telangiectasia.

History of the patient with haematemesis

The first fact that needs to be established is whether it is a true haematemesis.
- Haemoptysis is coughing of blood and can sometimes be confused with haematemesis.
- Epistaxis (nose bleed), especially if it is severe where the blood is often swallowed, can be difficult to differentiate from true haematemesis.
- Melaena should always follow a true haematemesis, but must not be confused with bleeding from the colon or rectum, which produces dark or bright red blood, respectively.

There are a few clues to help to decide the cause of bleeding. These are discussed below.

Volume of blood loss
Try to estimate this in terms that the patient can understand (i.e. 1/2 cupful, 2 cupfuls, etc.). Be aware that the amount of blood is often overestimated.
- A large haematemesis is indicative of a significant GI bleed and is more likely to be a result of bleeding from oesophageal varices or an arterial bleed from peptic ulceration.
- A small bleed may manifest itself as altered blood if it has been present in the stomach for some

time. The patient may complain of vomiting 'coffee grounds'.

Iron tablets can be confused with melaena, as they produce dark or black stool. However, iron stools have a sticky or grainy consistency unlike the tarry, runny nature of melaena. Melaena also has a characteristic odour!

Past medical history
Find out whether the patient suffers from chronic liver disease. Oesophageal variceal haemorrhage, consequent upon portal hypertension, is then more likely, although these patients also get peptic ulcers.

There may be a personal or family history of recurrent GI bleeds due to hereditary haemorrhagic telangiectasia.

Drug history
Pay particular attention to non-steroidal anti-inflammatory drugs, including low-dose aspirin. These drugs predispose to reflux oesophagitis, gastritis, and gastric erosions, especially in elderly people, causing both occult or manifest haemorrhage. Corticosteroid tablets (e.g. Prednisolone) increase this risk if administered concurrently.

Patients anticoagulated with warfarin for venous thromboses, atrial fibrillation or prosthetic heart valves may have large haemorrhages from very minor gastric erosions.

Associated features
Vigorous vomiting or retching preceding the haematemesis is suggestive of a Mallory–Weiss tear of the mucosa across the gastro-oesophageal junction. This can result in significant haemorrhage, although it is usually self-limiting.

An antecedent history of upper abdominal pain is suggestive of peptic ulcer disease or gastritis.

Heartburn may be due to acid reflux causing reflux oesophagitis.

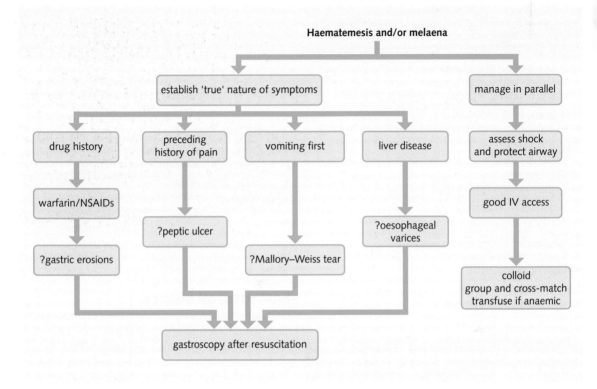

Fig. 8.1 Algorithm for investigation of upper gastrointestinal bleeding. (NSAIDs, non-steroidal anti-inflammatory drugs.)

Examining the patient with haematemesis

If the haemorrhage has been severe, it will be necessary to examine and resuscitate the patient concurrently, whilst trying to ascertain the cause. Important features to look for are:

- Hypotension—systolic blood pressure <100 mmHg (with or without alteration of consciousness).
- Tachycardic—heart rate >100 bpm.
- Pallor.
- Cold, clammy peripheries.

Features of liver disease suggesting the presence of oesophageal varices may be obvious such as:

- Jaundice.
- Parotitis.
- Spider naevi.
- Palmar erythema.
- Hepatosplenomegaly.
- Ascites.

Peri-oral telangiectasia may suggest hereditary haemorrhagic telangiectasia.

Rectal examination is imperative to establish the presence of melaena.

Remember to measure lying and standing blood pressure to look for evidence of postural hypotension. This an early sign of intravascular volume depletion, resultant upon a large bleed.

The priority in managing haematemesis is to make sure you have adequate intravenous access to resuscitate the patient, even before you take a full history. The airway should always be protected.

Investigating haematemesis

Endoscopy is the definitive test for all GI bleeding. If haematemesis and melaena are obvious or significant, then urgent endoscopy is indicated to establish the cause and stop the bleeding. However, the patient should always be resuscitated first.

Blood tests

Certain blood tests may give clues to the cause:

- Full blood count can be surprisingly normal until haemodilution occurs and should be rechecked once the patient is rehydrated.
- A low platelet count should alert one to the possibility of hypersplenism, due to portal hypertension, associated with bleeding oesophageal varices.

- Biochemistry may reveal an elevated urea disproportionate to serum creatinine. This is due to the 'high protein meal' provided by blood in the GI tract and is characteristic of upper GI bleeding.
- Liver enzymes may be abnormal, but can be normal even in the presence of cirrhosis. In chronic liver disease with oesophageal varices, hepatic synthetic function may be impaired and is reflected in a low serum albumin and a coagulopathy.

Summary

An algorithm summarizing the investigation of upper GI bleeding is shown in Fig 8.1.

9. Diarrhoea

Diarrhoea is broadly defined as an increased frequency or volume of bowel excretion. A more precise definition is the passage of 300 g of motion of altered consistency in 24 hours. It is a common condition which affects most people at some point in their lives. Most cases are due to an underlying infective cause, which is usually self-limiting and requires no treatment. However, more prolonged cases need further investigation to exclude a more serious pathology.

The possibilities include:
- Infection (i.e. viral, bacteria, protozoal, or parasitic).
- Malabsorption due to small bowel or pancreatic disease.
- Colonic carcinoma or polyps.
- Endocrine causes such as thyrotoxicosis, adrenal insufficiency, or endocrine tumours of the bowel.
- Neuropathic causes such as vagotomy or diabetic autonomic neuropathy.
- Drug-related (e.g. antibiotics, especially pseudomembranous colitis), purgative abuse.
- Radiation enteritis.
- Following surgery (e.g. postvagotomy), terminal ileal resection (including bile salt diarrhoea).
- Overflow diarrhoea (secondary to constipation).
- Graft versus host disease following bone marrow transplantation (or rarely blood transfusion) is an unusual but important cause

History of the patient with diarrhoea

It is essential to establish whether the patient's perception of diarrhoea is the same as yours. Often a patient presents to a gastroenterology clinic complaining of 'diarrhoea' when in reality the problem is that the frequency or consistency of stool, although within the normal range, has changed for that patient.

Features to consider are discussed below.

Onset

Acute onset of diarrhoea is usually of infective aetiology and, in the majority of cases, an underlying precipitant is identified, for example:

- Ingestion of suspicious food.
- Foreign travel.
- Contact with another person with similar symptoms.

Type of diarrhoea and associated features

Bloody diarrhoea with mucus is suggestive of mucosal inflammation, as seen in ulcerative colitis, radiation colitis, certain bacterial infections and pseudomembranous colitis. Colonic carcinoma can also give rise to blood-stained diarrhoea.

Pale, greasy diarrhoea due to a high fat content (steatorrhoea) is highly indicative of malabsorption, consequent upon small bowel disease or pancreatic insufficiency.

Ask the patient whether:
- There is a history of coeliac disease in the family.
- He or she has consumed excessive alcohol in the past.

There may be associated features that give some clue to the underlying diagnosis, such as:
- Joint pains, mouth ulcers, skin changes or uveitis in inflammatory bowel disease.
- Diabetes mellitus with evidence of peripheral neuropathy in autonomic bowel neuropathy.
- Scleroderma causing hypomotility with malabsorption.
- Jaundice with steatorrhoea due to pancreatitis or pancreatic carcinoma.

Diet

Has the patient's diet changed in any way recently:
- Increased ingestion of dairy produce.
- High-fibre cereals.
- Stimulants such as coffee.
- Increase in alcohol consumption.

It is surprising how often many patients fail to link intake to output!

Drug history

Diarrhoea commonly occurs with certain drugs:
- Metformin.
- Colchicine.

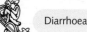

- Digoxin.
- Purgatives.

Broad-spectrum antibiotics such as the cephalosporins, the penicillins and macrolides (e.g. erythromycin) commonly cause diarrhoea as a result of alteration in gut flora and, in severe cases, pseudomembranous colitis occurs as a result of *Clostridium difficile* overgrowth.

Past medical and surgical history

Find out about:
- Gastric or intestinal surgical resection are relevant because they interfere with motility and absorption.
- Radiotherapy to the abdomen or pelvis for non-gastrointestinal malignancy, such as lymphoma, may not manifest its adverse gastrointestinal effects until many years later.
- Systemic conditions such as diabetes or collagen-vascular disease may also cause diarrhoea.
- HIV predisposes to atypical infections causing diarrhoea such as *Cryptosporidium* (fungal) and the *Cytomegalovirus*.

> Patients may forget, or omit to tell you that they have had previous intra-abdominal surgery. Remember to examine carefully for scars! Old surgical notes are sometimes valuable, for example:
> - Gastric surgery (vagotomy, gastrectomy) can produce diarrhoea
> - Pancreatectomy results in malabsorption
> - Cholecystectomy or right hemicolectomy can result in bile salt diarrhoea

Examining the patient with diarrhoea

General features to look for include:
- Dehydration is common in acute onset diarrhoea because gastroenteritis is usually associated with vomiting and hence a substantial fluid loss. Large

amounts of electrolyte-rich fluid can also be lost in severe diarrhoea seen in inflammatory bowel disease and VIPomas (tumours that secrete vasoactive intestinal peptide).
- Pallor due to anaemia may be seen in inflammatory bowel disease and colonic malignancy due to chronic blood loss, or reflecting the anaemia of chronic disease. Malabsorption can also result in anaemia due to deficiency of iron and vitamin B_{12} or folate.
- Weight loss associated with chronic diarrhoea is a common feature of malabsorption from all causes. Underlying malignancy should also be excluded.
- Associated features of inflammatory bowel disease may be apparent, such as aphthous mouth ulcers, pyoderma gangrenosum, and uveitis.
- Associated features of endocrine disease include skin pigmentation in adrenal insufficiency, proptosis or exophthalmos in thyrotoxicosis, and peripheral neuropathy in diabetes.
- Clinical features of alcoholic liver disease or of cystic fibrosis may suggest pancreatic insufficiency.

The discovery of abdominal scars from previous surgery may suggest postvagotomy diarrhoea, or terminal ileal resection for Crohn's disease which predisposes to bile salt diarrhoea. Previous surgery for intra-abdominal malignancy (e.g. ovarian) may be followed by radiotherapy causing radiation enteritis (skin burns may be present) (see Fig. 22.10).

Palpate for abdominal masses or tenderness. Most gastroenteritis will have associated abdominal discomfort. A mass in the right iliac fossa may be present in Crohn's disease as well as caecal carcinoma.

Rectal examination must be carried out in all patients presenting with diarrhoea, especially in elderly people, because overflow diarrhoea is a common cause. Faecal impaction or a rectal mass due to rectal carcinoma may be palpated.

Investigating diarrhoea

The extent of investigation is guided by the severity of diarrhoea and by the information gleaned from the history and examination. As always, correct interpretation of results in the clinical context is most important.

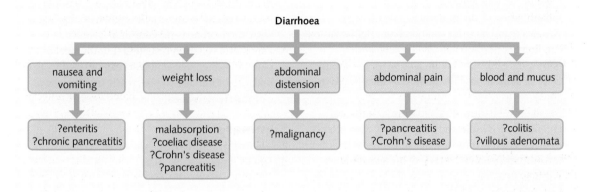

Fig. 9.1 Algorithm for the investigation of diarrhoea.

Haematology

Haematology tests may aid diagnosis:

- Full blood count may demonstrate a microcytic hypochromic picture of iron deficiency or macrocytic anaemia resultant upon vitamin B_{12} or folate deficiency (a combined deficiency can produce a normocytic anaemia).
- Microcytic anaemia with rectal bleeding and mucus associated with the diarrhoea favours a diagnosis of inflammatory bowel disease.
- Steatorrhoea with iron deficiency may suggest coeliac disease.

Biochemistry

Consider the following tests:

- Electrocytes may be disrupted if diarrhoea has been severe and prolonged or is caused by adrenal insufficiency.
- Urea is low if malabsorption or malnutrition is present. It is mildly raised in dehydration or in the presence of melaena.
- Iron studies, ferritin, vitamin B_{12}, and folate levels may help to interpret associated anaemia (for anaemia, see Chapter 11).
- Thyroid function tests should be performed for any patients who do not clearly have a gastrointestinal cause for the diarrhoea.
- Urinary 5-hydroxyindole acetic acid (5HIAA) is a metabolite of serotonin, which is elevated in carcinoid syndrome (see p. 95).
- Abnormal liver biochemistry may be associated with pancreatic insufficiency, particularly if secondary to chronic alcohol excess.

Microbiology

Stool culture is necessary to exclude an underlying infective cause. However, since most infective causes are viral and self-limiting, viral cultures are only carried out in particular circumstances, such as in the immunosuppressed patient. Stool microscopy can be performed to look for ova and cysts seen in parasitic infections such as *Giardia*.

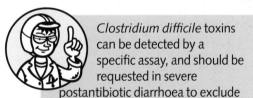

Clostridium difficile toxins can be detected by a specific assay, and should be requested in severe postantibiotic diarrhoea to exclude pseudomembranous colitis.

Radiology

Plain abdominal radiograph can be undertaken:

- To confirm faecal impaction.
- More commonly, to see whether there is a megacolon associated with inflammatory ulcerative colitis, especially if the patient is clinically unwell.

Calcification of the pancreas is suggestive of pancreatic insufficiency in patients with steatorrhoea secondary to chronic pancreatitis.

Further investigation at this point is usually guided by the clinical presentation and results of the above enquiry. Investigations to consider include:

- Rigid or flexible sigmoidoscopy, where inflammation of the mucosa can be directly visualized and biopsies can be taken. Rectosigmoid carcinoma or polyps can also be seen and appropriate biopsies taken. Extensive melanosis coli can sometimes be seen in chronic purgative abuse.
- Small bowel barium study, barium enema, or colonoscopy is indicated for patients with bloody diarrhoea and iron-deficiency anaemia to look for inflammatory bowel disease. This investigation will also detect underlying colonic malignancy, but bloody diarrhoea is rare.
- Duodenal biopsy is performed to look for coeliac disease, which usually presents with steatorrhoea associated with folate deficiency and anaemia.

- Breath tests using ^{14}C-glycholate or lactulose are used to exclude bacterial overgrowth in patients with steatorrhoea and vitamin B_{12} deficiency.
- Pancreatic function tests (e.g. Lundh meal or the para-aminobenzoic acid test) can be used to assess malabsorption due to pancreatic insufficiency causing steatorrhoea.

Summary

An algorithm summarizing the investigation of diarrhoea is given in Fig. 9.1.

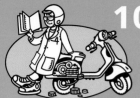

10. Rectal Bleeding

Rectal bleeding usually refers to bright red bleeding, and is usually due to anorectal pathology. A clear precise history will determine the site and the underlying cause in most cases.

Any rectal bleeding other than bright red blood indicates that the blood has been altered by bacterial or enzymatic digestion higher up in the colon or small bowel. The importance of distinguishing altered blood from just rectal bleeding cannot be overemphasized.

Causes of bright red rectal bleeding include:
- Haemorrhoids.
- Anal fissure.
- Anorectal carcinoma or polyps.
- Angiodysplasia.
- Diverticular disease.
- Inflammatory bowel disease.

History of the patient with rectal bleeding

Establish the relationship between the onset of rectal bleeding and passage of stool, as this will give important clues about the aetiology:
- 'Spotting' of bright red blood appearing on toilet paper only after the passage of stool is highly suggestive of haemorrhoids or anal fissure if there is associated pain on defaecation.
- Presence of blood that is separate from faeces (often noticed as bright red fresh blood in the toilet pan) is associated with low rectal lesions such as haemorrhoids and anorectal carcinoma, where passage of mucus is also common. Pain is not usually a feature, except where anal fissure is also present with the haemorrhoids.

- Passage of dark red blood mixed in with the stool is suggestive of a high rectal lesion such as carcinoma, angiodysplasia, or an inflamed diverticula.

Associated features such as weight loss, diarrhoea, or abdominal pain suggest serious pathology rather than simple anorectal conditions.

Examining the patient with rectal bleeding

A general examination looking for evidence of anaemia, cachexia or lymphadenopathy is followed by an abdominal examination. Faecal masses may be palpable if there is significant constipation, which predisposes to haemorrhoids and anal fissure. Left iliac fossa tenderness, with or without guarding, is suggestive of inflamed diverticula.
- Rectal examination is mandatory in this situation; take particular note of the external, peri-anal area. Anal tags suggest previously thrombosed haemorrhoids.
- Mucus discharge may be seen in inflammatory bowel disease and anorectal carcinoma.
- Increased anal tone and pain on rectal examination is highly indicative of anal fissure.
- Hard faeces in the rectum may suggest chronic constipation or anal fissure.
- Masses due to rectal carcinoma or polyp can also be palpated on rectal examination.

Proctoscopy enables examination of the position of haemorrhoids, which may be treated with sclerotherapy. Anal fissures can also be seen, although it is unlikely that the patient with this painful condition will tolerate the passage of a proctoscope.

Rigid sigmoidoscopy can visualize up to 15–20 cm from the anal margin, and biopsies can be taken of any suspicious lesion to detect carcinoma or inflammatory bowel disease.

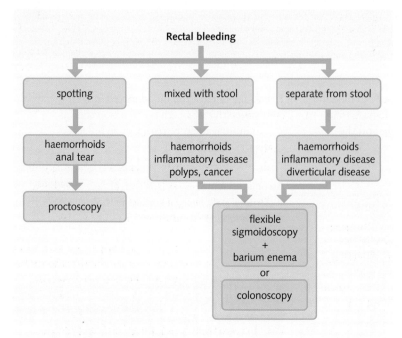

Fig. 10.1 Investigation of rectal bleeding.

Blood loss from haemorrhoids is usually not severe enough to cause anaemia. Rectal bleeding with anaemia is more likely to be due to carcinoma, angiodysplasia or inflammatory bowel disease.

Investigating rectal bleeding

The majority of conditions can be diagnosed with a careful history and examination with proctoscopy and sigmoidoscopy. However, further investigation may be required if the diagnosis is equivocal:

- Full blood count is essential to establish whether anaemia is present.
- Colonoscopy or flexible sigmoidoscopy allow higher sigmoid lesions, and many vascular lesions such as angiodysplasia to be seen. More than two-thirds of all colonic polyps and tumours occur within 60cm of the anal margin.
- Angiography can be performed to locate the site of bleeding from angiodysplasia. However, this is reserved for circumstances where there is a high index of suspicion and the patient has evidence of active bleeding.

Summary
An algorithm summarizing the investigation of rectal bleeding is shown in Fig. 10.1.

11. Anaemia

Anaemia is a low haemoglobin concentration in plasma, due to a low red cell mass. The symptoms of anaemia occur as a result of the reduced oxygen-carrying capacity of blood and therefore the reduced delivery of oxygen to tissues. Gastrointestinal causes of anaemia include:

- Reduced intake (e.g. dietary deficiencies of iron, folate, and vitamin B_{12}).
- Reduced absorption (e.g. pernicious anaemia, small bowel disease such as Crohn's, coeliac disease, or bacterial overgrowth, achlorhydria following gastrectomy).
- Gastrointestinal blood loss (e.g. from peptic ulcer disease, oesophagitis, occult carcinoma, or angiodysplasia).

History of the patient with anaemia

Depending on the severity of anaemia and the presence of concurrent pathology, the patient can present with symptoms of anaemia such as:

- Fatigue.
- Palpitations.
- Shortness of breath.
- Angina pectoris.

Frequently, the detection of anaemia is an incidental finding on a routine blood test when the patient presents with unrelated symptoms.

Symptoms of anaemia such as fatigue are thought to require a reduction in haemoglobin concentration of about 25%. For practical purposes this means that symptoms are uncommon unless haemoglobin is <8 g/dl (females) or <10 g/dl (males)

The following aspects of history should be considered in detail.

Diet
Check whether the patient has a well-balanced diet:

- Meat contains haem iron, which is more readily bioavailable than non-haem iron.
- Strict vegans are particularly at risk of iron deficiency.
- Fresh vegetables and fruit are important sources of the reductants (e.g. vitamin C) necessary to make iron bioavailable, resulting in the conversion of Fe^{3+} to Fe^{2+}.

Past medical and surgical history
Clearly, previous surgical procedures may be pertinent, such as:

- Partial gastrectomy resulting in achlorhydria and thus preventing reduction of iron.
- Terminal ileal resection, leading to vitamin B_{12} malabsorption.

Previous medical history is important for similar reasons:

- Long-term antisecretory medication could theoretically precipitate anaemia if iron stores were already low.
- Crohn's disease or tuberculosis can affect terminal ileal absorption.
- Use of non-steroidal anti-inflammatory agents, including low dose aspirin, is associated with chronic occult blood loss.

Associated features
Consider the following associated features:

- Diarrhoea with anaemia is a common manifestation of malabsorption. Chronic diarrhoea due to giardiasis or hookworm infestation is a common cause of anaemia worldwide. Coeliac disease is possibly the most common cause of malabsorption presenting with anaemia in the Western world.
- Abdominal pain or dyspepsia may be present, suggesting acid reflux or peptic ulcer disease causing chronic gastrointestinal blood loss,

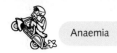

although these are not common causes of anaemia. Pain may also be present if a luminal tumour is the cause.

- Haematemesis is not usually ignored by patients but melaena occasionally is. This may be caused by gastric ulcer or erosion, angiodysplasia of the stomach, or a right-sided colonic tumour.

Examining the patient with anaemia

Look for features of anaemia such as:
- Pallor.
- Koilonychia.
- Atrophic glossitis.
- Tachycardia, or cardiac failure.

Check whether there are any abdominal scars from surgery (see Fig. 22.10). The patient may have forgotten about operations, so consider particularly:
- Midline scar of gastric surgery.
- Right lower abdominal or midline scar from a ileal resection.

Can you elicit any abdominal tenderness and does its position suggest underlying peptic ulcer disease or a caecal carcinoma (see Fig. 21.1)?

Is there palpable splenomegaly? This may be consequent upon portal hypertension or present as a feature of a myeloproliferative or lymphoproliferative disorder.

Are there features of chronic liver disease such as spider naevi, parotitis or gynaecomastia which may alert you to underlying oesophageal varices or portal hypertensive gastropathy?

A rectal examination is mandatory in any patient presenting with iron deficiency anaemia to exclude anorectal carcinoma. It also serves to confirm or refute a recent history of melaena.

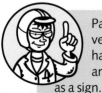

Pale conjunctivae correlate very poorly with haemoglobin concentration and cannot be relied upon as a sign.

Investigating anaemia

The full blood count is necessary not only to confirm the presence of anaemia, but also as an important key to its subsequent investigation. The severity of the anaemia is determined by haemoglobin and haematocrit. Important clues to the aetiology are often given by the red blood cell size and haemoglobin content. Thus:
- Microcytic hypochromic picture is due to iron deficiency. This can result from dietary deficiency, failure of absorption, or blood loss. A blood film may demonstrate anisocytosis and poikilocytosis (variation in size and shape of the red cell, respectively).
- Normocytic normochromic picture is commonly associated with chronic inflammatory disease, in which iron stores are adequate but not utilized effectively.
- Macrocytic picture, which can be due to folate or vitamin B_{12} deficiency, alcohol, hypothyroidism or certain drugs (e.g. phenytoin—antifolate action), or hydroxyurea.

Further investigation therefore, is dependent on the full blood count indices.

Because full blood counts are automated, macrocytosis can be spurious if there are increased numbers of larger red cells such as reticulocytes present. If in doubt, a reticulocyte count and a blood film examination should be performed.

Biochemistry
Biochemistry tests may aid diagnosis (Fig. 11.1):
- Serum iron is used to confirm iron deficiency.
- Serum ferritin is the most sensitive test to reflect iron stores but, as an 'acute phase protein', it may be falsely elevated in the presence of a concomitant inflammatory condition.

- Serum folate should be measured in any patient with macrocytosis. Deficiency is usually due to malabsorption (most commonly coeliac disease), poor dietary intake, excessive use as in pregnancy, or increased cell turnover in malignancy or red cell haemolysis. Antifolate drugs, such as methotrexate, and antibiotics, such as trimethoprim, also cause folate deficiency.
- Vitamin B_{12} must also be measured in patients with macrocytosis. If deficient, a Schilling test

(see Chapter 24) may be helpful in deciding the cause.
- Blood urea can be a useful, albeit rather unreliable, indicator of nutrition—low levels occur in malabsorption.
- Faeces can be tested for occult blood loss, although both false positive and false negative results can be obtained.

Parameters to differentiate iron-deficiency anaemia from anaemia of chronic disease		
	Anaemia of chronic disease	Iron deficiency
MCV	↓/normal	↓
Serum iron	↓	↓
TIBC	↓	↑
Ferritin	↓/normal/↑	↓
Iron stores in bone marrow (Perl's stain)	normal	↓/absent
Iron in red-cell precursors	↓	↓/absent

Fig. 11.1 Parameters to differentiate iron-deficiency anaemia from anaemia of chronic disease.

If macrocytic anaemia is due to vitamin B_{12} deficiency because of bacterial overgrowth, serum folate will be elevated as a consequence of bacterial metabolism. Otherwise, folate is often also deficient.

Endoscopy

Gastroscopy should be undertaken in all cases of iron deficiency anaemia, unless there is clearly an alternative explanation, to exclude oesophagitis, gastric ulcer or erosions, and carcinoma.

The presence of a duodenal ulcer is an insufficient explanation for iron deficiency anaemia. A biopsy of

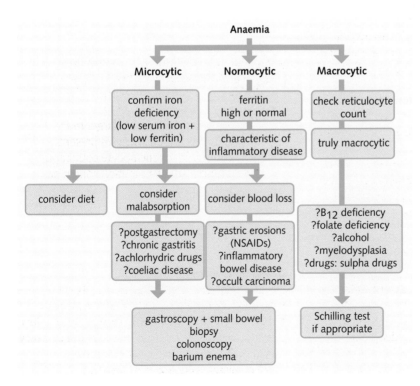

Fig. 11.2 Algorithm for the gastrointestinal investigation of anaemia. (NSAIDs, non-steroidal anti-inflammatory drugs.)

the second part of the duodenum should be taken at the same time, to exclude coeliac disease.

Colonoscopy is the preferred large bowel investigation because it should identify all lesions resulting in blood loss, including angiodysplasia. When it is not practical, barium examination should be undertaken.

Radiology

A barium meal is indicated if there is suspicion of gastric carcinoma and gastroscopy is not possible. Similarly, a barium enema will demonstrate the presence of diverticular disease, polyps, and carcinoma, but endoscopy is preferable in order to ascribe the cause of bleeding to a particular lesion or to identify angiodysplasia.

Angiography is helpful in the presence of active bleeding, but is not generally rewarding in the investigation of chronic anaemia.

Other tests for anaemia

Other tests may be useful:

- A Schilling test may help differentiate the different causes of vitamin B_{12} deficiency (see Chapter 24).
- A ^{14}C-glycocholic acid breath test or a lactulose hydrogen breath test may be used to investigate bacterial overgrowth (see Chapter 24).
- A ^{99}Tc radioisotope scan is helpful if a Meckel's diverticulum is suspected of causing chronic anaemia in a young patient.
- A ^{51}Cr-labelled red cell scan may give a clue to the general location of occult blood loss, but is not helpful to identify the nature of the lesion or the precise anatomical location.

Summary

An algorithm summarizing the investigation of anaemia is given in Fig. 11.2.

12. Jaundice

Jaundice is a yellow colouring of the skin and sclerae due to elevated levels of bilirubin in plasma. Jaundice is usually clinically evident if serum bilirubin exceeds 40 mmol/L (about twice the normal upper limit). There are numerous causes of jaundice, and a careful history and examination is vital so that unnecessary invasive investigations can be avoided.

The more common causes include:

- Haemolytic anaemias or ineffective erythropoesis such as autoimmune haemolytic anaemia or haemoglobinopathies, respectively.
- Congenital hyperbilirubinaemia due to enzyme defects, most commonly Gilbert's syndrome.
- Extra-hepatic bile duct obstruction due to gallstones, pancreatitis, or pancreatic cancer.
- Sclerosing cholangitis.
- Intra-hepatic cholestasis due to drugs, alcohol, hepatitis, or chronic liver disease.

History of the patient with jaundice

All aspects of the history should be taken with care as there are times when certain facts can appear to be trivial, yet may later become vital in the diagnosis. The following features help to differentiate causes of jaundice (Fig. 12.1).

Age
Younger patients are more likely to have congenital hyperbilirubinaemia or viral hepatitis than carcinoma of the pancreas, which rarely affects those aged under 60 years.

Onset of symptoms
The onset of symptoms may give clues to the diagnosis:

- An acute onset is more likely to be of infective or drug induced aetiology.
- A slow insidious onset is more likely to be due to chronic active hepatitis (e.g. caused by autoimmune disease or alcohol).

Infectious contact and risk behaviour
It is important to establish whether the patient has any risk factors for developing jaundice:

- Find out whether there has been contact with other people with jaundice, such as occurs in epidemics of hepatitis A and E or infectious mononucleosis (Epstein–Barr virus).
- Has there been high-risk behaviour for exposure to hepatitis B (promiscuous sexual activity or shared needles)?
- A history of recent travel abroad is also essential: ingestion of seafood abroad is a common source of infectious hepatitis. Do not forget exotic causes such as yellow fever from Africa!
- Occupational or recreational history may be relevant: sewage and farm workers are at risk of leptospirosis, as well as windsurfers and people who go pot-holing.
- A history of excess alcohol consumption must be excluded and tactful discussion with relatives may be necessary.

The most common mode for transmission of hepatitis B worldwide is not sexual or intravenous drugs but 'vertical' transmission from mother to baby. This takes place in the birth canal and presents the best opportunity to prevent transmission of hepatitis B virus by immunizing the neonate.

Past medical history
This may immediately suggest a diagnosis. For example:

- Previous cholecystectomy could suggest a bile duct stone or stricture.
- Ulcerative colitis can predispose to sclerosing cholangitis.
- Anaesthetic agents such as halothane can precipitate jaundice.
- Patients often forget that they have had antibiotics or other drugs recently.

Fig. 12.1 Causes of jaundice.

Causes of jaundice		Drugs
Pre-hepatic	• haemolysis • ineffective erythropoesis • Gilbert's and Crigler–Najjar syndromes	

Hepatic	• viruses: Hep A, B, C, E
	   Epstein–Barr
	   cytomegalovirus
	   herpes simplex/zoster
	• leptospirosis/toxoplasmosis
	• autoimmune hepatitis
	• cirrhosis
	• Wilson's disease
	• rotor/Dubin–Johnson syndrome
		• isoniazid
		• paracetamol excess
		• halothane
		• chlorpromazine

Post-hepatic (obstructive)	• intra-hepatic: primary biliary cirrhosis
	   primary sclerosing
	   cholangitis
	   cholangiocarcinoma
	   + same causes listed
	   under Hepatic
	• extra-hepatic: gallstones
	   carcinoma of head of
	   pancreas
	   enlarged lymph nodes
	   at porta hepatis
		• oral contraceptive pill
		
		• flucloxacillin
		   or co-amoxiclav

Drugs

Many drugs are metabolized in the liver, and some cause idiosyncratic reactions, resulting in jaundice. Others have a dose-related effect, resulting in liver damage and jaundice. Important drugs to consider include:

- Antibiotics such as co-amoxiclav or flucloxacillin.
- Antifungal agents such as Fluconazole.
- Allopurinol can occasionally cause profound jaundice.
- Antituberculous drugs such as isoniazid or rifampicin.
- Neuroleptics such as chlorpromazine.
- Paracetamol in excess of therapeutic dose.
- Anabolic steroids—these are occasionally illegally used by bodybuilders and cause jaundice.

Family history

A history of intermittent jaundice in the family suggests congenital hyperbilirubinaemia. Also enquire about Wilson's disease and alpha-1-antitrypsin deficiency.

Associated features

A number of features may suggest underlying pathology, such as:

- Presence of abdominal pain, particularly if localized to right upper quadrant, suggests bile duct stones or pain originating from the liver capsule.
- Acute onset abdominal distension with jaundice may indicate acute hepatitis or hepatic vein thrombosis (resulting in ascites).
- Painless jaundice in conjunction with weight loss in older patients is suggestive of carcinoma of the pancreas or enlarged metastatic lymph nodes at the porta hepatis.
- Signs of cardiac failure, especially elevated jugular venous pressure and peripheral oedema, may indicate a congested liver with jaundice.

Acholuric jaundice is the term given to jaundice without dark urine and pale stool. The presence of these features indicates that the jaundice is cholestatic in nature. Obstructive jaundice is only one cause of cholestatic jaundice.

Examining the patient with jaundice

Assess the severity of the jaundice clinically:
- Acute jaundice has a bright yellow hue.
- Chronic jaundice has a dusky appearance and if severe, the patient may look green.

Look for signs of anaemia, which may indicate underlying haemolysis.

Generalized lymphadenopathy may be due to Epstein–Barr, cytomegalovirus (CMV), or toxoplasmosis.

Are there features of chronic liver disease or cirrhosis (see Chapter 18) such as:
- Parotitis.
- Spider naevi.
- Gynaecomastia and loss of secondary sexual characterisitics.
- Palmar erythema.
- Splenomegaly (think of infections, haemolysis or portal hypertension).
- Hepatomegaly.
- Ascites (may be acute in Budd–Chiari syndrome).

The gall bladder may be palpated in a patient with progressive painless jaundice due to obstruction. If, in painless jaundice, the gall bladder is palpable, the cause will not be gallstones (Courvoisier's law). In elderly patients, this is commonly due to carcinoma of the head of the pancreas.

Associated systemic signs may suggest particular syndromes with liver involvement:
- Chronic respiratory disease with jaundice may occur with cystic fibrosis or alpha-1-antitrypsin deficiency.
- Neurological signs, particular those of Parkinsonism, with jaundice may suggest hepatolenticular degeneration (Wilson's disease).

Kayser–Fleischer rings are present in 70% of patients with Wilson's disease. They are seen as a brown ring around in the periphery of the cornea, most often at the top. Slit lamp examination may be necessary.

Investigating jaundice

Abdominal ultrasound is the key investigation in a patient with jaundice because it will differentiate obstructive jaundice from other causes, and the subsequent approaches to management are different. If the bile ducts are not dilated, then blood tests become useful to differentiate causes of jaundice:
- Urine testing for bilirubin and urobilinogen is an inexpensive and useful test to investigate the potential aetiologies. Unconjugated jaundice (e.g. Gilbert's or haemolysis) will result in an absence of bilirubin in the urine. Biliary obstruction will demonstrate increased urinary bilirubin and absent or reduced urobilinogen. If there is active red cell haemolysis, then urinary haemosiderin may be detectable.
- Liver biochemistry is helpful to confirm jaundice and to confirm unconjugated hyperbilirubinaemia in cases of congenital or haemolytic jaundice. A high alkaline phosphatase is indicative of cholestasis, whereas high levels of transaminases are suggestive of a hepatitic cause. However, a mixed picture is often the case; hence, too much emphasis should not be given to blood results alone.
- Prothrombin time is the most easily available test that gives some indication of hepatic synthetic function because all of the clotting factors are made in the liver. It correlates well with outcome in acute liver failure.

Prothrombin time is influenced by vitamin K, as this is a required co-factor for coagulation factors II, VII, IX, and X. Because vitamin K is a fat-soluble vitamin, its absorption is reduced in bilary duct obstruction, when sufficient bile fails to reach the small intestine. In this situation, a single dose of intravenous vitamin K may correct the prothrombin time; it will have no effect if the coagulopathy is due to deficient synthesis of coagulation factors, as in parenchymal liver diseases.

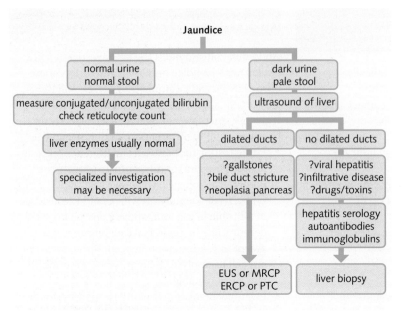

Fig. 12.2 Algorithm for the investigation of a patient with jaundice.

- Albumin, also synthesized in the liver, is reduced in any 'sick' state and correlates less well with severity of liver dysfunction. Similarly, blood urea is usually low but not very informative.
- Serum bilirubin does not necessarily reflect the degree of liver damage, particularly in the acute situation. In chronic liver disease, it gives a reasonable indication of the stage of progression.
- Full blood count may reveal anaemia. This may be spuriously macrocytic if accompanied by a significant reticulocytosis, as in haemolytic disease. Reticulocyte count should be checked. Macrocytosis with low platelets is suggestive of hypersplenism associated with the portal hypertension of chronic liver disease. A blood film may be appropriate to look for signs of haemolysis, sickle cells, or atypical lymphocytes seen in Epstein–Barr virus infection (or other viral infections).
- Serology should be reserved to look for viral markers of acute hepatitis A to E, and for Epstein–Barr, CMV, and toxoplasmosis. A monospot test can give a rapid diagnosis of infectious mononucleosis. Markers for leptospirosis should also be done if clinically indicated.
- Autoantibodies to nuclear proteins and smooth muscle indicate an acute autoimmune hepatitis. They will usually be accompanied by elevated immunoglobulin (Ig)G levels. IgA is commonly elevated in alcoholic hepatitis. IgM (specifically M_2 subtype) is elevated in primary biliary cirrhosis.
- Elevated urinary copper and low serum caeruloplasmin levels indicate the possibility of Wilson's disease which is fatal if undetected and untreated.
- Percutaneous liver biopsy can provide valuable information regarding both the cause and extent of parenchymal liver damage. It is usually performed under ultrasound guidance, and the prothrombin time must be checked pre-biopsy. Special staining for copper and alpha-1-antitrypsin can be performed on histological sections.
- A computed tomography scan of the abdomen is mainly used to assess pancreatic masses and nodes at the porta hepatis when obstructive jaundice has been confirmed by ultrasound.
- Magnetic resonance cholangiography or endoscopic ultrasound are useful examinations for assessment of the bile duct, whilst obviating the serious risk of acute pancreatitis which exists with an endoscopic retrograde cholangiopancreatography (ERCP).
- ERCP or percutaneous transhepatic cholangiography is useful for further assessment and therapy if obstruction is identified.

Summary

An algorithm summarizing the investigation of a patient with jaundice is shown in Fig. 12.2.

13. Abnormal Liver Biochemistry

Patients are commonly referred to the gastroenterology clinic for investigation of abnormal liver biochemistry. This may have been detected whilst investigating pertinent symptoms, or discovered incidentally during investigation of other complaints. The four enzymes involved are:

- Alanine aminotransferase (ALT or SGPT in older texts).
- Aspartate aminotransferase (AST or SGOT in older texts).
- Alkaline phosphatase (AlkPhos).
- Gamma-glutamyl transferase (GGT).

Often these tests are referred to as liver 'function' tests. This is misleading because the elevation of liver enzymes does not reflect hepatic function.

Abnormal liver enzymes in the absence of jaundice may be commonly due to:

- Acute or chronic liver disease.
- Cirrhosis.
- Drugs, including alcohol.
- Liver metastasis.
- Cardiac causes such as acute myocardial infarction, cardiac failure, and constrictive pericarditis.
- Bony metastasis or Paget's disease can cause elevation of AlkPhos, as can pregnancy.
- AlkPhos can also rise as part of an acute inflammatory response, e.g. in autoimmune disease.
- Hypothyroidism or pernicious anaemia occasionally present with elevated transaminases.
- Severe sepsis or atypical pneumonias can result in deranged liver enzymes.

History of the patient with abnormal liver biochemistry

It is first essential to establish the chronology of the abnormalities. When were the results last normal? Assess the trend of abnormalities and attempt to correlate this with relevant drug interventions and medical history.

Patients are usually asymptomatic when referred to outpatient clinics, or tests may have been carried out for vague symptoms such as malaise or fatigue. Hence it is important to interpret the results in context, in order to focus appropriate investigation and avoid further unnecessary tests.

The following points usually help.

Drug history

Prescribed medication is the most common cause of abnormal liver biochemistry in the general population, apart from alcohol:

- Antibiotics such as flucloxacillin or co-amoxiclav can result in elevated transaminases, that can remain elevated for several weeks after their cessation.
- Many anti-arthritis drugs and anti-epileptic drugs (such as phenytoin or carbamazepine) can induce liver enzymes.

Alcohol

Alcohol is often the first thing that comes to mind in relation to liver disease. However, as an aetiological agent, it accounts for less than 20% of patients with liver disease attending outpatients.

There is no specific pattern to liver enzymes with alcohol use:

- GGT is easily induced and the most common liver abnormality to be seen.
- As an isolated abnormality, GGT is of little significance; its most useful role is indicating that a raised AlkPhos is of liver origin.
- An AST to ALT ratio of 2 or more is said to be specific for alcoholic hepatitis, but it is not a sensitive indicator.

Past medical history and surgical history

A history of biliary tract surgery, including cholecystectomy, is particularly relevant. Otherwise, history should concentrate on those aspects discussed in Chapter 12.

Be alert to those patients with a history of malignant disease, with a new finding of elevated AlkPhos. This may imply either bony or liver metastases.

common causes in the absence of jaundice are drugs, cholangitis, and primary biliary cirrhosis. Antimitochondrial antibodies may be helpful.

 Drug-induced abnormalities do not require further investigation if, following cessation of the offending drug (including reducing alcohol intake), the biochemistry returns to normal within 8–12 weeks.

Examining the patient with abnormal liver biochemistry

A general physical examination is clearly important, but in particular, signs of liver disease should be sought as discussed in Chapter 12. Other medical conditions can also be associated with raised liver enzymes:

- Hypothyroidism.
- Pernicious anaemia.
- Congestive cardiac failure.
- Lymphoma.
- Diabetes mellitus or hypercholesterolaemia.

Investigating abnormal liver biochemistry

The investigation largely depends on the pattern of abnormality produced by the elevated enzymes. The following is simply intended as a guide and in clinical practice often it is difficult (sometimes impossible) to decipher the 'picture' of abnormality presented.

Liver chemistry tests

These tests may aid diagnosis:

- If all four liver enzymes are raised, this would imply that significant liver pathology is present.
- A predominantly hepatitic abnormality is suggested if AST, ALT and, to a lesser extent GGT, are the most prominently raised enzymes. These may be only slightly elevated in certain conditions such as hepatitis C, haemochromatosis, or alpha-1-antitrypsin deficiency.
- A predominantly cholestatic abnormality is suggested by raised AlkPhos and GGT with or without elevation of serum bilirubin. In this situation, think of intra-hepatic or extra-hepatic cholestasis. If the bilirubin is also elevated, then an extra-hepatic cause is more likely. The most

Other blood tests

The following may help direct further investigation:

- Full blood count may demonstrate macrocytosis, which in association with an elevated GGT implies alcohol as a causative factor. Thrombocytopaenia may indicate hypersplenism due to portal hypertension and cirrhosis.
- Serology for the hepatitis viruses (see Chapter 18) is necessary, especially if ALT and AST (with or without elevation of bilirubin) are primarily affected.
- An autoantibody screen may be appropriate if the demographics of the patient and the clinical picture is suggestive of autoimmune disease (see Chapter 18).
- A polyclonal increase in immunoglobulins, although not always specific, can be useful. Elevated immunoglobulin (Ig)A can be associated with alcohol mediated damage. Raised IgM can indicate primary biliary cirrhosis and IgG is associated with chronic active hepatitis.

Imaging

Ultrasound of the liver is essential to exclude bile duct dilatation, liver metastasis or other focal abnormality and hepatic congestion.

Biopsy

Liver biopsy may be necessary if no other explanation is found for the abnormal liver biochemistry. It can also be performed to establish the underlying cause of cirrhosis if suspected on ultrasound. Be sure to measure the prothrombin time first!

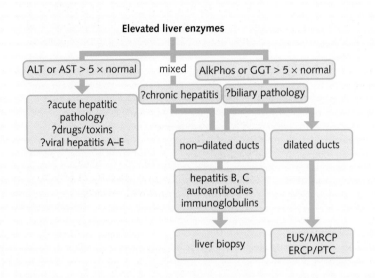

Fig 13.1 Algorithm for the investigation of a patient referred with abnormal liver enzymes. (ERCP, endoscopic retrograde cholangiopancreatography; EUS, endoscopic ultrasound; MRCP, magnetic resonance cholangiopancreatogram; PTC, percutaneous transhepatic cholangiography.)

Cirrhosis is a histological diagnosis which cannot be made on ultrasound scanning alone, although there are features such as irregular margins and nodules that may suggest the diagnosis. Metastatic disease is occasionally confused with cirrhosis on ultrasound scans.

Exceptions to consider
Note the following:
• Raised GGT alone is highly suggestive of alcohol consumption or drugs that induce hepatic enzymes such as anticonvulsants; hence, further investigation is usually unnecessary.
• Raised AlkPhos alone may suggest a non-hepatic origin, such as bone, placenta, or very occasionally

intestine. Isoenzymes can be measured if necessary, to establish the origin.
• AST is also produced by heart and striated muscle. It can be raised in myocardial infarction, hypothyroidism, and pernicious anaemia, hence its sole elevation should alert one to other medical conditions.
• ALT is much more specific for liver disease. A minor elevation on its own is probably of no consequence but, if raised in association with AlkPhos, it is usually an indication for further investigation including liver biopsy.
• There is no correlation between liver enzyme abnormalities and the extent of cirrhosis. The enzymes may be entirely normal even in advanced cirrhosis.

Summary
An algorithm summarizing the investigation of a patient referred with abnormal liver enzymes is shown in Fig. 13.1.

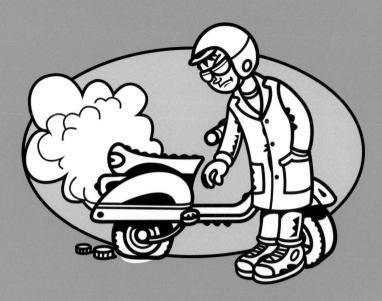

DISEASES AND DISORDERS

14. Oesophagus

Anatomy, physiology and function of the oesophagus

The oesophagus is a muscular tube composed of two layers:
- An outer longitudinal layer.
- An inner circular muscle layer.

The oesophagus connects the pharynx to the stomach. Striated (voluntary) muscle in the upper portion gradually changes to smooth muscle in the lower part and then becomes continuous with the muscle layer of the stomach. The lining of the oesophagus also changes from a stratified squamous epithelium to columnar epithelium at the gastro-oesophageal junction (Fig. 14.1).

When a food bolus is propelled into the pharynx by the tongue, the upper oesophageal sphincter (controlled by cricopharyngeus muscle) relaxes, allowing the passage of food into the oesophagus. A primary peristaltic wave starts from the pharynx and continues down along the length of the oesophagus. Secondary peristalsis occurs locally due to distension of the oesophagus by a food bolus. The lower oesophageal sphincter (LOS) relaxes prior to peristaltic contractions when swallowing is initiated. The progression of a peristaltic swallow wave can be followed by placing pressure transducers at intervals along the oesophagus (oesophageal manometry; see Figs 24.9 and 24.10).

Preventing regurgitation of the stomach contents back in to the oesophagus is dependent on:
- Gravity.
- LOS pressure.
- The oblique course of the gastro-oesophageal junction.
- The diaphragmatic crura wrapped around the oesophagus.
- The physiological emptying of the stomach contents into the duodenum through the pylorus.

Inflammatory conditions

Reflux oesophagitis
Incidence
A common condition of which the incidence increases with age. This is probably multifactorial, but may be related to the fact that hiatus hernias are found more commonly in elderly people.

Clinical features
A variety of symptoms are associated with the reflux of gastric acid contents to the oesophagus. When the symptoms produce upper abdominal pain, belching, or heartburn, they are referred to collectively as dyspepsia (see Chapter 1). Otherwise, more specific terms should be used to describe them:
- Heartburn is the most common presenting symptom due to reflux of gastric acid into the oesophagus. This can cause erosive oesophagitis. Correlation between symptoms and extent of oesophagitis is poor.
- Retrosternal chest pain can be due to spasm of the distal oesophageal muscle or from inflammation.
- Vomiting of blood (haematemesis) can present in association with severe oesophagitis.
- Iron deficiency anaemia can occur due to insidious blood loss from chronic inflammation.
- Nocturnal cough and early morning bronchospasm, producing a dip in peak flow readings, may occur as a result of reflux with microaspiration into the trachea. There is some evidence that acid in the oesophagus can precipitate reflex bronchospasm (see Figure 1.1).

Do not forget to consider medication as a cause or precipitant for dyspepsic/reflux-type symptoms. Many drugs can be implicated—especially those with anticholinergic effects. If in doubt, look in the British National Formulary!

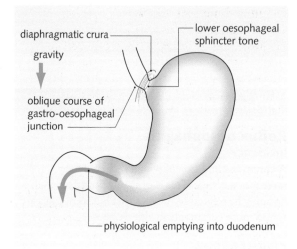

diaphragmatic crura

gravity

lower oesophageal
sphincter tone

oblique course of
gastro-oesophageal
junction

physiological emptying into duodenum

Fig. 14.1 Anatomical relations of the oesophagus.

Diagnosis and investigation
Endoscopy
This may show the varying grades of oesophagitis and in severe cases, ulceration. However, normal endoscopy does not exclude reflux oesophagitis and a biopsy may be necessary.

Twenty-four hour intraluminal pH monitoring
This is probably the most accurate way of detecting reflux disease because there is a reasonable correlation between low pH (<4) occurring within the 24-hour period and symptoms of reflux (see Figs 24.11 and 24.12).

Barium swallow
This is still used, but is only significant when a free reflux of barium is demonstrated.

Aetiology and pathogenesis
A reduction in tone of the LOS is the main factor contributing to acid reflux. This normally occurs when the patient lies down or if there is raised intra-abdominal pressure (e.g. pregnancy, obesity, weight lifting, chronic constipation). Reduction in the resistance of the oesophageal mucosa to acid and delayed gastric emptying will also predispose to acid reflux. Any drug with an anticholinergic action (e.g. tricyclic antidepressants, anti-psychotics, oxybutynin, theophylline) may aggravate symptoms of reflux. Non-steroidal anti-inflammatory drugs can also contribute to symptoms.

Alcohol and smoking have also been implicated in its pathogenesis: smoking reduces LOS tone and alcohol stimulates gastric acid production.

A sliding-type hiatus hernia, where the gastro-oesophageal junction lies above the diaphragm, is associated with oesophageal reflux. However, its presence alone is not diagnostic because not all patients with hiatus hernia will develop symptoms.

Complications
Stricture
Stricture occurs after long-standing acid reflux, causing stricture of the lower oesophagus, producing symptoms of dysphagia.

Barrett's oesophagus
Columnarization of squamous epithelium (metaplasia) occurs with chronic reflux. Cells that develop other abnormal features may become dysplastic with potential for malignant transformation. This may be prevented or possibly even reversed by antireflux therapy.

Prognosis
Over 50% of patients will have significant improvement with only conservative treatment.

Aims of treatment
Treatment is mainly for symptom control. Barrett's oesophagus should be treated and surveillance for development of dysplastic features should be undertaken by endoscopy.

Treatment
Treatment may include:
- Conservative treatments, such as weight reduction, cessation of smoking, and reduction in alcohol consumption, will help symptoms in mild cases. If reflux is mainly nocturnal, then raising the head of the bed may be of benefit. Regular meals and avoidance of fatty food is important.
- Antacids, such as magnesium trisilicate or alginate-containing compounds (Gaviscon), coat the mucosa and will abolish symptoms in most mild cases.
- H_2-receptor antagonists (e.g. nizatidine or ranitidine) work by reducing gastric acid output as a result of histamine H_2-receptor blockade.
- Proton pump inhibitors (PPIs) (e.g. omeprazole or lansoprazole) are potent inhibitors of acid production. This is achieved by blocking the hydrogen-potassium ATP enzyme system (the 'proton-pump') of the gastric parietal cell. They are the drug class of choice for severe symptoms

and Barrett's oesophagus because there is almost complete inhibition of acid production from the stomach.

- Prokinetic drugs (e.g. domperidone) can enhance gut motility, probably by increasing the release of dopamine or acetylcholine. (Cisapride was a similar drug that improved gastric emptying and concomitantly increased LOS pressure, but has now been withdrawn as it predisposed toward dangerous cardiac arrhythmias.)
- Surgery—tightening the lower oesophagus by wrapping the fundus of the stomach around it (fundoplication) is reserved for patients who are symptomatic despite conforming with conservative and pharmacological treatment. This procedure can be performed safely and successfully via laparoscopy, but patients should be carefully selected. Too tight a wrap results in dysphagia.

The National Institute for Clinical Excellence (NICE) has provided guidance on the use of PPIs. In the context of GORD, they are indicated for severe symptoms (reduce dose when symptoms abate), and in disease complicated by stricture, ulceration or haemorrhage.

Barrett's oesophagus
Incidence
About 15% of patients with prolonged reflux of acid into the lower oesophagus have Barrett's oesophagus.

Aetiology and pathogenesis
Prolonged irritation causes the transformation (metaplasia) from squamous epithelium to columnar-type intestinal epithelium, which is covered by mucin (Fig. 14.2). Intestinal metaplastic change is occasionally followed by dysplastic change predisposing to malignant transformation.

Clinical features
The clinical features are the same as for reflux oesophagitis.

Diagnosis and investigation
Seen at endoscopy, where normal squamous epithelium is replaced by columnar epithelium (metaplasia). Barrett's oesophagus manifests endoscopically as a change of colour, from pink to slightly orange, and of texture. Histological examination will confirm the diagnosis, revealing varying grades of cellular change, from metaplasia through to severe dysplasia.

Complications
Barrett's oesophagus predisposes to adenocarcinoma of the oesophagus. This tumour has an increasing prevalence throughout the developed world. It is thought to carry up to a 40-fold risk of adenocarcinoma. Absence of the tumour suppressor gene p53 may have aetiological relevance.

Prognosis
Dependent on grade of dysplasia, cessation of reflux and endoscopic surveillance. Adequate treatment with a proton pump inhibitor abolishes symptoms of reflux and may allow columnar epithelium to return to normal squamous epithelium, thus avoiding premalignant change.

Treatment
Proton pump inhibitors such as omeprazole may be given long-term to prevent recurrence. Repeated endoscopies may be required to monitor dysplastic change if present. Techniques such as epithelial laser ablation or photodynamic therapy intend to result in resolution of metaplasia, but the long-term outcome is not known.

Oesophageal strictures
Incidence
Benign strictures secondary to acid reflux are becoming less common amongst those with GORD because of the availability of H_2 antagonists and proton pump inhibitors.

Clinical features
Dysphagia, or difficulty in swallowing, is the main presenting symptom. This can be progressive from solids to liquids as fibrosis worsens.

Weight loss can be marked because the patient may have difficulty maintaining the required caloric intake. The patient may often give a history of preceding reflux that disappeared before the onset of dysphagia. This happens because the development of

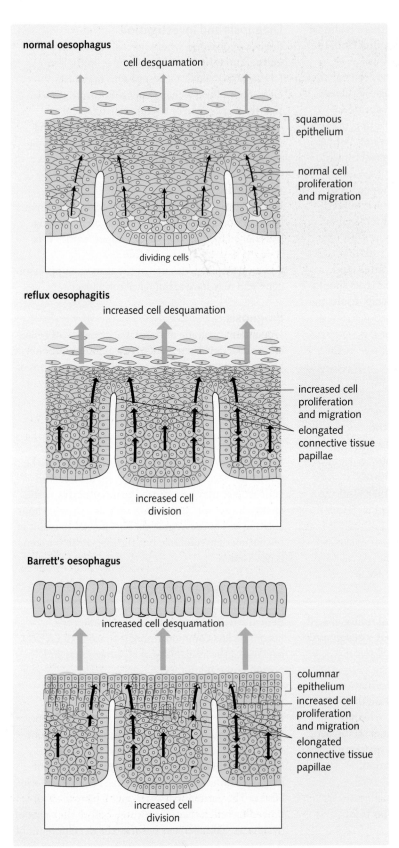

normal oesophagus

cell desquamation

squamous epithelium

normal cell proliferation and migration

dividing cells

reflux oesophagitis

increased cell desquamation

increased cell proliferation and migration

elongated connective tissue papillae

increased cell division

Barrett's oesophagus

increased cell desquamation

columnar epithelium

increased cell proliferation and migration

elongated connective tissue papillae

increased cell division

Fig. 14.2 Changes in Barrett's mucosa: the normal squamous epithelium is replaced by columnar epithelium. Cells with abnormal nuclear material constitute dysplastic change and herald malignant transformation.

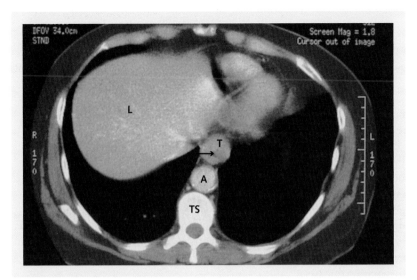

Fig. 14.3 Computed tomography scan demonstrating malignant infiltration from an oesophageal stricture. Only a pinhole lumen remains of the oesophagus (arrow), which is surrounded by tumour (T). (A, aorta; L, liver; TS, thoracic spine.)

a fibrotic stricture can impair further reflux of acid. Symptoms can mimic malignant stricture, although benign strictures tend to have a longer symptomatic history.

Diagnosis and investigation
Consider the following investigations:
- Endoscopy can show extensive scarring of the oesophagus, and biopsy is necessary to exclude malignant disease.
- Barium swallow is an alternative if the patient cannot tolerate endoscopy. A smooth diffuse stricture can be seen usually without shouldering.
- Imaging by endoluminal ultrasound or a spiral computed tomography (CT) scan may be necessary to exclude malignant infiltration (Fig. 14.3).

Aetiology and pathogenesis
Long-standing acid reflux causes permanent scarring and fibrosis. Other causes include:
- Ingestion of caustic substance.
- Previous radiotherapy.
- Previous sclerotherapy for oesophageal varices.

Prolonged intubation of a nasogastric tube can also give rise to benign strictures.

Complications
There is an increased incidence of malignant change in benign strictures, but this may reflect the underlying pathology.

Prognosis
Once a stricture has formed, the condition is likely to remain throughout life.

Aim of treatment
Purely for symptomatic relief of dysphagia. Reflux should also be treated to prevent worsening of the condition.

Treatment
Treatment may include:
- Dilatation is undertaken endoscopically with graduated tubes of increasing sizes inserted through the affected part of the oesophagus to widen the lumen. The procedure often needs to be repeated because re-narrowing of the lumen can occur over a period of time. Endoscopic balloon dilatation is an alternative which is probably safer. Oesophageal perforation is a small but significant procedure-related risk.
- Surgery—required if dilatation fails to control symptoms of dysphagia.

Neoplasia

Carcinoma of oesophagus
Incidence
Occurs in approximately 10 out of 100 000 people in the UK. A higher rate is seen in parts of China and Africa, possibly related to local diet.

Clinical features

Dysphagia is the most common presenting symptom, and is progressive from solids to liquids. This can occur relatively rapidly over a period of weeks to months.

Other features include:
- Weight loss—consequent upon anorexia, dysphagia, and possibly mediated by release of tumour cytokines.
- Anaemia due to ulceration of the lesion is common, and may cause insidious blood loss, resulting in iron deficiency anaemia.
- Pain on swallowing (odynophagia) occurs in advanced stages; local infiltration by the tumour causes diffuse, persistent, retrosternal pain.
- Dyspnoea and cough, due to aspiration of pharyngeal secretions. In advanced cases, this may be due to oesophagotracheal fistulae or tracheal encasement.

Diagnosis and investigation

Consider the following investigations:
- Full blood count may demonstrate iron-deficiency anaemia or rarely pancytopaenia from metastatic bone marrow infiltration by tumour.
- Derangement of liver biochemistry or hypercalcaemia may be seen if metastases are present.
- Urea and electrolytes often reveal dehydration, as a result of dysphagia.
- Endoscopy—the investigation of choice because it allows direct visualization of the lesion and an opportunity for biopsy and histological confirmation.
- Barium swallow—reserved for patients who cannot tolerate an endoscopy, or those suspected of having a high-level stricture. Malignant strictures characteristically have a shouldered appearance (see Fig. 2.3B).
- Endoscopic ultrasound and spiral CT scan of thorax—used for staging if surgery is under consideration. Commonly, this is precluded by the frailty of the patient, late presentation with advanced malignancy or concomitant medical conditions.

Aetiology and pathogenesis

Rarely occur under age of 50 years. Two histological types are seen:

- Squamous carcinoma.
- Adenocarcinoma.

Squamous carcinoma:
- 90% of all oesophageal cancer is squamous in nature.
- 50% of all squamous cancers occur in the lower third of oesophagus.
- Higher incidence in China, which may suggest a dietary aetiology.
- More common in men, particularly with high alcohol intake and cigarette smoking.
- More unusual predisposing factors include achalasia, Plummer–Vinson syndrome, and tylosis (hyperkeratosis of palms and soles inherited as an rare autosomal dominant condition).

Adenocarcinoma:
- Usually as a result of malignant transformation of Barrett's oesophagus.
- Occasionally, it arises as an extension from adenocarcinoma of gastric cardia.

Complications

The tumour may invade adjacent anatomical structures:
- Through the oesophageal wall and into a bronchus, creating an oesophageal–bronchial fistula, resulting in recurrent pneumonia (note that aspiration pneumonia may occur as a result of severe dysphagia, in the absence of a fistula).
- Into the thoracic aorta, resulting in rapid exsanguination.

Prognosis

To some extent, this is dependent on stage of the tumour and fitness of the patient. However, the prognosis is usually exceptionally poor, with an overall survival of 2% at 5 years.

Treatment

Mainly palliative because curative treatment is rarely possible due to late presentation of the disease. Consider:
- Surgery—provides the only possible cure but carries an operative mortality of 5–10%. Less than 40% of patients are suitable for surgical resection at presentation, but these patients are often

elderly and frail with medical co-morbidity precluding radical surgery.

- Radiotherapy—reduces the bulk of the tumour and may relieve dysphagia. Fistula formation is more common after radiotherapy treatment.
- Laser therapy—high-energy thermal laser ablation is used to burn through the bulk of tumour and restore oesophageal lumen. An alternative for smaller tumours is photodynamic therapy, using a lower energy laser light in combination with a chemical photosensitizer which is selectively taken up by tumour tissue. Repeated administration of either modality may be required.
- Endoscopic placement of a plastic or expanding metal hollow stent (endoprosthesis) across the obstructing lesion can give palliative relief of dysphagia. This carries a risk of perforation in up to 10% of patients.

Tumour–node–metastasis (TNM) classification of tumours

The approach to management of many malignant tumours depends on their stage. In addition, a comparison of treatment strategies is heavily reliant on making sure that like is compared with like.

An internationally accepted classification for tumours is the TNM staging system. This system varies for different organs and tissues but follows the general principle shown in Fig. 14.4:

- 'T' refers to the extent of the tumour itself: T0 usually indicates no detectable tumour, T1 is confined to mucosa, and T3+ is infiltrating deeper layers or surrounding structures depending on the site.
- Similarily, 'N' refers to lymph node involvement, N0 meaning no node involvement, N1 is usually confined to local nodes and N2+ is confined to more distant nodes specified for that tumour type.
- Very distant nodes are usually classified as 'M' for metastatic. M0 means no metastases detected, Mn indicates distant spread, again 'n' having a specific meaning for each tumour type.

Thus, T4N2M2 is a tumour with:
- Extensive local infiltration.
- Distant lymph node involvement.
- Metastatic spread to other sites.

Anatomical and functional problems

Pharyngeal pouch and oesophageal diverticulum
Incidence
Usually discovered coincidentally whilst a barium meal is performed for other reasons.

Clinical features
The majority are asymptomatic, although they can cause regurgitation of food and are a rare cause of dysphagia.

Diagnosis and investigation
Barium swallow demonstrates the size and location of the lesion (Fig. 14.5).

Aetiology and pathogenesis
Probably related to dysmotility of cricopharyngeus muscle and inferior constrictor forming a mucosal outpouching (pharyngeal pouch). Diverticulae may also occur in the mid-oesophagus due to traction by mediastinal lymph node inflammation (traction diverticulum), or just above the lower oesophageal sphincter (epiphrenic diverticulum).

Complications
Occur rarely—perforation may occur when endoscopy is performed for investigation of dysphagia, as the pouch may be mistaken for the oesophageal lumen!

Treatment
Surgical resection is reserved for pouches that are problematic.

Oesophageal webs
Incidence
Oesophageal web is often a coincidental finding on barium meal. Those associated with iron deficiency anaemia are rare.

Clinical features
Usually the patient is asymptomatic, but high level dysphagia may occur when tough fibrous food is swallowed without care. There may be a history of a persistent cough, due to the aspiration of pharyngeal secretions.

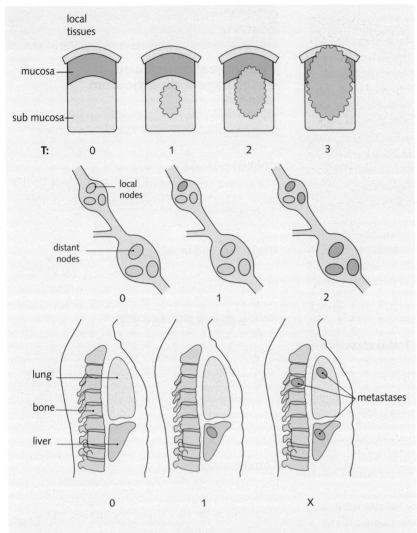

Fig. 14.4 Graphic illustration of the Tumour–node–metastasis (TNM) classification of mucosal malignant disease. T0, no evidence of primary tumour; T1, tumour confined to mucosa; T2, infiltration through sub mucosa but not penetrating through the muscularis; T3, extends through muscularis to serosa; T4, extends to local tissues; N0, no lymph node involvement; N1, local lymph node involvement; N2, distant lymph node involvement.

T = graded 0–4, refers to the primary tumour according to its depth of involvement
T0 = no evidence of primary tumour

N = 0–2, refers to lymph nodes involved; increasing score indicates higher numbers of lymph node involvment

M = 0 or 1 refers to presence and absence of metastases. The example shown might be for carcinoma of the colon

Anaemia may present as part of the Plummer–Vinson syndrome (see below).

Diagnosis and investigation
- Barium swallow—demonstrates narrowing of the oesophagus by fibrous tissue. Proximal part of the oesophagus may be distended with barium.
- Endoscopy—webs may be difficult to see, especially those in the postcricoid area.

Aetiology and pathogenesis
Unknown aetiology—different clinical outcome depending on site of the web. Two types are commonly recognized:
- Postcricoid web.
- Lower oesophageal web.

Postcricoid web:
- Is also know as Plummer–Vinson or Paterson–Brown–Kelly syndrome.

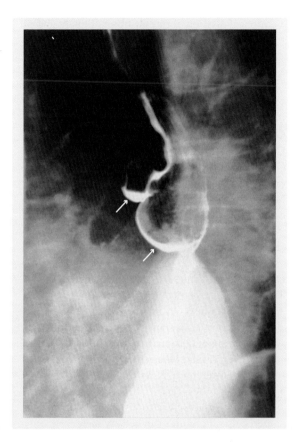

Fig. 14.5 Lateral view of oesophageal diverticulum (arrows) in the upper oesophagus seen on barium swallow. Note the fluid levels.

- Is associated with iron deficiency anaemia and atrophic glossitis.

Lower oesophageal web:
- Is also known as Schatzki ring, where there is a small, fibromuscular band that originates from the diaphragm.
- Is often associated with a hiatus hernia.

Complications
There is an increased risk of developing postcricoid carcinoma of the pharynx associated with Plummer–Vinson syndrome.

Treatment
Dilatation of the obstruction is rarely needed.

Oral iron supplementation may be required if iron-deficiency anaemia, associated with Plummer–Vinson syndrome, is present.

Achalasia
Incidence
Achalasia is a rare condition with a prevalence of approximately 1:100 000.

Clinical features
These include:
- Intermittent dysphagia—usually a long history with both liquids and solids. Presentation in childhood is rare.
- Regurgitation—common; may result in aspiration pneumonia if it occurs at night-time. Dysphagia can sometimes be overcome by drinking large quantities of fluid; hence, increases risk of aspiration.
- Chest pain—this is common and is typically retrosternal and occasionally severe, due to non-peristaltic contraction of oesophageal muscles. Often mistaken for cardiac pain, especially when dysphagic symptoms are mild.

Diagnosis and investigation
The following investigations should be considered:
- Chest X-ray—may show a double cardiac shadow with a fluid level behind the heart. Evidence of pneumonia, or atelectasis implying previous infection, may also be present. Aspiration classically occurs down the right main bronchus, into the right middle and lower lobes.
- Barium swallow—dilatation of the oesophagus is seen with a narrowed lower portion (beak appearance) due to lack of relaxation by the lower oesophageal sphincter (Fig. 14.6). Reduced peristaltic contraction is also seen.
- Endoscopy—usually passes through the narrowed region without resistance, and is therefore often missed. Biopsy is taken to confirm the diagnosis and exclude underlying malignancy.
- Motility studies—used to confirm lack of peristalsis along the oesophagus and failure of relaxation by the lower oesophageal sphincter (see Fig. 24.10b).
- Endoscopic ultrasound—may be helpful in excluding submucosal malignant infiltration and can show characteristic muscle thickening.

Aetiology and pathogenesis
Unknown aetiology—characterized by lack of peristalsis and failure of relaxation by the lower oesophageal sphincter after swallowing.

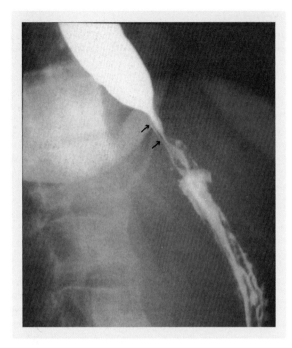

Fig. 14.6 Barium swallow showing 'bird's beak' appearance of achalasia.

Histology shows a reduction of Auerbach plexus ganglia cells in the oesophageal walls.

Infection with *Trypanosoma cruzi* (Chagas' disease or American trypanosomiasis) will produce a similar appearance.

Complications and prognosis

There is an increased risk of developing oesophageal carcinoma (up to 10% higher than normal population).

Reflux oesophagitis is a major complication after treatment.

Treatment

Treatment may include:
• Dilatation with high pressure balloons—this is undertaken endoscopically and is successful in over two-thirds of cases.

• Surgical division of muscle fibres at lower end of oesophagus (cardiomyotomy)—can now be performed laparoscopically.
• Calcium antagonists (e.g. nifedipine) reduce oesophageal spasm and may be used by elderly patients who are unsuitable for procedures.

Oesophageal spasm
Clinical features

Chest pain is retrosternal and severe, and often radiates to the back. It can be relieved by nitrates; hence, it is difficult to distinguish from ischaemic cardiac pain.

Dysphagia can occur due to marked contraction of oesophageal muscles.

Diagnosis and investigation

The following investigations may be used:
• Barium swallow—characteristically demonstrates a 'corkscrew' appearance due to uncoordinated contraction of oesophageal muscles (see Fig. 1.5). However, similar changes may be seen in elderly people without any symptoms.
• Motility studies—show diffuse contraction of oesophageal muscle without progression of peristalsis. Pressures can be very high ('nutcracker' oesophagus).

Aetiology and pathogenesis

Unknown aetiology—after swallowing, the oesophagus contracts diffusely in an uncoordinated fashion without peristalsis; hence, the onset of dysphagia and chest pain.

Complications

Formation of diverticula is commonly associated with oesophageal spasm. Cricopharyngeal spasm is closely related to formation of pharyngeal pouches.

Treatment

Drugs such as antispasmodics, calcium channel antagonists, or nitrates may be of help. Surgery, such as myotomy, may be required in exceptional cases.

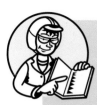

- What are the physiological mechanisms that normally prevent regurgitation of stomach contents into the oesophagus?
- What are the factors predisposing to acid reflux? Name some drugs that might exacerbate reflux and explain why this occurs.
- What is the pathophysiology of Barrett's oesophagus?
- What is the role of surgery in reflux oesophagitis?
- What are the treatment options for a patient with oesophageal cancer, and which factors influence the choice?

15. Stomach

Anatomy, physiology and function of the stomach

The stomach is divided into:
- An upper portion known as the fundus.
- The body of the stomach.
- The antrum, which extends to form the pyloric region, encompassing the pyloric sphincter (Fig. 15.1).

Three muscle layers form the stomach: outer longitudinal, middle circular, and inner oblique. The thickened circular layer at the pyloric area forms the pyloric sphincter.

The upper two-thirds of the stomach contains:
- Parietal cells which secrete acid (hydrochloric acid).
- Chief cells which secrete pepsinogen.

The antrum secretes gastrin from G-cells which stimulates acid production.

Acid secretion consists of three different phases (Fig. 15.2):
- Cephalic-mediated via the vagus stimulated by sight or smell of food.
- Gastric distension of the stomach by food directly stimulates secretory cells.
- Intestinal hormones are released as food is passed into small intestine, stimulating acid release.

A low pH in the stomach is required to activate enzymes required for digestion and to act as a barrier to bacteria. Other functions of the stomach include secretion of intrinsic factor and, of minor importance, absorption of glucose and amino acids.

As the stomach is a port of entry to the body, ingestion of unsuitable agents can be problematic. These manifest as nausea, vomiting, or pathologically, as acute gastritis. Other entities are categorized according to pathological mechanisms.

Acute gastritis

Incidence
A very common condition with a variety of causes.

Clinical features
These include:
- Nausea and vomiting are the most likely presenting symptoms, together with indigestion.
- Acute gastrointestinal (GI) bleed if gastritis is severe.
- Asymptomatic.

Diagnosis and investigation
The diagnosis is often made on clinical grounds (e.g. history of non-steroidal anti-inflammatory drugs, NSAIDs), heavy alcohol consumption, etc. There may be epigastric tenderness but this is not a discriminating sign.

Endoscopic appearance can vary from superficial erosions to haemorrhage secondary to acute ulceration.

Aetiology and pathogenesis
The pathological appearance is that of an acute inflammatory infiltrate in the superficial mucosa, predominantly of neutrophils. Occasionally, superficial ulceration can be seen. Drugs such as aspirin and other NSAIDs reduce the production of prostaglandin and interfere with cytoprotection. Alcohol damages the mucosal mucus layer and causes gastritis. *Helicobacter pylori* can also cause acute gastritis, but is more commonly associated with chronic gastritis.

Superficial ulceration can develop in acutely ill patients (e.g. acute renal failure, liver disease, sepsis, etc.). The exact mechanism is unknown but may be related to the alteration in the mucus barrier.

Prognosis and treatment
Patients usually recover without any long-term complications. The removal of the offending cause is usually all that is required. An acute GI bleed should be treated in the conventional way. An H_2 antagonist may be of help in some cases.

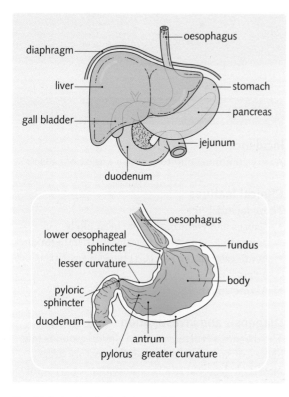

Fig. 15.1 Anatomical relations of the stomach.

Peptic ulcer disease

Under this heading, we include gastritis, gastric ulcer, and duodenal ulcer, which is dealt with here rather than in Chapter 16. These conditions are all associated with *H. pylori* infection.

Helicobacter pylori infection
Incidence
It is estimated that, in developed countries, 50% of the population over the age of 50 years are infected with the spiral-shaped Gram-negative bacterium. The incidence is declining with improved sanitation, and there is evidence that infection is most often acquired in childhood. In certain parts of the world (e.g. South America), the majority of the population is infected.

Clinical features
Asymptomatic infection is often discovered incidentally. Furthermore, the high prevalence of *H. pylori* infection in certain populations (e.g. Nigeria), without a concomitant, active disease process such as

duodenal ulceration, indicates that host factors also have a role in producing pathology and symptoms.

Symptoms suggestive of acute gastiris, chronic gastritis or peptic ulcer disease usually unmask the presence of *H. pylori* (Fig. 15.3).

Epidemiological data suggest that there is an increased risk of gastric carcinoma, and long-standing gastritis increases the risk of gastric lymphoma.

Diagnosis and investigation
The following investigations may be useful:
- Endoscopy may demonstrate a blotchy mucosal appearance and a biopsy can be taken for urease test, histology, or culture to confirm the presence of *H. pylori*.
- Urease test—an antral biopsy is added to a pre-prepared urea solution containing a colour reagent. If bacterial urease is present, ammonia is produced and reacts with the reagent to produce a colour change which is indicative of the presence of the bacterium.
- Histology—the bacteria can be detected histologically by routine staining and section.
- Culture—can be achieved in special medium.
- Urea breath test: ^{14}C or ^{13}C radiolabelled urea is given orally and in the presence of *H. pylori* will break down to ammonia and radiolabelled CO_2, which is absorbed and subsequently measured in the exhaled breath (see Fig. 24.8).
- Serology: a relatively specific antibody (immunoglobulin G class) can now be measured in serum using an enzyme-linked immunosorbent assay technique, but its clinical value is limited because it confirms past exposure rather than current infection and it is not helpful in confirming eradication.

Aetiology and pathogenesis
The exact mechanism remains obscure but it is thought that people infected with *H. pylori* have an elevated level of gastrin due to G-cell hyperplasia in the antrum, which, in turn, predisposes to gastric and duodenal ulceration. There may also be an increase in parietal cell mass and pepsinogen production.

Normal gastric mucosa concentrates vitamin C, and its secretion is suppressed by *H. pylori*. This may account for the increased incidence of gastric lymphoma and carcinoma that can occur due to loss of antioxidant activity mediated by ascorbic acid.

Most people are infected during childhood and have been associated with overcrowded living

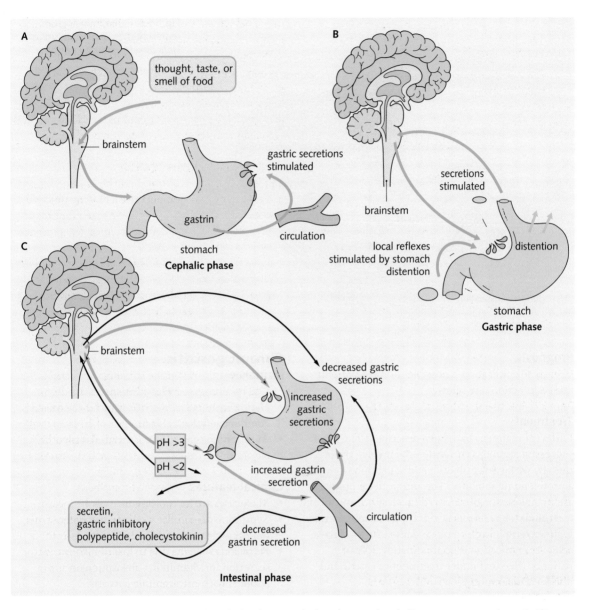

Fig. 15.2 Physiology of acid secretion. (A) Cephalic phase in which taste, visual and olfactory senses act through the brainstem and parasympathetic system to cause gastrin secretion, which in turn stimulates acid production. (B) Gastric phase in which ingested food distends the stomach and stretch receptors act through brainstem reflexes to increase gastric secretions. (C) Food in the intestine has different effects depending upon the pH. At higher pH, the pathways are stimulatory and increase gastric secretion further (green lines); at lower pH negative and inhibitory factors come into play to reduce gastric secretion (black lines).

conditions. The incidence of infection in many countries is falling as a result of improved living conditions.

Complications

- Acute GI bleed, due to peptic ulcer disease.
- Gastric lymphoma of a particular variety

'Maltoma' has been associated with Helicobacter infection. This is a proliferative disease of the mucosa-associated lymphoid tissue (MALT). Reports of regression following *H. pylori* eradication therapy have been published.

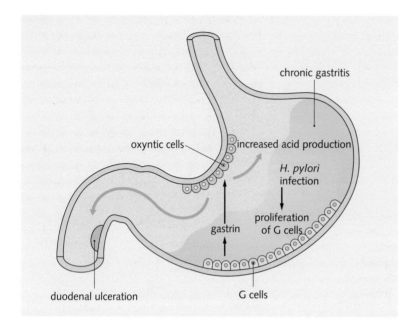

Fig. 15.3 Pathophysiological representation of mechanisms of *Helicobacter*-induced gastritis.

Labels in figure: chronic gastritis; oxyntic cells; increased acid production; *H. pylori* infection; gastrin; proliferation of G cells; duodenal ulceration; G cells

Prognosis
Complete eradication is possible for most patients and re-infection rate is low.

Treatment
Different regimens have been described. The most successful regimens currently used involve triple therapy with two antibiotics and acid inhibition with a proton pump inhibitor. The antibiotics employed are a combination of amoxycillin, clarithromycin, and metronidazole. Currently, this type of triple therapy regimen, employed as a twice-daily dose for 7 days, achieves eradication in approximately 90% of patients. (See text under treatment of gastric and duodenal ulceration.)

Any patient receiving metronidazole must avoid alcohol because the drug can inhibit acetaldehyde dehydrogenase and produce unpleasant histamine-induced symptoms if this metabolite builds up. This can manifest as facial flushing, headache, palpitations, vomiting and even cardiac arrhythmias.

Chronic gastritis
Incidence
- Can be a progression of acute gastritis.
- *Helicobacter pylori* gastritis is by far the most common aetiological factor.
- Autoimmune gastritis is associated with other autoimmune diseases.

Clinical features
- Most cases are asymptomatic.
- Symptoms are similar to those of acute gastritis, but occurring over a period of time.
- Pernicious anaemia due to loss of intrinsic factor secretion for vitamin B_{12} absorption occurs in patients with autoimmune gastritis.

Diagnosis and investigation
Endoscopy reveals an atrophic mucosa. Intrinsic factor autoantibodies and antiparietal cell antibodies are positive in patients with pernicious anaemia.

Aetiology and pathogenesis
Helicobacter pylori is the most common cause of chronic gastritis. Chronic ingestion of alcohol and NSAIDs may also be contributory, and reflux of bile has also been implicated.

There is loss of parietal and chief cells together with an infiltration of the lamina propria with plasma cells and lymphocytes. Chronic atrophic changes cause intestinal metaplasia.

Autoantibodies to parietal cells and intrinsic factor cause achlorhydria and pernicious anaemia with atrophic changes seen in the stomach.

Complications
Intestinal metaplasia predisposes to malignancy.

Treatment
The aim is to treat the underlying cause:
- Eradication therapy for *H. pylori*.
- Vitamin B_{12} is given intramuscularly if pernicious anaemia is present.

Gastric ulcer
Incidence
More commonly seen in the elderly population, gastric ulceration is less common than duodenal ulceration by a ratio of 1:4. Peak incidence occurs between 50 and 60 years of age.

Clinical features
Epigastric pain can be the main presenting feature. Classically, pain with gastric ulcer is associated with food, whereas duodenal ulcers tend to cause symptoms at night, or with an empty stomach, and are relieved by food. However, in the majority of cases, the discriminating value of these histories is poor and not helpful in the diagnosis.

Temporary relief with antacids is usually reported.

Associated features include: nausea, heartburn, anorexia, and weight loss. These symptoms also occur with gastric carcinoma.

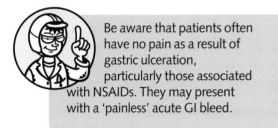

Be aware that patients often have no pain as a result of gastric ulceration, particularly those associated with NSAIDs. They may present with a 'painless' acute GI bleed.

Diagnosis and investigation
Investigations include:
- Endoscopy—the investigation of choice as biopsy enables differentiation of benign from malignant ulcers. During an acute bleed from a vessel, an injection of adrenaline may halt the bleeding.
- Barium meal—will also demonstrate gastric and duodenal ulceration, but biopsies cannot be taken to exclude underlying malignancy.

Aetiology and pathogenesis
The exact aetiology is unknown, but *H. pylori* is present in 70% and most of the remainder are associated with NSAIDs. Some patients with gastric ulcers have normal or low acid output, especially ulcers occurring at the lesser curve. Theories regarding pathogenesis include:
- A possible defect in the mucosal barrier usually maintained by bicarbonate secretion by the gastric epithelium.
- Prostaglandin-mediated cytoprotection has also been postulated to be deficient.

This may account for the higher incidence seen in elderly people because this cytoprotective mechanism diminishes with age.

Pre-pyloric ulcers are associated with a high acid output and behave more like a duodenal ulcer.

Differences between malignant and benign gastric ulcers are shown in Fig. 15.4.

Complications
Iron deficiency anaemia is common. Acute GI bleed, perforation, or erosion can occur. Pre-pyloric ulcers may cause pyloric stenosis and resultant gastric outlet obstruction, but this is more commonly seen with duodenal ulcers.

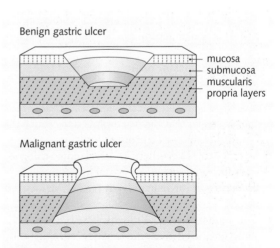

Fig. 15.4 Differences between malignant and benign gastric ulcers. Usually benign ulcers are more superficial. Malignant ulcers have more heaped edges. Multiple biopsy is essential.

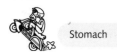

Prognosis

Fifty per cent of gastric ulcers recur within 1 year. It has been suggested that long-term antisecretory medication with H_2 receptor antagonists or proton pump inhibitors (PPI) should be used.

Treatment

For *H. pylori* positive ulcers, a triple therapy eradication regimen, with acid suppression, is used. There is no known single best eradication regimen, but the following regimes are recommended by the British Society of Gastroenterology.

First line, one week duration: PPI (standard dose twice daily) plus Amoxicillin (1 g twice daily) or Metronidazole (400 mg twice daily), plus Clarithromycin (500 mg twice daily). It is sensible to avoid metronidazole if the patient has had a previous course of treatment with this agent.

Second line, quadruple therapy: PPI (standard dose twice daily), plus Bismuth Subcitrate (poorly tolerated), plus metronidazole (three times daily), plus tetracycline four times daily. Compliance with treatment has been shown to be very important in determining the success of triple therapy regimens. The eradication course should be followed by anti-secretory therapy for 2 months as gastric ulcers tend to take longer to heal than duodenal ulcers.

Helicobacter pylori negative ulcers should be treated with standard anti-secretory therapy for 2 months with cessation of NSAIDs where possible (see below).

Other strategies to aid healing include:

- Sulcralfate, which acts by mucosal protection against action of pepsin, can be useful in resistant cases.
- Discourage smoking because it is linked to increased acid production.

Where NSAID use is clinically desirable, there are certain strategies that can be employed to reduce the risk of further mucosal damage:

- Misoprostol is a synthetic prostaglandin analogue with anti-secretory and mucosal protective properties. It can help prevent NSAID-associated ulcers.
- Concomitant use of a PPI with NSAIDs is sometimes used in clinical practice, although this strategy is only recommended for those patients with a documented NSAID-induced ulcer who must unavoidably continue with NSAID therapy (e.g. severe rheumatoid arthritis) (as guided by National Institute for Clinical Excellence: NICE).

- Cyclo-oxygenase 2 selective ('COX-2') inhibitors (e.g. celecoxib, rofecoxib) have a significantly lower, but not zero, incidence of adverse upper GI effects. However, they should be reserved for specific indications (e.g. those patients with a history of peptic ulceration or at high risk—aged over 65 years or concomitant medications predisposing to peptic ulceration) of developing the same.
- There is no evidence to justify the combination of PPIs and COX-2 inhibitors as an additional strategy to prevent adverse gastric effects.

Surgical treatment, such as partial gastrectomy and vagotomy, is reserved for complications of ulceration such as perforation or uncontrolled bleeding.

 Repeat endoscopy with biopsies is essential until a gastric ulcer has completely healed, because of the small risk of neoplasia. If the ulcer remains unhealed for 6 months, then surgery should be considered.

Duodenal ulcer

Incidence

Approximately 15% of the population will have suffered from duodenal ulceration at some time.

Clinical features

The history is one of predominantly epigastric pain, and often intermittent. Classically, duodenal ulcers are said to be be relieved by food or antacids and made worse by hunger. The patient can sometimes point to a specific site of pain in the epigastrium. They can also present with an acute GI bleed.

Diagnosis and investigation

As for gastric ulceration (i.e. endoscopy and biopsy, etc.). Tests for *H. pylori* infection should also be performed.

Aetiology and pathogenesis

Similar to that described for gastric ulceration (i.e. acid production, reduction in cytoprotection, etc.). The relationship between *H. pylori* infection and duodenal ulcers is more closely linked because 95% of patients with duodenal ulcers are infected with *H. pylori*. The exact pathogenic mechanism remains uncertain.

High acid output states are associated with duodenal ulceration as seen in Zollinger–Ellison syndrome. However over two-thirds of patients have acid secretion within normal limits, which suggests that other factors, such as mucosal barrier and prostaglandin cytoprotection, are involved in its pathogenesis.

Environmental factors such as smoking and psychological stress are associated with increased basal output of acid and NSAIDs reduce prostaglandin production, hence predisposing to ulceration.

First degree relatives are at three times the normal risk of developing duodenal ulceration. Blood group O has a 40% increase in risk compared to the general population, especially those who do not secrete group O-related antigen in their gastric mucus glycoprotein.

Complications

Acute GI bleed, especially if there is an erosion of an artery. Perforation can present as an acute abdominal emergency and gastric outlet obstruction can occur with chronic disease.

Prognosis

Typically a recurrent disease, approximately 80% of patients relapse within 1 year if no maintenance or eradication therapy is given. Follow-up is not usually necessary in asymptomatic patients.

Treatment

The strategies taken are similar to those for gastric ulceration.

Confirmation of *H. pylori* infection is preferable before an eradication scheme is embarked upon. However, some authorities advocate eradication therapy should be given to all patients with duodenal ulceration because the correlation with *H. pylori* infection is so high.

Iron deficiency (hypochromic, microcytic) anaemia due to chronic blood loss is unusual in duodenal ulcers and if present, coexisting pathology must be sought, such as carcinoma of the colon.

Neoplasia of the stomach

Gastric polyps

Incidence

Rare—discovered, often coincidentally, during approximately 2% of endoscopies.

Clinical features

Majority are asymptomatic. Occasionally, they may ulcerate and bleed.

Diagnosis and investigation

Investigations that may be of use include:
- Endoscopy for dyspepsia or abdominal pain often identifies polyps incidentally. If multiple polyps are present, then conditions such as Peutz–Jeghers and familial polyposis coli should be considered. The latter has particular significance because of its malignant potential.
- Biopsy for histological examination will usually confirm the nature of the polyp.
- Endoscopic ultrasound may be necessary to exclude submucosal malignant infiltration.

Aetiology and pathogenesis

- Over 90% of polyps are hyperplastic and they are usually non-sinister.
- Approximately 5% of polyps are adenomas and have similar pre-malignant potential as those found in the colon.

Rarely, patients with pernicious anaemia have polyps in the fundus, which subsequently turn out to be carcinoid tumours. These may be due to the trophic effects of gastrin secondary to achlorhydria.

Complications

Bleeding and malignant change are the usual complications.

Prognosis and treatment

Resection of the polyp will abolish the malignant risk. They can be removed endoscopically via a snare, but those that are large or sessile may not be suitable, hence multiple biopsies are usually taken and local surgical resection may be required. Hyperplastic polyps are usually left alone unless the patient is symptomatic (Fig. 15.5).

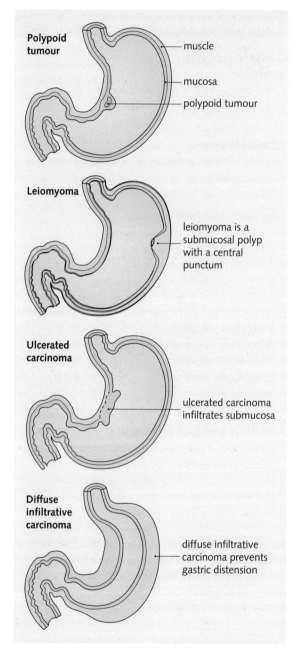

Fig. 15.5 Types of gastric polyps and contrast with leiomyoma and carcinoma.

Gastric leiomyoma
Incidence
This is the commonest tumour of the stomach. Autopsy studies have shown the tumour to be present in up to 50% of the population over the age of 50 years.

Clinical features
Small tumours are asymptomatic. Larger tumours may ulcerate or bleed causing abdominal pain which can be mistaken for peptic ulcer disease.

Diagnosis and investigation
A leiomyoma is often identified incidentally during an endoscopy carried out for other reasons such as epigastric pain or anaemia.

Aetiology and pathogenesis
A benign tumour of the smooth muscle cells which are submucosal and covered by intact mucosa. Underlying aetiology is unknown.

Treatment
Local resection is curative.

Leiomyosarcoma
Incidence
This accounts for 1% of gastric malignancy.

Clinical features
Similar to those of leiomyoma, except weight loss can be a marked feature. A palpable mass in the epigastrium can be demonstrated in approximately 50% of cases. Larger tumours are more likely to have metastasized at the time of diagnosis to local lymph nodes and lungs.

Treatment
Surgical resection is the treatment of choice.

Ménétrièr's disease
Incidence
Rare.

Clinical features
These include:
- Abdominal pain, vomiting, or bleeding similar to those of chronic gastritis.
- Hypoalbuminaemia due to protein loss from the gastric mucosa.

Diagnosis and investigation
Endoscopy demonstrates the typical appearance of enlarged thickened folds of mucosa.

Aetiology and pathogenesis
Unknown aetiology—normal gastric mucosa is replaced by hypertrophied epithelium producing a

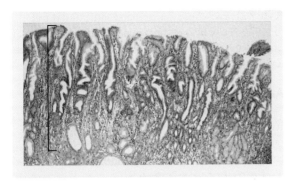

Fig. 15.6 Ménétrièr's disease. The gastric mucosa is grossly thickened due to hypertrophy. Note elongated crypts (C).

characteristic appearance. It is not a true 'neoplasia', but can be very difficult to differentiate, macroscopically, from infiltrating neoplasms.

Histologically, there is hyperplasia of the mucin-producing glands with glandular proliferation, together with loss of parietal and chief cells (Fig. 15.6). Excessive protein loss occurs through the gastric mucosa as a consequence of mucus secretion.

Complications
The condition is possibly pre-malignant but the risk is poorly characterized.

Treatment
Treatment includes:
- Anti-secretory medication—may be of help to some patients.
- Partial gastrectomy—may be required to ameliorate the amount of protein loss.

Gastric carcinoma
Incidence
The frequency of gastric carcinoma increases with age and affects approximately 15 out of 100 000 people in the UK. There is a higher incidence in Japan and the Far East for which dietary factors have been implicated.

Clinical features
These include:
- Abdominal pain with a nature similar to that of peptic ulceration, but progressive and severe if local invasion has occurred.
- Weight loss—often profound and may be the only presenting complaint.

- Nausea, vomiting, and anorexia—these are common features. If the tumour is close to the pylorus, then vomiting can be marked due to gastric outlet obstruction.
- Anaemia—this can be iron deficient as a result of occult blood loss, reflect chronic disease, or rarely bone marrow infiltration with metastases.
- Distant metastases (e.g. to brain, bone, liver, and lung) produce symptoms and variable clinical presentations according to site.

Up to 50% of patients will have a palpable epigastric mass at presentation. Supraclavicular lymph nodes behind the left sternomastoid muscle (Virchow's node) can be palpated in one-third of patients. Other physical signs (all suggestive of incurable disease) include hepatomegaly, jaundice, ascites and paraneoplastic skin manifestations such as acanthosis nigricans.

Diagnosis and investigation
Relevant investigations include:
- Endoscopy—this is the investigation of choice. Care should be taken for biopsy of benign-looking gastric ulcers as negative biopsies can occur.
- Barium meal—in the investigation of dyspepsia, barium meal may show a gastric ulcer, or a diffuse infiltrative type of gastric cancer may be seen as a rigid, contracted stomach.

In proven or suspected cases a chest radiograph, liver ultrasound, and computed tomography (CT) scan, to look for evidence of local or metastatic spread, may be necessary if surgery is contemplated. Biochemical tests may demonstrate derangement of liver enzymes or hypercalcaemia suggesting distant metastases.

Aetiology and pathogenesis
Chronic gastritis leading to metaplasia is a strong risk factor and may be due to *H. pylori* infection. Epidemiological studies demonstrate a higher incidence in lower socio-economic groups, although *H. pylori* infection may be a confounding factor in this regard.

Dietary factors have been implicated, especially nitrites, which are converted by bacteria at neutral pH to nitrosamines—known to be carcinogenic in animals. Pernicious anaemia is also associated with an increased risk of gastric carcinoma, and this may be partly due to achlorhydria and hence neutral pH in the stomach.

Patients with previous partial gastrectomy are at an increased risk after 20 years.

Genetic predisposition has been described with an increased incidence in people with blood group A.

Gastric polyps are rare, but malignant changes can occur in them and they should be removed.

Two histological types of gastric cancer have been described:

- Glandular adenocarcinoma, similar to that seen throughout the intestine with well-differentiated glandular formation or acini which secrete mucin.
- Diffuse, spreading-type adenocarcinoma with a fibrous stroma giving a fibrotic appearance to the stomach (linitis plastica or 'leather-bottle' stomach).

Prognosis

Carcinomas that are confined to the mucosa (rare) have a 90% 5-year survival compared with invasive lesions, which have less than 10% 5-year survival. Early detection appears to be possible in screening programmes such as those in Japan, where gastric carcinoma is common.

Treatment

This includes:

- Surgery—this is the only treatment that can offer a cure. This ranges from partial gastrectomy to radical resection with local lymph node clearance, but is only suitable for patients without widespread metastases. Palliative procedures to relieve outlet obstruction may be apposite.
- Chemotherapy and radiotherapy—these are not usually of use but may be helpful for control of symptoms due to tumour bulk.
- Symptom control with opiate analgesia and anti-emetics—can be difficult to achieve.

Gastric lymphoma
Incidence
Accounts for 5–10% of all gastric malignancy in UK.

Clinical features
Similar to those of gastric carcinoma, although drenching night sweats may also be a prominent feature.

Diagnosis and investigation
Endoscopy and biopsy will provide a histological diagnosis. CT of thorax, abdomen and pelvis looks for extra-GI lymphadenopathy and splenomegaly.

Bone marrow biopsy, particularly indicated if full blood count (FBC) is abnormal, provides evidence of marrow involvement with lymphoma. Serum lactate dehydrogenase may be elevated.

Aetiology and pathogenesis
Nearly all are of non-Hodgkin's B cell type arising from mucosal-associated lymphoid tissue (MALT), rather than a primary lymph node tumour. These tumours are associated with *H. pylori*.

Prognosis
Very good, with 80–90% survival depending on the type of lymphoma. Complete excision of the tumour can be curative.

Treatment
Treatment options include:

- Eradication therapy for *H. pylori*, which can produce regression of certain types.
- Chemotherapy and radiotherapy, which may be necessary for aggressive 'high-grade' transformation or relapsed disease.
- Surgical resection of the tumour.
- Endoscopic surveillance to monitor response to treatment or for interval biopsies is undertaken by some clinicians.

Gastroparesis
Clinical features
Vomiting and nausea are the main symptoms. Weight loss may ensue if the patient avoids eating.

Diagnosis and investigation
Investigations include:

- Barium meal—demonstrates distension of the stomach with markedly reduced passage of barium into the duodenum.
- Radio-isotope scan—this is an alternative to barium meal.

Aetiology and pathogenesis
Characterized by reduced motility of the stomach. Causes include previous surgical vagotomy (now rarely performed) or autonomic neuropathy complicating diabetes mellitus. In some cases, no identifiable cause is found.

Complications
Are those associated with prolonged vomiting (hypokalaemia, aspiration pneumonia), and malnutrition.

Treatment

Anti-emetics with a prokinetic action such as domperidone or metoclopramide are often used to enhance gastric emptying. In severe cases, a motilin analogue such as erythromycin may be required. Clearly, the underlying cause should be addressed where possible.

Gastric outlet obstruction
Incidence

Affects up to 3% of patients with duodenal or pre-pyloric ulceration.

Clinical features

These include:

- Vomiting—this is the main complaint. Classically, the vomiting is projectile and contains undigested food.
- Pain—which is unusual because the ulcer would have started to heal or scarring has already occurred.
- An epigastric succussion splash—may be elicited due to distension of stomach with fluid.

Diagnosis and investigation

Investigations should include:

- Barium meal—to demonstrate slow or absent passage of barium into the small intestine.
- Endoscopy—which may also identify the obstruction.

Electrolyte disturbance such as a hypokalaemic, metabolic alkalosis can occur because of prolonged vomiting.

Aetiology and pathogenesis

Mainly occurs as a result of long-standing peptic ulcer disease affecting the pre-pyloric, pylorus, or duodenal area, resulting in scarring and narrowing of the gastric outlet. Gastric outlet obstruction affecting the pylorus is known as pyloric stenosis, which is not to be confused with the congenital type due to hypertrophy of the fibromuscular layer.

Occasionally, the obstruction may be a result of oedema due to an ulcer and this is usually transient.

Gastric outlet obstruction can also be due to external compression from lymph nodes or pancreatic carcinoma, or due to underlying gastric malignancy.

Complications

Those associated with prolonged vomiting (i.e. aspiration pneumonia, electrolyte imbalance, malnutrition).

Treatment

Management should include:

- Correction of dehydration, electrolyte imbalance and metabolic alkalosis with intravenous fluids.
- Nasogastric tube to aspirate gastric contents and prevent further vomiting.
- Surgical intervention is required unless the obstruction is due to oedema.

Complications following gastric surgery

Gastric surgery for peptic ulcer disease is now a rare occurrence and is reserved for perforation, uncontrolled bleeding or obstruction. However, patients who have previously had surgery commonly re-present with upper GI symptoms.

Recurrent ulceration
Incidence

Occurs in approximately 5% of patients after gastric surgery and is more common in those with duodenal ulcer.

Clinical features

Similar to those found with duodenal ulceration. Complications such as anaemia and perforation appear to be more common than with primary peptic ulcers.

Diagnosis and investigation

Endoscopy is preferred to barium meal due to distorted anatomy.

Aetiology and pathogenesis

As a result of continuing acid production, patients with partial gastrectomy without vagotomy are at a higher risk of developing recurrent ulceration compared with patients who had a highly selective vagotomy (only gastric branches are severed).

Retained antrum after a Billroth II resection (Fig. 15.7) may be the cause for recurrent ulceration. The antrum may not have been completely resected and

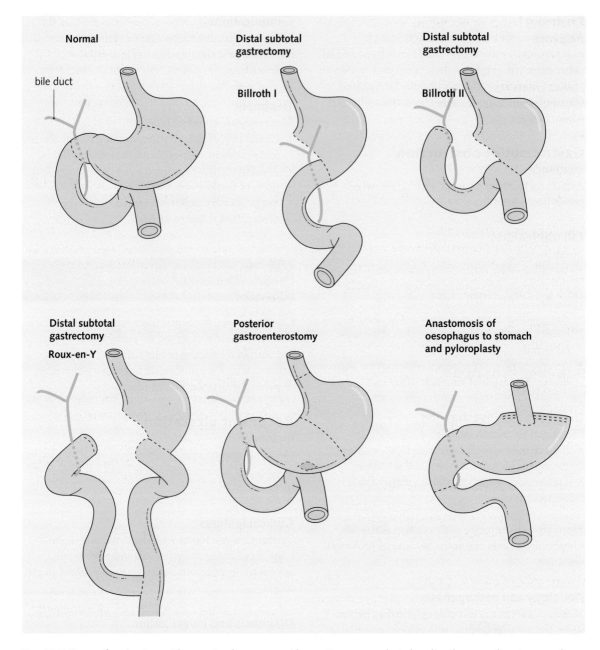

Fig. 15.7 Types of gastrectomy. These not only remove acid-secreting mucosa but also alter the normal anatomy and motility to produce a variety of symptoms. Some re-routing of the duodenum is usually necessary with gastrectomy in order to preserve its relationship to the bile duct.

continues to produce gastrin because its usual inhibition mechanism is lost (low pH in the antrum inhibits gastrin production). A similar picture may be seen with Zollinger–Ellison syndrome, but this can be distinguished by a lack of gastrin suppression following intravenous administration of secretin.

Treatment

Treatment options:

- Eradication of *H. pylori* if present.
- H_2 antagonists or proton pump inhibitors are often effective.
- Surgery may be required for retained antrum.

Afferent loop syndrome

Incidence
A rare complication.

Clinical features
Abdominal pain usually occurs up to 1 hour after meals, associated with distension, nausea, and vomiting. Symptoms are relieved with vomiting.

Diagnosis and investigation
Diagnosis can be difficult, but HIDA scan (see p. 198) may demonstrate bile stasis in the afferent loop.

Aetiology and pathogenesis
Thought to be due to partial obstruction and hence distension of the afferent loop of bowel, resulting in incomplete drainage of bile and pancreatic secretions which are stimulated by eating.

Treatment
Surgical revision of the loop is usually required.

Dumping syndrome

Clinical features
Two types have been described:
- Early dumping—usually occurs within 30 minutes after a meal and causes palpitations, lightheadedness, postural hypotension, and sometimes abdominal discomfort.
- Late dumping—typically occurs between 90 minutes and 3 hours after a meal. Similar symptoms of lightheadedness, palpitation, hypotension, and sweating are experienced. Syncope may also be seen.

Diagnosis and investigation
The diagnosis is often made on clinical grounds alone. Measurement of serum glucose, electrolytes, and blood pressure during an attack is usually sufficient for diagnosis.

Aetiology and pathogenesis
Early dumping syndrome is thought to be caused by a vasovagal response to a rapid emptying of gastric contents into the small intestine, resulting in a depletion of intravascular volume secondary to the change in osmotic gradient. Hypokalaemia is noted during such an attack. However, fluid and potassium replacement does not appear to abolish these attacks and there may be some other underlying mechanism involving a complex release of gut hormones.

Late dumping syndrome appears to be caused by hypoglycaemia due to an excessive release of insulin. The insulin release is thought to be precipitated by transient hyperglycaemia, secondary to a rapid emptying of carbohydrate-rich substances in the small intestine. A glucose tolerance test shows an acute hyperglycaemic phase followed by hypoglycaemia.

Treatment
Dietary advice such as small frequent meals may be all that is required in mild cases.

Symptoms in severe cases are very difficult to control. Some have derived symptomatic relief from octreotide (somatostatin analogue) injections but the cost has restricted its use in clinical practice.

Diarrhoea

Incidence
Up to 50% of patients can be affected following gastrectomy.

Aetiology and pathogenesis
The exact mechanism is unknown, but patients with truncal vagotomy are affected more commonly, suggesting autonomic dysfunction.

Other aetiological factors include bile salts and bacterial overgrowth especially in Polya gastrectomy.

Loss of pyloric regulatory emptying mechanism may contribute to diarrhoea.

Treatment
Note that:
- Bile salt diarrhoea can be treated with colestyramine.
- Bacterial overgrowth can be confirmed with a hydrogen breath test and treated with antibiotics.

Anaemia

Incidence
Often presenting late, this is a common complication of gastrectomy.

Aetiology and pathogenesis
Iron-deficiency anaemia is the most common type to be seen and may be related to a reduced production of hydrochloric acid which promotes iron solubility.

Ascorbic acid is also secreted in the normal stomach and aids iron absorption by reducing Fe^{3+} to Fe^{2+}. Supplementing the diet with vitamin C after gastrectomy can correct the iron deficiency and improve the anaemia.

A lack of intrinsic factor and bacterial overgrowth will cause macrocytic anaemia due to vitamin B_{12} deficiency.

Diagnosis and investigation
An underlying GI malignancy, whether in the gastric remnant or in the colon, must be excluded when a patient presents with iron-deficiency anaemia.

Tests to perform include:
- Serum B_{12} measurement.
- Hydrogen breath test for bacterial overgrowth causing B_{12} deficiency.

Treatment
Oral iron supplements should be given together with ascorbic acid to promote absorption.

Intramuscular B_{12} is given 3-monthly, the reticulocyte count and FBC can be measured to monitor response. Be aware that B_{12} replacement can result in hypokalaemia.

Malabsorption
Incidence
Common, and it may contribute to weight loss seen in over 50% of patients after gastrectomy.

Clinical features
The following features may present:
- Weight loss (often multifactorial).
- Steatorrhoea (in severe cases).
- Anaemia is common, as discussed.
- Osteomalacia (due to reduced absorption of vitamin D).

Diagnosis and investigation
Dependent upon clinical presentation.

Mild malabsorption may unmask a subclinical condition such as coeliac disease and chronic pancreatitis, so appropriate investigation should be initiated.

Aetiology and pathogenesis
No single factor accounts for malabsorption seen. The following causes have all been implicated:
- Rapid gastric emptying.
- Reduced capacity of the stomach.
- Reduced bile concentrations in the intestinal lumen.
- Increased gut transit time.

Bacterial overgrowth causing steatorrhoea and reduced absorption of fat soluble vitamins is probably the most important factor.

Treatment
This involves replacement of trace elements and deficient vitamins and treatment of bacterial overgrowth if identified.

Carcinoma
Incidence
There is a two-fold increase in the risk of adenocarcinoma at the site of the anastomosis 20 years after gastrectomy. In the interim, the risk of gastric carcinoma is less as the stomach has been removed.

Clinical features
Recurrence of epigastric pain or weight loss in patients who have previously had surgery.

Diagnosis and investigation
Endoscopy, with biopsy of suspicious lesions.

Aetiology and pathogenesis
Bile reflux and *H. pylori* infection have been postulated as potential aetiological factors.

Treatment
Resection of the tumour is required.

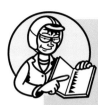

- What are the main physiological functions of the stomach?
- What investigations can be employed to detect the presence of *Helicobacter pylori*?
- Why do NSAIDs predispose toward peptic ulceration?
- Describe the mechanism of action of proton pump inhibitors and H_2 antagonists.
- How would you manage a patient in the first few hours following an acute upper gastrointestinal bleed?
- What strategies can be used in a patient with a history of peptic ulceration, who requires NSAIDs for another condition?
- Why may a patient be anaemic following gastrectomy?

16. Small Intestine

Anatomy, physiology and function of the small intestine

The small intestine extends from the duodenum to the terminal ileum where it joins the caecum. The surface area is markedly increased by mucosal folds in the form of villi and microvilli. Each villus contains a core of blood vessels and lymphatic lacteals (Fig. 16.1).

Its main function is absorption of nutrients (i.e. carbohydrate, protein, fat, vitamins, etc.). It also secretes immunoglobulin (Ig)A as a local defence mechanism against infection.

Absorption is achieved by the following mechanisms:
- Simple diffusion.
- Active transport (e.g. Na^+/K^+ ATPase for absorption of glucose).
- Facilitated diffusion (a carrier-mediated transport system to allow faster absorption compared with simple diffusion, e.g. proteins).

Disease of the small intestine is usually manifest as malabsorption with resultant mineral or vitamin deficiency, weight loss, or diarrhoea.

Immune-related problems

Coeliac disease
Incidence
More commonly seen in the west of Ireland, where it occurs in 1 out of 500 compared with an average prevalence in the UK of 1 out of 2000 people. It is rarely seen in Black Africans. Although it may present at any age, there is a peak incidence in the third decade with a smaller peak in the fifth and sixth decades.

Clinical features
The manifestations are protean, but common clinical features include:
- Diarrhoea, steatorrhoea and iron deficiency are the most common presentations in adults.

- Abdominal pain and weight loss are associated with general malaise.
- Failure to thrive is the most common presentation in young children.
- Dermatitis herpetiformis is an intensely itchy, blistering condition of the skin associated with coeliac disease, occurring particularly on knees, elbows and scalp. It is characterized by the finding of granular IgA at the dermo–epidermal junction of uninvolved skin on biopsy.
- Hyposplenism is relatively common.
- Howell–Jolly bodies may be seen on a blood film.

Features of mineral and vitamin deficiency may be present (e.g. iron-deficiency anaemia, vitamin D deficiency and osteomalacia).

 In cases of unexplained iron-deficiency anaemia, always consider coeliac disease. A duodenal biopsy can be performed at the same time as an upper GI endoscopy.

Diagnosis and investigation
Anaemia can be due to folate or iron deficiency. The blood film may have a dimorphic picture (i.e. both macrocytic and microcytic red cells) if both are deficient.

Blood tests may aid diagnosis:
- Biochemistry may show low calcium with a normal or low phosphate indicative of osteomalacia. Hypoalbuminaemia is seen in severe malabsorption.
- Low urea is usual in any malabsorption.
- Slight increase in liver transaminases is common.
- If malabsorption is severe, a coagulopathy may be seen due to vitamin K deficiency.
- Anti-endomysial antibody is the most reliable marker for coeliac disease, with sensitivity up to 90% and enough specificity to be of clinical value. Anti-gliadin antibody is less useful but can be found in two-thirds of patients.

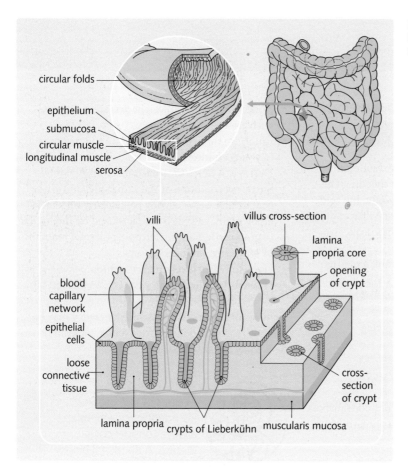

Duodenal biopsy is the investigation of choice and nowadays is carried out by endoscopy. Partial or subtotal villous atrophy with an infiltrate of intraepithelial lymphocytes is diagnostic (Fig. 16.2).

Aetiology and pathogenesis

This is a gluten-sensitive enteropathy characterized by villous atrophy of the jejunum, which morphologically and symptomatically responds to institution of a gluten-free diet. Gluten is a high molecular weight compound that is cleaved to alpha, beta-, and gamma gliadin peptides. Alpha-gliadin is said to be toxic to the small bowel and possibly the other forms to a lesser degree.

An immunological basis is likely because of the increased incidence in patients with certain HLA types, namely A1, B8, DR3, DR7, and DQW2. Moreover, other autoimmune conditions occur more frequently in patients with coeliac disease.

Viral infections have also been implicated as an aetiological influence, and there may be a history of a preceding episode of gastroenteritis.

Complications

Features of mineral and vitamin deficiency can occur. Severe malnutrition in some cases can result in severe hypoalbuminaemia with consequent ascites and peripheral oedema.

Osteopaenia is a well recognized long-term complication that should be addressed.

Hyposplenism can predispose to infection, particularly with capsulated organisms such as *Pneumococcus*.

There is an increased risk of developing T-cell lymphoma of the small intestine compared to the normal population but the risk may be reduced by a gluten-free diet. An overall increase in other gastrointestinal (GI) malignancies, such as colonic adenocarcinoma, is also seen.

Fig. 16.2 Subtotal villous atrophy in coeliac disease (A) recovers completely with a gluten-free diet (B). Note the increased number of intraepithelial lymphocytes (IEL) and decreased villous height in (A).

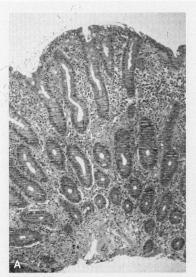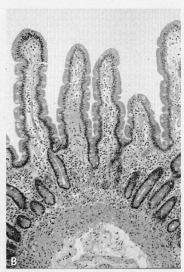

A patient with stable coeliac disease who has recurrence of diarrhoea or weight loss may be unknowingly ingesting gluten or may have developed an intestinal lymphoma.

Treatment

Treatment options include:

- Elimination of gluten-containing food (e.g. wheat, rye, barley) from the diet will usually provide symptomatic and histological improvement. Non-compliance is usually the cause of relapse or lack of improvement.
- Replacement of deficient vitamins may be needed in the initial stages, but long-term replacement is usually not required.
- Strategies for bone density protection range from calcium supplementation to bisphosphonates or hormone replacement therapy in women.
- Re-introduction of gluten to the diet will result in a re-emergence of symptoms and villous atrophy and repeat biopsy can be used to confirm the diagnosis in doubtful cases.

Dermatitis herpetiformis will usually resolve with a gluten-free diet. Resistant cases can be treated with dapsone.

Crohn's disease

Incidence

Average of 4 out of 100 000 each year in the UK. Rare in people of Afro-Caribbean origin.

Clinical features

Patients with Crohn's disease have recurrent attacks, with acute 'flares' of disease activity interspersed between periods of remission.

The main symptoms are:

- Abdominal pain.
- Diarrhoea.
- Weight loss.

General malaise, anorexia, and fever are also common.

Acute ileitis mimics acute appendicitis with pain in the right iliac fossa.

Extra-GI manifestations such as uveitis, oligoarthritis, and erythema nodosum can also be seen (Fig. 16.3).

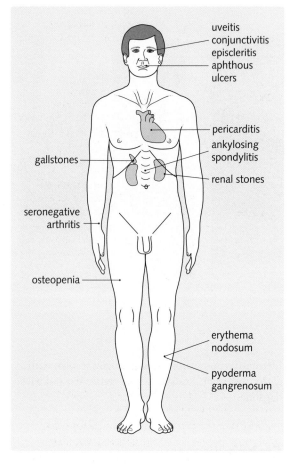

uveitis
conjunctivitis
episcleritis
aphthous
ulcers

pericarditis
ankylosing
spondylitis

gallstones

renal stones

seronegative
arthritis

osteopenia

erythema
nodosum

pyoderma
gangrenosum

Fig. 16.3 Systemic manifestations of Crohn's disease.

- Low albumin levels indicate severe disease. Liver enzymes are less commonly deranged compared with ulcerative colitis.
- Blood cultures are vital if there is any evidence of sepsis.
- Stool cultures should be routinely done for patients presenting with diarrhoea as concomitant infection is not uncommon.
- Small bowel enema/follow-through is used to visualize the small bowel to locate the affected area and determine extent of disease (see Fig. 24.24).
- Colonoscopy is preferred if diarrhoea is the predominant symptom rather than pain, as then colitis is more likely and biopsies can be taken to distinguish from ulcerative colitis.
- Computed tomography (CT) or magnetic resonance scan of abdomen is helpful if fistula or abscesses are suspected. Magnetic resonance scan may be more sensitive.

> C-reactive protein is elevated during acute attacks, mirroring inflammatory activity in Crohn's disease, and is useful for monitoring response to treatment.

> A severe exacerbation of inflammatory bowel disease is suggested by signs of systemic upset such as tachycardia, fever, anaemia and low albumin.

Diagnosis and investigation

On investigating Crohn's disease, note the following:

- Anaemia is common and can be of normocytic, normochromic type of chronic disease or secondary to iron/folate deficiency due to blood loss/malabsorption. A thrombocytosis is seen and reflects inflammatory activity.
- CRP is a sensitive acute phase protein rising in the first 6 hours after initiation of inflammation. ESR can also be useful but is less sensitive.

Aetiology and pathogenesis

This is a chronic inflammatory condition characterized by the presence of non-caseating granulomas which can affect any part of the bowel from mouth to anus, but are most commonly seen in the terminal ileum. Another feature is that of 'skip lesions', where normal bowel is interposed between diseased sections of bowel. Affected bowel wall is usually thickened and narrowed, producing a clinical scenario of bowel obstruction. Deep ulceration and fissuring is also seen producing a 'cobblestone' appearance macroscopically.

Inflammation is described as transmural (affects all layers of the bowel), unlike ulcerative colitis, and there are non-caseating granulomas with typical chronic inflammatory infiltrates. Crypt abscesses may also be seen in colonic disease (Fig. 16.4).

The exact aetiology is unknown, but the epidemiology suggests an environmental agent with a genetic predisposition. Up to 10% of patients'

Fig. 16.4 Gastrointestinal features of Crohn's disease.

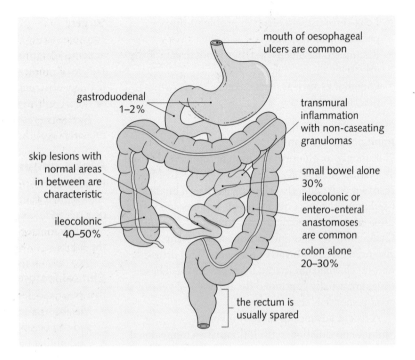

relatives have either Crohn's or ulcerative colitis and some investigators believe that the two diseases represent a spectrum of a single pathological process.

Tobacco smoking is associated with increased risk of Crohn's, whereas non-smokers or ex-smokers are more likely to develop ulcerative colitis.

An infective cause has been postulated, but there is no clear evidence to support such a hypothesis. Similarly, immunological abnormalities have been noted but it is uncertain whether these changes are a primary or secondary phenomenon.

Complications

Fistulae can form between bowel and bladder (entero-vesical), another segment of intestine (entero-enteral), skin (sinus), or vagina (entero-vaginal). This process can produce very disabling symptoms and the patient may be embarrassed to volunteer their presence.

Secondary amyloidosis can occur over time, consequent upon high levels of acute-phase proteins produced during inflammatory episodes.

There is an increased risk of developing adenocarcinoma.

Treatment

The cessation of smoking should, of course, be encouraged.

Corticosteroids

These are used empirically for acute attacks to suppress symptoms, but there is little evidence to suggest that the prognosis improves with treatment. Maintenance steroids should be avoided if at all possible due to the long-term deleterious effects such as osteoporosis. Localized rectal Crohn's can be treated by steroid suppositories or enemas to reduce the systemic side-effects.

Salicylates

Salazopyrine is a 5-aminosalicylic acid (5-ASA) attached to sulfapyridine and is broken down in the colon by bacteria to release the active compound 5-ASA. Unlike ulcerative colitis in which the drug is very effective, the beneficial effect in Crohn's is more uncertain.

Newer compounds such as mesalazine and olsalazine are now available which have fewer toxic side effects because they do not have a sulphonamide component. They have all shown to be beneficial for colonic disease but for small intestinal Crohn's disease, mesalazine tends to be used.

Antibiotics

Antibiotics to note:
- Metronidazole is used for peri-anal disease in which anaerobic infections are common and its use often has to be prolonged to be effective.

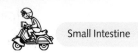

Long-term use can result in problems due to peripheral neuropathy.

- Rifampicin has been used, but is not dramatically effective.
- Quinolones such as ciprofloxacin are showing promise.

Immunosuppression

Commonly, azathioprine or mercaptopurine are used as 'steroid-sparing' agents and can be effective for resistant or frequently relapsing disease. The predominant toxic effect is myelosuppression (often dose-related) although hepatic toxicity is recognized. Cyclosporin A, a potent immunosuppressant, has also been given with variable success. This drug is non-myelotoxic but markedly nephrotoxic. These drugs are usually continued for at least 1–2 years if a good response is seen.

A recent advance in therapy involves 'immunomodulation' with Infliximab, a monoclonal antibody which inhibits the pro-inflammatory cytokine: tumour necrosis factor-α. This drug is indicated in certain circumstances, as guided by the National Institute for Clinical Excellence. These include:

- Severe active disease, with or without the formation of new fistulae or extra-intestinal manifestations.
- Disease that is refractory to immunosuppressive drugs described above, or patients who have suffered toxicity from, or been intolerant of, their adverse effects.
- Patients in whom surgery is considered inappropriate (e.g. because of diffuse disease).

It is noteworthy that Infliximab has been associated with the development of tuberculosis (often in extra-pulmonary sites).

Elemental diets

Enteral or parenteral feeding can induce remission, especially in small bowel disease. The bowel is allowed to 'rest' and hence reduce inflammation and exposure to potential antigens.

Parenteral feeding via a central venous line may be necessary for patients who are severely malnourished or for whom enteral feeding is not suitable (e.g. fistula formation). Unfortunately, over half of the patients relapse when a normal diet is re-introduced.

Surgery

Approximately 80% of patients will require surgery at some juncture. This is usually indicated because of failure of medical therapy, complications such as fistulae, obstruction from strictures, toxic dilatation, or failure to thrive in children.

Extensive resection should be avoided because recurrence of the disease is common.

Alpha chain disease
Incidence

Also known as immunoproliferative small intestinal disease, this condition is predominantly seen in Mediterranean countries, Africa, South America, and the Far East.

Clinical features

Symptoms include:
- Malabsorption is the commonest manifestation, and can be severe.
- Abdominal pain.
- Anaemia.
- Finger clubbing—often seen.

Diagnosis and investigation

IgA alpha chains can be detected in urine and serum. These can also be detected by immunofluorescence of gut mucosa.

Aetiology and pathogenesis

The underlying aetiology is unknown. There is a proliferation of the plasma cells in the lamina propria which produces the heavy or alpha chain of IgA molecules without the light chains, probably as a result of long-standing antigenic stimulation. Subsequently, there is a defect in the IgA secretory function resulting in bacterial overgrowth, villous atrophy, and malabsorption. The disease is associated with low socio-economic groups in areas where poor hygiene and chronic intestinal infestation are common.

Complications

The condition is considered to be pre-malignant, with progression to small bowel B-cell lymphoma.

Treatment

In early stages, tetracycline will give some improvement in the condition. Once invasive lymphoma has occurred then surgery and radio/chemotherapy is required.

Neoplastic problems

Intestinal lymphomas
Incidence
Non-Hodgkin's lymphomas are a relatively rare intestinal malignancy.

Clinical features
Symptoms include:
- Abdominal pain.
- Intestinal obstruction.
- Diarrhoea.
- Anorexia and weight loss.
- Night sweats.
- Anaemia (which may be iron deficiency due to blood loss).

The symptoms are similar to those of any tumour in the small intestine or colon. A palpable mass may occasionally be present.

Diagnosis and investigation
Consider:
- Small bowel enema or follow-through will detect most lesions but is unlikely to distinguish it from other tumours.
- A CT of the abdomen will visualize the lesion and show enlargement of local lymph nodes, which is commonly seen in small bowel lymphomas. Biopsy will confirm the diagnosis.

Aetiology and pathogenesis
More frequently found in the ileum. Majority are of the non-Hodgkin's B cell type arising from mucosa-associated lymphoid tissues (MALT). They tend to be of annular or polypoid masses in the terminal ileum. T-cell lymphomas are seen in patients with coeliac disease and are characteristically ulcerated plaques or strictures in the proximal small bowel.

Complications
Extensive involvement will result in malabsorption.

Prognosis
Small tumours with surgical resection have a good prognosis of 75% at 5 years depending on the grade of lymphoma. T-cell lymphomas have a poorer outcome, with an overall survival of 25% at 5 years.

Treatment
Surgery followed by radiotherapy and/or chemotherapy. *Helicobacter pylori* should be eradicated.

Adenocarcinoma of small intestine
Incidence
Rare, but accounts for 50% of all tumours found in small intestine.

Clinical features
Most commonly presents with anaemia, abdominal pain, weight loss, and diarrhoea.

Diagnosis and investigation
Consider:
- Barium follow-through/enema usually demonstrates a stricture.
- A CT of the abdomen demonstrates local invasion and any local lymph node involvement can also be detected.

Aetiology and pathogenesis
Both coeliac and Crohn's disease show a higher incidence of adenocarcinoma of small bowel. The exact mechanism is unknown.

Treatment
Surgical resection of the tumour is undertaken. Radiotherapy and chemotherapy are of limited value.

Carcinoid tumours
Incidence
Account for up to 10% of small intestinal tumours.

Clinical features
Most are asymptomatic. Approximately 10% are found incidentally following appendicectomy for acute appendicitis. Occasionally, patients can present with an acute abdomen secondary to obstruction by the tumour.

Carcinoid syndrome
This is seen in 5% of patients with carcinoid tumours when liver metastases are present. Characteristic features are:
- Facial flushing.
- Abdominal pain.
- Chronic diarrhoea (Fig. 16.5).

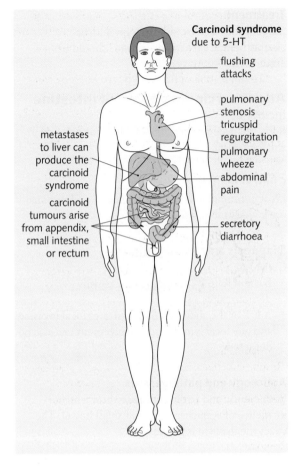

Carcinoid syndrome
due to 5-HT

flushing attacks

pulmonary stenosis
tricuspid regurgitation
pulmonary wheeze
abdominal pain

metastases to liver can produce the carcinoid syndrome

carcinoid tumours arise from appendix, small intestine or rectum

secretory diarrhoea

Fig. 16.5 Clinical features of carcinoid syndrome.

Right-sided cardiac lesions (i.e. tricuspid regurgitation or pulmonary stenosis) are found in half of the patients with carcinoid syndrome.

Diagnosis and investigation

Primary tumours are only diagnosed on histological specimens.

Liver ultrasound or CT scan confirms the presence of liver metastases. These deposits usually take up radiolabelled metaiodobenzylguanidine (MIBG) or octreotide if the diagnosis is uncertain.

Urinary 5-hydroxyindole acetic acid, the major metabolite of 5-hydroxytryptamine (serotonin, 5-HT), is increased in the urine.

Aetiology and pathogenesis

Originates from APUD (amine precursor uptake and decarboxylation) cells and the most common

primary sites include the appendix, terminal ileum, and rectum.

The tumours secrete a number of vasoactive peptides, including 5-HT, bradykinin, and histamines, which cause the facial flushing, GI symptoms, and cardiac lesions.

> Primary carcinoid tumours may secrete hormone (usually 5-HT, but also bradykinin and histamine), but the serum concentration is reduced by hepatic metabolism on 'first pass' via the portal circulation from the gut. Once the tumour metastasizes to the liver, this 'protection' is bypassed and massive amounts of hormone reach the systemic circulation, whereupon symptoms of the carcinoid syndrome are manifest.

Prognosis

Most patients survive up to 5–10 years after diagnosis.

Treatment

Octreotide, a somatostatin analogue, is the standard treatment. It inhibits gut hormone release and consequently stops the flushing and diarrhoea. Inhibition of tumour growth can occur in some patients. Some tumours secrete other hormones, producing different clinical syndromes e.g. adrenocorticotropic hormone excess resulting in Cushing's. Consequently, treatment should be tailored to the manifestations.

Peutz–Jeghers syndrome
Clinical features

Mucocutaneous pigmentation of the face, hands, and feet with multiple polyps along the intestine. The polyps can manifest with bleeding and occasionally intussusception.

Diagnosis and investigation

Barium enema or barium follow-through is carried out to demonstrate the extent of polyposis with confirmation by biopsy taken at colonoscopy or enteroscopy.

Aetiology and pathogenesis

Inherited as an autosomal dominant trait. The polyps are hamartomas and can occur anywhere along the GI tract, but particularly in the small bowel.

Complications

There is a small but a definite risk of malignant change of hamartomas.

Treatment

Polypectomies should be carried out along the bowel to look for dysplastic features but bowel resection should be avoided if possible. Regular endoscopic and histological surveillance is necessary, the frequency of which can be guided by the grade of dysplasia.

Bacterial overgrowth
Clinical features

Malabsorption tends to be the predominant feature (i.e. diarrhoea, steatorrhoea and vitamin deficiency, especially B_{12}).

Diagnosis and investigation

Investigations of value include:

- Hydrogen breath test—oral lactulose or glucose is ingested and metabolized by the bacteria to hydrogen, which can be detected in expiration (Fig. 24.8). However, interpretation can be difficult because there are bacteria present in the oral cavity and rapid transit time will allow bacteria in the large intestine to break down lactulose.
- ^{14}C glycocholic acid breath test—^{14}C-labelled bile salt is ingested and bacteria deconjugates the bile salts releasing $^{14}CO_2$, which can be detected in exhaled breath. Rapid transit time will also cause a rise in radioactivity due to substrate reaching bacteria in the large intestines.
- Small intestinal aspiration—direct aspiration followed by aerobic and anaerobic cultures can be an alternative method for diagnosing bacterial overgrowth.

Aetiology and pathogenesis

Gastric acid normally kills most bacteria and intestinal motility keeps the jejunum free of bacteria. The terminal ileum usually contains faecal type of bacteria (e.g. *Escherichia coli*, *enterococci* and anaerobes such as *Bacteroides*).

Bacterial overgrowth occurs as a result of structural abnormality (i.e. Polya gastrectomy, small intestinal diverticulosis, strictures, or where stasis exists), allowing bacteria to grow. The condition can also be seen in elderly people and in scleroderma (due to hypomotility).

Deconjugation of bile salts by the bacteria can result in fat malabsorption (steatorrhoea) and deficiency of the fat soluble vitamins A, D, E, and K. The bacteria can also metabolize vitamin B_{12} and interfere with its binding to intrinsic factor, hence causing B_{12} deficiency. Folate levels tend to be elevated consequent upon bacterial metabolism.

Patients with vitamin B_{12} deficiency due to bacterial overgrowth often have a high serum folate, due to its absorption following production by the bacteria.

Complications

Result from malabsorption of vitamin B_{12} and fat-soluble vitamins causing macrocytic anaemia, peripheral neuropathy (rarely), osteomalacia, coagulopathy, etc.

Treatment

Treatment of underlying cause (e.g. strictures, blind loop in Polya gastrectomy, etc.) should be addressed, which may require surgical resection. Multiple diverticula and other conditions may not be amenable to surgery. Prolonged or cyclical courses of antibiotics are usually required, in an attempt to re-establish normal intestinal flora. Anti-bacterial agents such as metronidazole and tetracycline, or ciprofloxacin, are found to be effective. Vitamin deficiency should be corrected.

Tropical sprue
Clinical features

These consist of:

- Diarrhoea— with malabsorption and nutritional deficiency.
- Weight loss.
- Anorexia.

Diagnosis is reserved for people resident in epidemic areas such as Asia, South America, and parts of the Caribbean. Often, there is a preceding enteric infection.

Diagnosis
Investigations to aid diagnosis include:
- Stool culture is necessary to exclude other causes of infective diarrhoea (e.g. giardiasis).
- Jejunal biopsy shows partial villous atrophy but it is usually less severe than that of coeliac disease.

Aetiology and pathogenesis
Likely to be an infective cause, but the exact aetiology is unknown. A number of pathogens have been implicated but conclusive evidence is unavailable. There could be geographic variation with differing precipitants from country to country.

Complications
Folate deficiency is common. Complications are a result of vitamin deficiency seen in any malabsorptive state.

Treatment
Improvement of symptoms is frequently seen upon leaving the endemic area.

Most patients will require antibiotics (e.g. tetracycline) for up to 6 months. Folic acid and other vitamin supplements are also required.

Whipple's disease
Incidence
Rare—particularly affects middle-aged males.

Clinical features
These include:
- Steatorrhoea.
- Abdominal pain.
- Fever.
- Weight loss.

Peripheral lymphadenopathy, migratory arthritis and pigmentation may also be seen.

Involvement of the brain causes chronic encephalitis and may be the dominant feature.

Diagnosis and investigation
Jejunal biopsy typically demonstrates the cells of the lamina propria replaced with periodic acid–Schiff positive macrophages, which represent the remains of dead bacteria. There is usually only minimal villous atrophy.

Aetiology and pathogenesis
The bacteria responsible have been identified as *Tropheryma Whippeli* and are thought to be of low infectivity. Exact mechanism of the disease is uncertain, but may involve a type of immunodeficiency.

Treatment
Prolonged antibiotics therapy with agents such as penicillin, tetracycline, or chloramphenicol, are effective and improvement can be dramatic. Supplements of relevant vitamins and minerals may be required for patients with severe malabsorption.

Tuberculosis
Incidence
Rare in the UK but should be suspected in areas where it is more common (e.g. Asia), and in the context of known HIV infection.

Clinical features
These are similar to those of Crohn's disease (i.e. weight loss, abdominal pain, anorexia, anaemia, etc.) (Fig. 16.6). Intestinal obstruction may occur. A right iliac fossa mass may be palpable. It can also manifest as tuberculous (exudative) ascites, which may mimic malignant disease. B_{12} deficiency may exist as a result of terminal ileal involvement.

Diagnosis and investigation
Consider:
- Abdominal ultrasound—may show mesenteric thickening and lymph node involvement.
- Laparotomy for histological confirmation followed by bacteriological confirmation is the gold standard, but tuberculosis (TB) cultures can take up to 6 weeks.
- Chest radiograph—may demonstrate evidence of co-existent pulmonary TB and thus aid in the diagnosis of small intestine TB.

Aetiology and pathogenesis
Usually occurs as a consequence of reactivation of the primary disease caused by *Mycobacterium tuberculosis*. Bovine TB is very rare and is due to ingestion of unpasteurized milk. The ileocaecal area is the most commonly affected. Typical caseating granulomas are seen histologically.

Treatment
Similar anti-bacterials are employed as for pulmonary TB (e.g triple therapy of isoniazid, rifampicin, and pyrazinamide). Treatment is often extended for at least 9 months.

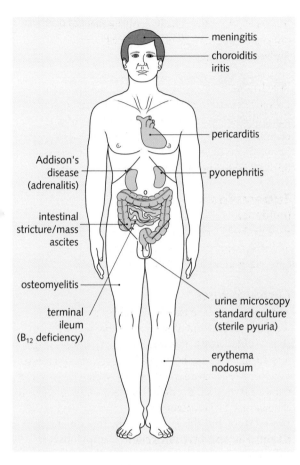

meningitis

choroiditis
iritis

pericarditis

Addison's
disease
(adrenalitis)

pyonephritis

intestinal
stricture/mass
ascites

osteomyelitis

terminal
ileum
(B$_{12}$ deficiency)

urine microscopy
standard culture
(sterile pyuria)

erythema
nodosum

Fig. 16.6 Body map of features seen in extra-pulmonary tuberculosis.

Yersinia infection
Clinical features
In adults, it causes an enterocolitis characterized by fever, diarrhoea, and abdominal pain. It can also give rise to terminal ileitis, which often clinically mistaken for appendicitis.

Reiter's syndrome (conjunctivitis, arthritis, and non-specific urethritis) can sometimes occur after infection with Yersinia. Manifestations such as erythema nodosum and seronegative arthritis are not uncommon and are probably related to circulating immune complexes.

In children, the infection is more likely to cause mesenteric adenitis, giving rise to abdominal pain.

Diagnosis
Not routinely confirmed, but occasionally made on tissue diagnosis or lymph node biopsy (e.g. after appendicectomy).

Aetiology and pathogenesis
The offending organisms are *Yersinia enterocolitica* (enterocolitis) and *Yersinia pseudotuberculosis* (terminal ileitis).

Treatment
Usually a self-limiting disease, and no specific treatment may be necessary. In severe cases, tetracycline may be given.

Giardiasis
Incidence
Common in the tropics and is an important cause of travellers' diarrhoea.

Clinical features
Typical symptoms include:
- Watery (non-bloody) diarrhoea.
- Nausea.
- Anorexia.
- Abdominal pain.
- Malabsorption and disaccharide intolerance may occur.

Asymptomatic carriage is also observed.

Diagnosis and investigation
Stool examination is important, but cysts can be seen only in fresh stool samples as they often die when stored.

Negative stool examination does not exclude the diagnosis because excretion of the parasite can be intermittent.

Duodenal aspirate/biopsy allows direct visualization of the parasite. Serology-specific IgG and IgM antibodies can be measured.

Aetiology and pathogenesis
Giardia lamblia is a flagellate protozoan that is found worldwide and epidemics have been reported in parts of Europe and North America.

Transmission is by the faecal–oral route and mainly via contaminated water supplies.

The organism colonizes within the small intestinal wall and can produce an asymptomatic infection. However, in most cases, villous atrophy ensues, causing diarrhoea and malabsorption.

The exact mechanism by which *Giardia* causes villous atrophy is unknown, but an immune-mediated response may be responsible. Bacterial overgrowth may account for some of the malabsorption seen.

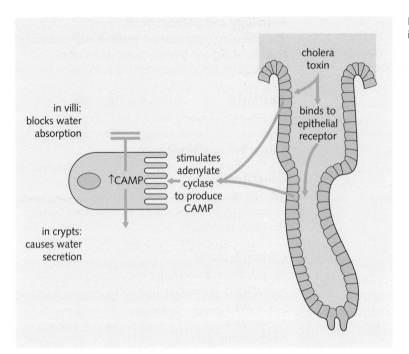

Fig. 16.7 Mechanisms of diarrhoea in cholera infection.

Complications

These are mainly due to malabsorption of vitamins and malnutrition seen in small bowel disease. If diarrhoea persists, consider lactose intolerance and recommend a trial of abstinence from milk.

Treatment

Metronidazole is the drug of choice given for 7–10 days with or without vitamin supplements.

Cholera
Clinical features

Incubation takes from a few hours to 6 days.

Diarrhoea is often profuse and watery (also painless). Classically likened to 'rice water' stool due to presence of mucus.

Circulatory collapse due to profound dehydration occurs in severe cases. As much as 1 litre of watery stool may be passed each hour. Consequently, acute renal failure and profound electrolyte disturbance may ensue.

Diagnosis and investigation

Diagnosis is mainly made on clinical grounds.

Stool examination is helpful. The flagellate, actively motile, organism can be seen in freshly passed stool, but this is not specific for cholera, as a similar appearance can occur in Campylobacter infections. Stool cultures will normally confirm the diagnosis.

Aetiology and pathogenesis

Transmission of the Gram-negative bacillus *Vibrio cholerae* is achieved by the faecal–oral route, via contaminated water supplies and food sources. Exotoxins produced by the bacteria bind irreversibly to epithelial receptors along the small intestine that activate adenylate cyclase and, hence increase intracellular cAMP concentrations (Fig. 16.7). This, in turn, causes the stimulation of salt and water secretion into the intestinal lumen, resulting in a devastating loss of fluid and electrolytes. Reabsorption of fluid in the small intestine is also inhibited, contributing to the fluid loss.

Treatment

Fluid and electrolyte replacement either intravenously or orally is the mainstay of treatment.

Antibiotics such as tetracycline will shorten the duration of the illness but drug resistance is an increasing problem. Oral vaccines (live and killed) are emerging as effective preventative measures.

Strongyloidiasis
Clinical features
These include:
- Local skin erythema and itching where the larvae have gained entry.
- Respiratory symptoms, such as cough and rarely pneumonitis, approximately 7–10 days after initial penetration.
- Abdominal discomfort, intermittent diarrhoea, and constipation are seen approximately 3 weeks later when intestinal colonization occurs. Heavy infestation may result in more marked manifestations including steatorrhoea and intestinal malabsorption.

Diagnosis and investigation
An eosinophilia is commonly seen on full blood count.

Larvae can be detected in fresh stool sample or duodenal aspirate.

Aetiology and pathogenesis
Due to infection with *Strongyloides stercoralis*, found especially in South America and Asia. Infection can persist for decades and new cases are still diagnosed on war veterans who were infected while abroad.

Adult worms reside in the crypts of the small intestine, provoking an inflammatory response with consequent mucosal damage. The worms are excreted in the stool and auto-infection is common.

Complications
Disseminated strongyloidiasis is rare and often a fatal condition seen in those who are immunocompromised.

Treatment
Thiabendazole or albendazole (fewer side-effects) are effective treatments.

Hookworm infection
Incidence
Seen worldwide, and is said to affect a quarter of the world's population.

Clinical features
These include:
- Local skin irritation where the worm gains entry.
- Mild respiratory symptoms may be seen approximately 2 weeks later.
- Iron-deficiency anaemia.

On a worldwide basis, hookworm infection is the commonest cause of iron-deficiency anaemia.

Diagnosis and investigation
Full blood count shows a microcytic, hypochromic anaemia. Eosinophilia may be seen early in the infection. Microscopy can demonstrate ova in a fresh stool sample.

Aetiology and pathogenesis
Ancylostoma duodenale is responsible for the cases found in Europe and Middle East, whereas *Necator americanus* causes the disease in South East Asia, Far East, and sub-Saharan Africa.

The adult worm attaches to the small intestinal mucosa by its buccal capsule and feeds off blood from the mucosa.

Treatment
The treatment of choice is Mebendazole, a broad spectrum anthelminthic that is effective against hookworms.

Roundworm infection
Incidence
Seen worldwide, but particularly prevalent in deprived, rural areas.

Clinical features
Often asymptomatic. Nausea, vomiting, abdominal discomfort, diarrhoea, and intestinal obstruction occur with heavy infections.

Invasion of appendix or biliary tree will cause appendicitis and biliary obstruction, respectively.

Larvae in lung will cause pulmonary eosinophilia.

Diagnosis and investigation
Eggs can be seen on microscopic preparations from fresh stool samples.

Adult worm may appear from mouth or anus.

Aetiology and pathogenesis
Due to *Ascaris lumbricoides*, which can grow to a considerable size, resulting in malnutrition in some cases. Eggs are ingested via a faecally contaminated source and hatch into larvae in the small intestine.

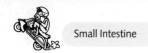

They can travel via the portal system to the liver and lungs, where they develop further. Pulmonary larvae may be expectorated, and then swallowed back into the intestine to grow into mature worms up to 20cm in length.

Treatment

Mebendazole is effective against the parasite. Surgical intervention may be needed for acute appendicitis and intestinal obstruction.

- What are the mechanisms that facilitate absorption of nutrients through the intestinal mucosa?
- What are the systemic manifestations of Crohn's disease?
- What investigations should be performed for a patient with an acute exacerbation of Crohn's disease?
- What maintenance pharmacological therapies should be considered for patients with frequently relapsing Crohn's disease?
- What are the clinical features of coeliac disease?
- What are the potential complications of bacterial overgrowth?
- Describe the mechanism of diarrhoea in cholera infection.

17. Colon

Anatomy and physiology of the colon and rectum

The colon starts at the ileocaecal valve and joins the rectum at the rectosigmoid junction (Fig. 17.1).

The muscle wall consists of an inner circular layer and an outer longitudinal layer which is incomplete and comes together to form taenia coli.

The anal canal has:

- An internal sphincter (involuntary control).
- An external sphincter (voluntary control).

The main role of the colon is absorption of water and electrolytes, which takes place mainly in the ascending colon.

Entry of faeces into the rectum produces relaxation of the internal sphincter and the urge to defecate. Defecation is brought about by voluntary relaxation of the external anal sphincter and an increase in intra-abdominal pressure.

Functional disorders

Irritable bowel syndrome
Incidence
This is a common condition that accounts for up to 40% of patients attending gastroenterology clinics. The majority of people affected are women.

Clinical features
These include:

- Abdominal pain that typically occurs in the left iliac fossa and is relieved by defecation and passage of wind.
- Alternating constipation and diarrhoea is common with passage of pellet-like stools or frequent small-volume bowel motions of a loose consistency. The patient may also complain of a sensation of incomplete emptying of the rectum.
- Abdominal distension and a subjective sensation of bloating is very suggestive of irritable bowel syndrome in the absence of bowel obstruction.
- Features suggestive of anxiety or depression may also be present.

Diagnosis and investigation
Diagnosis is predominantly made on clinical grounds. Investigations such as routine full blood count, biochemistry and inflammatory markers will be normal. In some cases, it may be necessary to exclude Crohn's disease or coeliac disease (see Chapter 16).

Further investigations such as sigmoidoscopy and barium enema are usually only necessary if there is a suspicion of an underlying pathology, especially in patients presenting over about 40 years of age.

Aetiology and pathogenesis
Precise aetiology is unclear, but it appears to be closely linked to psychological stress and patients often describe worsening of symptoms with high stress levels. The condition more commonly affects young females.

Intraluminal pressure readings are normal during symptom-free periods and pain is associated with increased force of contraction in the small intestine and colon during an attack, which may reflect an exaggerated response of the intestine to psychological stress. Depression may be an important contributory factor.

Raised intraluminal pressure is associated with reduced intestinal bulk and development of diverticulosis, but increased fibre intake does not always improve symptoms and may make the condition worse, particularly if fluid intake is not concomitantly increased.

Complications
There is an increased incidence of diverticular disease in later life, probably due to longstanding increased intraluminal pressure.

Treatment
Reassurance and tactful explanation are pivotal to the management of these patients, and it must be emphasized that the disorder is a functional one rather than one with a pathological cause. It is essential to relate your explanation to the patient's symptoms. High-fibre diets may benefit those with constipation as a dominant feature.

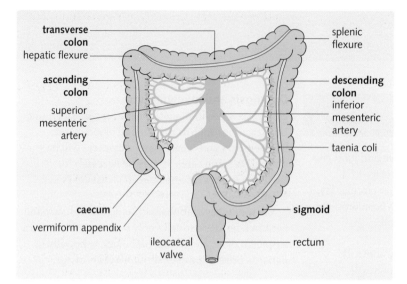

Fig. 17.1 Anatomy of the large intestine.

Antispasmodics (e.g. mebeverine) can be given for relief of painful, episodic spasms. Opioid drugs such as those containing codeine should be avoided, as they impede bowel transit and exacerbate the condition.

Megacolon
Clinical features
Constipation is characteristic, with a long, protracted history possibly with faecal impaction and soiling at a young age. Reduced rectal sensation is usual and anal tone may be increased on rectal examination.

Diagnosis and investigation
Investigations to consider:
- Barium enema or plain abdominal X-ray shows a dilated proximal colon (Fig. 17.2). A narrowed distal colon may be seen in Hirschsprung's disease.
- Deep mucosal rectal biopsy is necessary, especially in young patients, to confirm or exclude Hirschsprung's disease in which a segment of the rectum has absent or reduced ganglion cells in the submucosa.
- Manometry shows failure of internal sphincter relaxation in response to rectal distension.

Aetiology and pathogenesis
The condition can be congenital or acquired.

Congenital type is known as Hirschsprung's disease, which usually presents in childhood with chronic constipation and faecal soiling. Rectal biopsy shows an absence of ganglion cells in the submucosal

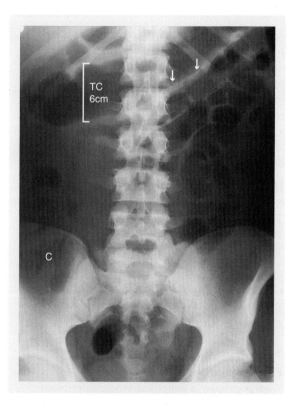

Fig. 17.2 Plain abdominal X-ray showing megacolon. Note the transverse colon (TC) 6cm and thumbprinting in the caecum (C), indicating severe mucosal oedema, which can also be seen between bowel layers (arrows).

Causes of chronic constipation
Low residue diet
Drugs, e.g. opioids, iron, anti-depressants
Metabolic conditions: hypothyroidism, hypercalcaemia
Neuropsychiatric conditions: Parkinson's, depression, stroke (immobility)
Obstruction and pseudo-obstruction
Painful anorectal conditions, e.g. fissure
Carcinoma of the colon

Fig. 17.3 Causes of chronic constipation.

plexus. Adults presenting with the condition may have segmental disease, hence initial biopsy may be normal and a deeper biopsy or a full thickness biopsy is required.

The most common cause of acquired megacolon is chronic constipation with or without laxative abuse. Causes of chronic constipation are many (Fig. 17.3). Chronic ingestion of laxatives results in depletion of ganglion cells.

Complications
Subacute or acute bowel obstruction can ensue.

Treatment
Hirschsprung's disease is primarily treated by surgical resection of the affected colon.

Acquired megacolon is more difficult to treat because patients may have been taking laxatives for some time. Frequent enemas or manual evacuations may be needed. In severe cases, surgical intervention is required.

Pseudo-obstruction
Clinical features
Similar to those of bowel obstruction (i.e. vomiting, distension, non-passage of flatus, etc.), but unlike true obstruction, bowel sounds are absent.

Aetiology and pathogenesis
Bowel paralysis is common after laparotomy due to manual handling and will return to normal within 2–3 days. Systemic conditions can also give rise to an adynamic bowel (e.g: drugs, electrolyte disturbance,

septicaemia). It is commonly seen in intensive care patients.

Treatment
Correction of the underlying abnormality will usually result in the return of normal peristalsis.

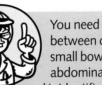

You need to distinguish between dilated large and small bowel on an abdominal X-ray. Small bowel is identified by valvulae conniventes that entirely cross the width of the lumen and the gas pattern tends to be central. Large bowel haustra do not cross all the lumen's width and gas can be seen in colon proximal to the obstruction (e.g. in the caecum).

Inflammatory bowel disease

Ulcerative colitis
Incidence
Average incidence is 5–8 out of 100 000 people in Europe and the USA.

Peak age of onset between 20–40 years of age. Women are affected more often than men.

Clinical features
Diarrhoea is the most prominent feature, usually associated with presence of blood and mucus. Patients may pass up to 20 loose motions per 24 hours during an acute attack, often accompanied by urgency and tenesmus.

Less specific features such as malaise, anorexia and weight loss are common, and there may be symptoms of anaemia or hypoalbuminaemia. Extra-intestinal manifestations also occur (Fig. 17.4).

Diagnosis and investigation
You should consider the following investigations:
- Full blood count, C-reactive protein, blood cultures, and stool cultures, as for Crohn's disease.
- Raised biliary enzymes suggest the presence of primary sclerosing cholangitis.

- A plain abdominal X-ray is essential to exclude colonic dilatation, particularly in the context of abdominal pain.
- A barium enema shows ulceration, and the extent of colonic involvement may be seen in active disease. In long-standing chronic cases, characteristic 'lead-pipe' colon can be demonstrated.

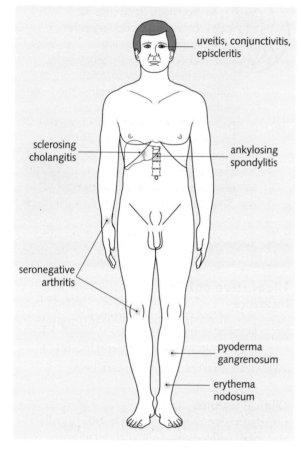

Fig. 17.4 Body map of extra-intestinal features of ulcerative colitis.

- Colonoscopy is the preferred investigation because it offers the advantage of biopsy to differentiate from Crohn's disease and other forms of colitis. Mucosa is inflamed, friable and bleeds easily.

Aetiology and pathogenesis

Unknown aetiology but there is an association with HLA-B27 and ankylosing spondylitis which is suggestive of a genetic basis but no conclusive evidence is yet available.

Histological features are similar to those seen in infectious diarrhoea but no agent has been shown to be responsible.

Perinuclear antineutrophil cytoplasmic antibodies (pANCA) can be found in 60% of patients with ulcerative colitis, which suggests an underlying immunological cause, but it is difficult to ascertain whether this autoantibody is a cause, or a result, of the disease.

Patients with ulcerative colitis are more likely to be non-smokers or ex-smokers compared to the general population but the significance of this observation is unclear. Conversely, Crohn's disease is associated with smoking.

Ulcerative colitis affects the rectum and may extend along the whole length of the colon. Small bowel involvement is not seen in contrast to Crohn's disease, except in patients with extensive disease affecting the terminal ileum ('backwash ileitis') (Fig. 17.5).

Macroscopically, the mucosa looks inflamed and bleeds easily. In severe disease, extensive ulceration is seen with neighbouring mucosa appearing like polyps ('pseudopolyps'). Fulminant colitis results in loss of the mucosal layer and involvement of the muscle layer, producing toxic dilatation.

Microscopically, the inflammation is limited to the mucosa and submucosa with inflammatory cells

Ulcerative colitis versus Crohn's disease		
	Ulcerative colitis	**Crohn's disease**
Clinical features	Bloody diarrhoea	Abdominal pain and weight loss
Macroscopic appearance	Usually confined to colon Rectum always involved Ulceration superficial and continuous	Most often terminal ileum but can affect anywhere in GI tract Patchy transmural ulceration and skip lesions are common
Microscopic appearance	Crypt abscesses	Granulomas are common

Fig. 17.5 Contrasting features between ulcerative colitis and Crohn's disease.

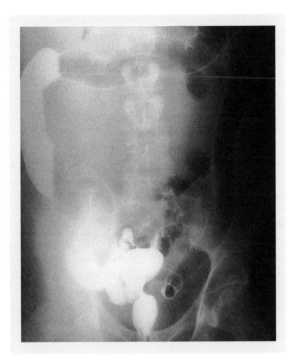

Fig. 17.6 Barium enema showing 'lead pipe' appearance in chronic ulcerative colitis.

accumulating in the lamina propria and colonic gland to form crypt abscesses. Goblet cell depletion is also seen. Long-standing colitis results in fibrosis of mucosa and submucosa, hence loss of haustral pattern and a shortened and featureless colon ('lead-pipe colon') (Fig. 17.6).

Complications

Toxic megacolon is seen on plain abdominal X-ray. Dilatation of 5 cm or greater is associated with a risk of perforation and peritonitis. The patient is usually unwell with fever, tachycardia and abdominal distension with tenderness (Figs 17.2 and 17.7). Shock with oliguric renal failure can occur as a consequence of sepsis and hypovolaemia.

The risk of developing adenocarcinoma after 10 years of colitis is approximately 5% higher than the general population. The risk is related to the extent of colon involved and the duration of the disease process. The current recommendations for screening in this regard are as follows:

- Time of initial screen should be at eight years for those with pan-colitis and for left-sided colitis, 15 years from onset of symptoms.

Features of severe ulcerative colitis
Stool frequency >8 times/day with blood
Abdominal pain and tenderness
Fever >37.5°C
Tachycardia >100 bpm
C-reactive protein >20 mg/l
ESR >35 mm/h
Haemoglobin <10 g/L
Albumin < 30 g/L

Fig. 17.7 Features indicating severity in ulcerative colitis.

- Colonoscopy (with biopsies every 10cm) should be performed on a 3-yearly basis in the second decade, 2-yearly in the third decade and annually thereafter.
- Haemorrhage is a potential complication, although blood transfusion is usually only required in severe attacks.
- Cholangiocarcinoma arises with increasing frequency in patients with ulcerative colitis when primary sclerosing cholangitis coexists.
- Secondary amyloidosis is probably related to high levels of circulating acute-phase protein during exacerbations.

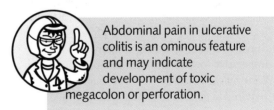

Abdominal pain in ulcerative colitis is an ominous feature and may indicate development of toxic megacolon or perforation.

Prognosis

The course of the disease is variable, but characteristically it is a chronic relapsing disease. Patients with proctitis alone have a good overall prognosis, with only 10% progressing to more extensive disease. By contrast, severe fulminant disease is associated with up to 25% mortality.

Treatment

Treatment options include:

- Corticosteroids given during an acute attack to gain remission. Topical treatment can be given for localized disease (proctitis) in the form of an enema. Long-term use of oral steroids should be avoided.
- Management of an acute, severe attack may necessitate intravenous steroids (e.g. hydrocortisone), intravenous fluid and electrolyte replacement and appropriate antibiotics for proven, or suspected coexistent infection. IV nutrition (total parenteral nutrition) may be required for protracted exacerbations and intramuscular vitamins are sometimes given.
- 5-aminosalicylic acid (5-ASA) compounds are effective in reducing acute inflammation and maintaining remission in ulcerative colitis. Sulfasalazine is attached to sulfapyridine, which is broken down by bacteria to active 5-ASA. Mesalazine (5-ASA alone) or olsalazine (two 5-ASA moeties) may be less toxic because they do not have a sulphur compound conjugated. These can also be given in enema form for localized proctitis.
- Immunosuppression with azathioprine can be used for patients who are not responding to steroids, or in frequently relapsing cases where long-term steroid use is undesirable. Azathioprine is an antiproliferative immunosuppressant with the rare but serious adverse effect of myelosuppression. Blood counts should be monitored closely for the first few weeks, and the patient should be warned to report immediately any signs or symptoms of bone marrow suppression, e.g. infections, bleeding or spontaneous bruising. Hepatic toxicity is also well recognized.
- Surgical resection, usually in form of colectomy, is imperative for patients with complications such as toxic megacolon or perforation, and may be required in patients not responding to medical treatment. Total surgical mortality is in the order of 5%; and in the acute situation with perforation, can be as high as 50%.

Crohn's colitis
Clinical features
Crohn's disease can affect any part of the intestine including the colon and is occasionally confined to the colon alone (Crohn's colitis).

It can be difficult to differentiate Crohn's colitis from ulcerative colitis and the two conditions can overlap (referred to as indeterminate colitis).

The clinical picture is of abdominal pain and diarrhoea. Pain is more common than in ulcerative colitis and bleeding is far less common.

Investigation and diagnosis
These are basically the same as for ulcerative colitis. Differentiation from ulcerative colitis can be difficult.

The presence of granulomas and deep inflammation is suggestive of Crohn's colitis, whereas paucity of mucin and crypt abscesses are more in favour of ulcerative colitis.

Aetiology and pathogenesis
Up to 15% of patients will have clinical features of ulcerative colitis, but the biopsy will reveal the presence of granulomas which are pathognomic of Crohn's disease, therefore making the diagnosis difficult.

Recent genetic studies have shown that a presence of certain genes occurring simultaneously predisposes an individual to developing inflammatory bowel disease. It is now thought that ulcerative colitis and Crohn's disease may represent opposite ends of a spectrum.

Treatment
Standard treatment remains the same. However, it is important to distinguish between Crohn's and ulcerative colitis because there are important implications in their treatment. For example, surgery is generally considered to be curative in ulcerative colitis, whereas this is clearly not the case for Crohn's disease.

See Chapter 16 for further details on Crohn's disease.

Collagenous colitis
Clinical features
Occurs more commonly in women and presents as intermittent chronic watery diarrhoea. Abdominal pain may also be present. Patients are asymptomatic during remission.

Diagnosis and investigation
Stool culture, inflammatory markers, and colonoscopy are usually normal.

Diagnosis is based on histology, which demonstrates the presence of a thickened subepithelial collagen layer (Fig. 17.8). There may also be intraepithelial lymphocytic infiltration, but

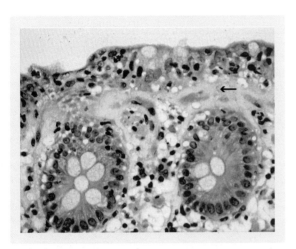

Fig. 17.8 Photomicrograph of collagenous colitis. Note the thickened amorphous layer just below the surface epithelial cells (arrow).

this is more commonly seen in microscopic colitis (see below).

Aetiology and pathogenesis

There is an association with long-term use of non-steroidal anti-inflammatory drugs (NSAIDs) but an underlying immunological cause has been postulated, as this condition is more commonly seen in people with seronegative arthritis, Raynaud's phenomenon and coeliac disease.

Treatment

NSAIDs should be stopped. Anti-diarrhoeal drugs are ineffective. Sulfasalazine and colestyramine have been tried with variable success rates. In persistent cases, short-term oral corticosteroids can be employed.

Microscopic colitis
Clinical features

Similar to collagenous colitis (i.e. intermittent diarrhoea, abdominal pain, etc.). Again, the condition is more commonly found in women.

Diagnosis and investigation

These are as for collagenous colitis, except the biopsy shows intraepithelial lymphocytic infiltration without thickening of the collagen layer.

Aetiology and pathogenesis

An immune aetiology has also been suggested because there is an association with:

- Increased frequency of patients who have HLA-A1 haplotype.
- Decreased frequency of HLA-A3.

In addition, a minority of patients have subsequently been found to have coeliac disease.

Treatment

As for collagenous colitis. Colestyramine may also be helpful.

Neoplastic disorders

Colonic polyps
Clinical features

Usually, these polyps are an incidental finding as part of an investigation for abdominal pain, rectal bleeding, altered bowel habit, etc. In addition:
- Obstruction and intussusception can occur, especially in infants.
- Iron deficiency anaemia may be present if the polyp ulcerates or bleeds.
- Diarrhoea is seen with the villous type and can be severe enough to cause hypokalaemia.

Diagnosis and investigation

Investigations include:
- Barium enema—may demonstrate either solitary or multiple polyps.
- Endoscopy—used to confirm and remove polyps for histological examination (Fig. 24.21).

Aetiology and pathogenesis

The majority of polyps are adenomas (tubular, tubulovillous, or villous).
   The malignant potential of any polyp is related to:
- Increasing polyp size.
- Polyp type (i.e. tubulovillous rather than metaplastic) (Fig. 17.9).

Polyps can be solitary or multiple. Genetic and environmental factors have been implicated because they are more commonly seen in the Western world (10% of population), but no definite cause has been found. Almost all colonic carcinomas originate from a polyp and 90% of patients with colonic carcinoma will have polyps elsewhere in the colon. Five per cent of polyps removed at sigmoidoscopies are found to have invasive carcinoma.

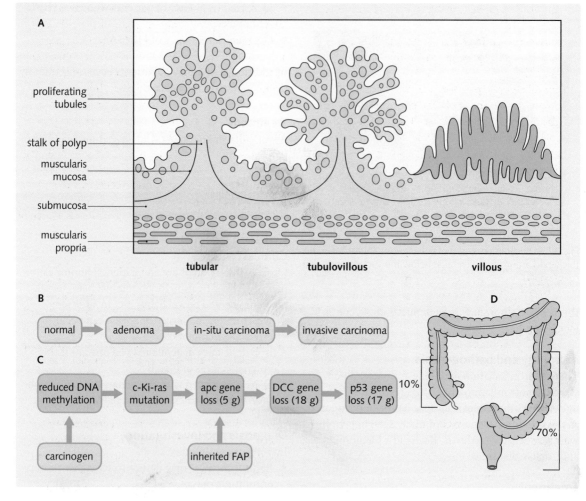

Fig. 17.9 (A) Types of colonic polyps. (B) A summary of the polyp cancer sequence in the colon. (C) Molecular changes involved. (D) Two-thirds of colon cancers occur within 60 cm of the anal verge and within reach of a flexible sigmoidoscope.

Familial polyposis coli is an inherited autosomal dominant condition involving a gene located on the long arm of chromosome 5. There are polyps throughout the gastrointestinal (GI) tract, especially in the colon, and patients commonly present in their teens. Hypertrophy and osteomas of the mandibles and long bones are commonly associated with this syndrome.

The other main type of polyps are the hamartomas such as Peutz–Jeghers syndrome (see Chapter 16). More commonly in children are juvenile polyps which histologically are shown to be mucus-retention cysts and mainly confined to the colon.

People who have Cronkhite–Canada syndrome have polyps similar to those of Peutz–Jeghers syndrome but in addition have ectodermal abnormalities such as nail dystrophy and skin pigmentation.

Complications
These include:
- Malignant change with increasing size.
- Bleeding, obstruction, and intussusception.

Prognosis
There is a 50% chance of recurrence after removal of an adenomatous polyp.

Treatment
This involves:
- Endoscopic removal of polyps—any lesions found on endoscopy or barium studies should ideally be

removed to prevent malignant transformation (Fig. 24.18).

- Surgical resection for patients with familial polyposis coli for whom individual polyps cannot be removed.
- Surveillance of patients who are at risk (i.e. polyposis coli and their first degree relatives).
- Colonoscopic screening for those who have had a colonic adenoma is undertaken according to size and number of polyps (assigned low, intermediate or high risk). For example, one or two adenomas measuring <1 cm may only need one screen after 5 years, whereas multiple large polyps require annual colonoscopy.

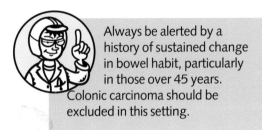

Always be alerted by a history of sustained change in bowel habit, particularly in those over 45 years. Colonic carcinoma should be excluded in this setting.

Colorectal carcinoma
Incidence
The second most common carcinoma in the UK affects approximately 20 out of 100 000 people. Mean age at diagnosis is between 60 and 65 years. Disease is rare in Africa and Asia and this is thought to be linked to environmental rather than genetic factors.

Aetiology and pathogenesis
Western diets of high animal fat and low fibre have been linked to colorectal carcinoma, possibly due to slow transit of intestinal content which increases contact time between potential carcinogens and the bowel wall.

Familial polyposis coli and inflammatory bowel disease are risk factors for the development of colonic tumours. The relationship between inflammatory bowel disease and carcinomas is not clearly defined, but it does not appear to be directly associated with chronicity of inflammation. It is possible that the risk for development of colonic carcinoma is an inherited one because the age of onset is more important than the severity of the disease and seems to be an independent risk factor.

Colonic carcinoma is now thought to be a result of a multiple genetic alterations that occur in a progressive, stepwise manner. Oncogenes that normally regulate cell division and differentiation may undergo mutation as a result of external stimuli. This produces hyperplasia, followed by metaplasia, and eventually dysplastic change and tumour. Most commonly associated with colonic carcinoma are the c-KRAS and c-MYC oncogenes. The APC gene on the long arm of chromosome 5 is responsible for familial polyposis coli, which may have a role in development of colonic carcinoma (Fig. 17.9).

Dukes' classification of colonic cancer is shown in Fig. 17.10.

Hereditary colonic carcinomas have been described, and the gene responsible is located on chromosome 2. These patients have tumours at an early age (i.e. peak incidence at 40 years), and typically have a right-sided lesion (Lynch syndrome type I). Some of these patients also have an increased incidence of other carcinomas such as endometrial, brain, and lung, as well as other GI carcinomas (Lynch syndrome type II).

Approximately two-thirds of tumours arise from the rectosigmoid colon and these tumours typically start off as a flat lesion and later become bulky, polypoid, and ulcerate. Similar types of lesions are found in the caecum and ascending colon. Lesions in the descending colon tend to be annular and produce the typical 'apple core' lesion on barium enema (Fig. 24.25).

The tumours produce a variable amount of mucin, and histologically signet ring cells can be seen where the nucleus is pushed to one side due to cytoplasmic mucus.

Clinical features
The main features are:
- Anaemia, weight loss, abdominal pain, or loose bowel motions are the most common features. A mass may be palpable in the right iliac fossa, especially with caecal lesions. Rectal bleeding or obstruction is more common with left-sided lesions (e.g. rectosigmoid).
- Altered bowel habits are seen in >50% of all patients.
- Perforation and abscess formation is not uncommon, and jaundice due to liver metastases can occur in advanced cases.

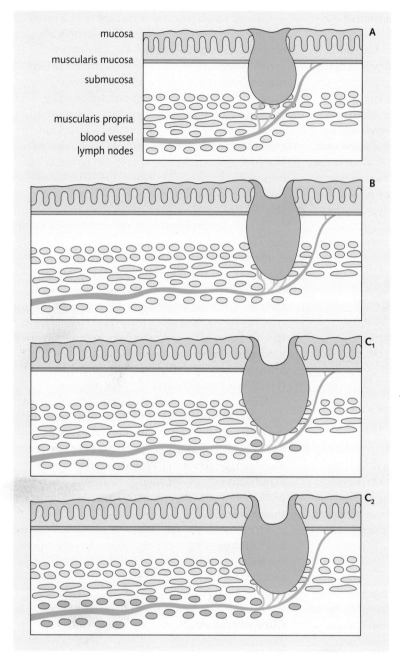

Fig. 17.10 Dukes' classification of colonic cancer. (A), the tumour is confined to the bowel wall; (B) it extends through the muscle coat but does not involve lymph nodes; (C) all layers are affected, with the proximal lymph node affected in C₁ and both the proximal and the highest resected nodes positive in C₂.

mucosa

muscularis mucosa

submucosa

muscularis propria

blood vessel

lymph nodes

A

B

C₁

C₂

 Rectal examination is a mandatory part of the examination as a tumour can often be palpated.

Diagnosis and investigation

Investigations of use include:

- Full blood count—may detect iron deficiency anaemia, which is common.
- Faecal occult blood—is often positive but can be seen in any cause of underlying GI bleed (e.g. duodenal ulceration).

- Barium enema—is still the investigation of choice in most centres. Poor bowel preparation can make interpretation difficult.
- Rigid sigmoidoscopy—is easily performed on an outpatient basis, but only identifies rectosigmoid tumours.
- Flexible sigmoidoscopy—can detect up to 70% of tumours and is a better investigation in combination with barium enema to examine the remainder of the colon. Colonoscopy is reserved for patients unsuitable for barium enema or in doubtful cases. Adequate bowel preparation is essential.
- Abdominal ultrasound—is sensitive for detecting metastases in the liver before surgical resection.

Treatment

The mainstays of management are:
- Surgical resection with end-to-end anastomosis or end colostomy depending on the site of the tumour.
- Chemotherapy with or without radiotherapy— given to patients with Dukes' B and C which can improve survival (Fig. 17.10). Chemotherapy can sometimes be given to patients with liver metastases, but the results are disappointing.

Prognosis

See Fig. 17.11. Overall survival is 30% at 5 years.

Angiodysplasia

Incidence

Relatively rare condition affecting the elderly population.

Clinical features

To note:
- Chronic iron-deficiency anaemia is due to chronic blood loss from the GI tract.
- Acute GI bleeding can occur, causing hypotension and shock in some patients.

Diagnosis and investigation

Diagnosis can be difficult and often involves repeated gastroscopy and colonoscopy to detect the lesion:
- Red cell radio-isotope-labelled scanning can be helpful to identify the site of blood loss.
- Selective angiography may demonstrate abnormal blood vessels or the site of active bleeding.

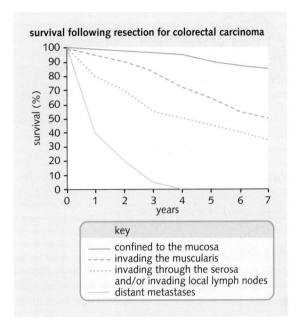

survival following resection for colorectal carcinoma

key
— confined to the mucosa
--- invading the muscularis
····· invading through the serosa and/or invading local lymph nodes
— distant metastases

Fig. 17.11 Survival following resection for colorectal carcinoma according to Dukes' staging. Note that survival is commensurate with that of the normal population if the tumour is confined to the mucosa.

Aetiology and pathogenesis

The underlying aetiology is unknown but the condition is most likely to be acquired because it affects mainly the elderly population. There is an association with aortic stenosis, and approximately half the patients will have some form of cardiac disease. It can exist anywhere along the GI tract, but is more commonly found in proximal colon, caecum, and terminal ileum.

Treatment

Diathermy during colonoscopy can be successful for small lesions. Larger proximal lesions will need surgical resection. Hormonal treatment with progesterone derivatives can result in regression of the lesions.

Anorectal conditions

Haemorrhoids
Clinical features

The main symptoms are:
- Rectal bleeding, which may coat the stools or drip into the toilet at the end of defecation.
- Peri-anal irritation and itching are also seen.

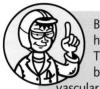

Bleeding from haemorrhoids is bright red. This is because it is capillary blood from the spongy vascular anal cushions. Piles are not 'varicose veins'.

Diagnosis and investigation
Proctoscopy reveals blood vessels classically seen at the 3, 7, and 11 o'clock positions.

Aetiology and pathogenesis
Haemorrhoids result from enlargement of the venous plexuses at the lower end of anal mucosa.

Raised intra-abdominal pressure inhibits venous return to the vena cava and hence causes venous engorgement. Common contributing factors are constipation, pregnancy, excessive straining to pass urine or stool, etc.

A minor degree of rectal prolapse is common. Oestrogen-related venous dilatation may also contribute to development of haemorrhoids in pregnancy.

Rectal bleeding occurs as a result of trauma by passage of hard stools. Symptoms are usually intermittent and exacerbated by constipation.

Mucus secreted by glandular epithelium can block skin pores, which causes secondary infection by bacteria and *Candida*, followed by local skin irritation. Haemorrhoids are classified as first, second and third degree as shown. They may be painful if they thrombose (Fig. 17.12).

Complications
Thrombosis of the haemorrhoids is painful and irreducible. However, it is a self-limiting condition that eventually results in atrophy and fibrosis of the thrombosed haemorrhoids, leaving visible anal tags.

Treatment
Mild cases can be improved simply by addressing the underlying constipation; a high-fibre diet may be all that is necessary.
- Injection of a sclerosant or elastic band ligation may be needed in more troublesome cases.
- Surgical resection is reserved for irreducible prolapsed and problematic cases.

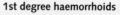

1st degree haemorrhoids   levator ani

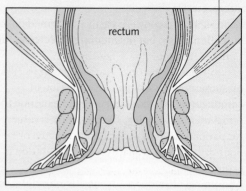

rectum

2nd degree haemorrhoids

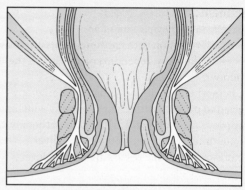

3rd degree haemorrhoids

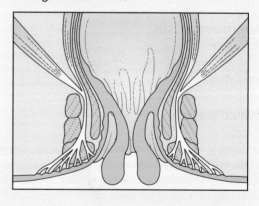

Fig. 17.12 Anatomical representation of haemorrhoid classification. In 1st degree haemorrhoids, the spongy vascular cushions remain within the rectum; 2nd degree piles prolapse through the anus on defecation but spontaneously reduce; 3rd degree piles require digital reduction or may remain persistently prolapsed.

Anal fissures
Clinical features
Rectal pain during defecation associated with rectal bleeding is the classic presentation. Pain, in turn, will cause anal spasm and aggravate the constipation that caused the condition originally.

Diagnosis
Often made on clinical grounds. Rectal examination is extremely painful and rarely possible. If rectal examination is required, then local or general anaesthesia may be used.

A small skin tag or sentinel pile may be seen at the anus and parting of the buttocks may reveal the fissure itself.

Aetiology and pathogenesis
Usually the result of passage of a large constipated stool causing a tear in the anal mucosa. Over 90% of cases are in the midline of the posterior margin and are perpetuated by internal sphincter spasm.

Treatment
Treatment depends on the type of fissure:
- Acute fissures can be treated with local anaesthesia and prevention of further constipation with either a bulking agent or osmotic laxative.
- Chronic fissuring may require surgical intervention in the form of anal stretch or more recently lateral internal sphincterotomy, which has a better result with regard to incontinence in later age. Glyceryl trinitrate ointment can improve pain and ischaemia caused by chronic fissuring and spasm, and may negate the need for surgery.

Pruritus ani
A common complaint. The majority of cases are secondary to poor hygiene and some degree of faecal incontinence, especially in elderly people. Associated conditions such as haemorrhoids, threadworm infestation, or fungal infection should be excluded.

In the absence of any underlying cause, treatment should include good personal hygiene and keeping the area dry. Use of topical steroids or antimicrobial creams should be avoided.

Rectal prolapse
Incidence
Common among elderly people and young children.

Clinical features
Tenesmus is a feeling of incomplete defecation which can be due to prolapse. Rectal bleeding can occur due to mucosal ulceration secondary to stool trauma. Incontinence of faeces may be seen.

Complete prolapse of the rectal wall can sometimes be seen through the anus (Fig. 17.13).

Diagnosis and investigation
Usually made on history and examination. However:
- Sigmoidoscopy may reveal a 'solitary' rectal ulcer approximately 8–10 cm above the anal verge, usually on the anterior rectal wall. These 'solitary' ulcers can also be multiple.
- Prolapse can often be seen when the patient is asked to voluntarily strain as if to pass a stool.
- Defecating proctogram is a very useful, albeit undignified, examination if the prolapse is internal but producing significant symptoms.
- Endoscopic ultrasound can be useful to determine whether muscle damage has occurred (possibly due to obstetric trauma) as this can be repaired surgically.

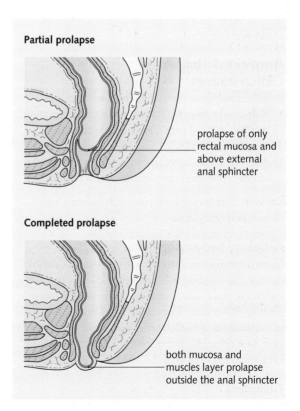

Partial prolapse

prolapse of only rectal mucosa and above external anal sphincter

Completed prolapse

both mucosa and muscles layer prolapse outside the anal sphincter

Fig. 17.13 Classification of rectal prolapse.

Aetiology and pathogenesis

The condition results from excessive straining when opening bowels. In the initial stages, the prolapse only occurs after defecation and returns spontaneously, but later the condition worsens and prolapse may appear on standing.

In early stages, prolapse of the mucosa or rectal wall may remain internal to the anal sphincter; hence, the patient may experience discomfort but no obvious abnormality can be seen.

Treatment

Rectal prolapse in childhood rarely requires surgical treatment. Parents should be reassured because the prolapse will almost always be reduced either spontaneously or with gentle manipulation. A high-fibre diet should be given, and the child taught not to strain at defecation.

Minor prolapses often do not require treatment because they reduce themselves and only appear after straining. General advice such as a high-fibre diet and avoidance of straining should be given. Patients with severe prolapse should be treated surgically by posterior fixation of the rectum to the sacral wall. Sphincter repair may also be necessary if problematic incontinence occurs as a result of weakened sphincter.

Anorectal abscesses
Clinical features

Pain depends upon the site of the abscess:
- A fluctuant mass sitting just beneath the inflamed skin is typical of peri-anal and ischiorectal abscesses.
- A tender mass on rectal examination may be due to intersphincteric or pararectal abscesses.

Systemic features of infection such as fever and neutrophilia may occur.

Aetiology and pathogenesis

More often seen in patients with diabetes, Crohn's disease and conditions or therapies leading to immunosuppression, but do occur in otherwise healthy individuals. The condition is due to infection of the anal glands which tends to spread along the anal duct through the external sphincter and its surrounding tissues (Fig. 17.14).

Treatment

Surgical drainage is required in all cases, except for those that are very minor for which antibiotics alone

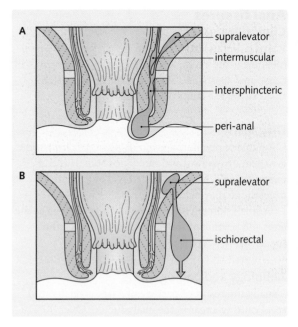

Fig. 17.14 Illustration showing how peri-anal infection can develop into abscess (A) or fistula (B).

can be given. Antibiotics to cover skin organisms, such as *Staphylococci*, and gut bacteria including anaerobes are routinely given after the drainage procedure.

Anal fistula
Clinical features

This is usually manifest as intermittent discharge over the peri-anal area from the fistula. The fistula itself can be seen as a small area of granulation tissue around the anal margin. It is often dismissed as incomplete healing of anorectal abscess. Underlying Crohn's disease should be excluded or confirmed.

Diagnosis and investigation

Examination under anaesthesia is usually required to establish the site of the proximal opening by a probe. Occasionally, a dye is injected into the distal orifice to identify the opening (fistulogram).

Aetiology and pathogenesis

Anal fistula is a common complication of anorectal abscesses as the anal gland infection spreads to form an abscess and drains externally in the form of a fistula. MR imaging demonstrating an anal fistula is shown in Fig. 17.15. Crohn's disease is also a cause of anal fistula, and they are often multiple.

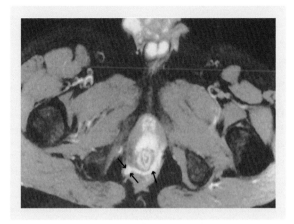

Fig. 17.15 Magnetic resonance scan demonstration of anal fistula tracking around the back of the anal canal and through the muscularis on the right side (arrows).

Treatment

Once the proximal opening has been identified, the fistula can be laid open and healing by secondary intention occurs, providing the fistula does not involve the anal sphincter.

Fistulae that involve the sphincter will require a specialist anorectal surgeon for preservation and repair of the sphincter to ensure continence.

Fistulae caused by Crohn's disease should be treated with conservative treatment as for active Crohn's disease. Surgical treatment usually involves an ileostomy.

Infections

Bacterial infection of the colon
Incidence

This is the most common cause of diarrhoea worldwide, especially afflicting travellers outside their own country.

Clinical features

These include:
- Diarrhoea, abdominal pain, fever, and vomiting.
- Leucocytosis may be seen on full blood count.

Clinical and biochemical evidence of dehydration is not uncommon, especially at extreme of ages (i.e. elderly and infants).

Diagnosis and investigation

Investigations of use include:
- Routine biochemistry and full blood count.
- Stool culture.
- Sigmoidoscopy and biopsy if diarrhoea is persistent.

Aetiology and pathogenesis

Common pathogens include species of *Escherichia coli*, *Shigella*, and *Salmonella* which are spread via faecal–oral route and are often the result of poor food hygiene. Invasion of the colonic epithelium occurs and in some cases with certain strains of *E. coli*, an enterotoxin is produced.

Clostridium difficile infection is typically seen after broad spectrum antibiotic therapy, but especially clindamycin. Disturbance of normal colonic flora caused by antibiotics allow proliferation of *C. difficile* and toxin production. On sigmoidoscopy, plaques of inflammatory exudates can be seen giving the appearance of pseudomembranes (pseudomembranous colitis). Direct person-to-person spread can also occur.

Diagnosis can be made by isolation of the toxins in the stool.

Escherichia coli serotype 0157 is associated with the development of a microangiopathic haemolytic anaemia, thrombocytopenia and renal failure, often requiring dialysis. This is termed HUS (Haemolytic Uraemic Syndrome) and has an associated mortality.

Treatment

Adequate rehydration and electrolyte correction is required either intravenously or orally.

Once stool cultures have confirmed the diagnosis, appropriate antibiotics should be started. If the patient is severely ill, ciprofloxacin can be started empirically once stool and blood cultures have been taken. If *C. difficile* is suspected or confirmed, then oral metronidazole or vancomycin are the drugs of choice.

Anti-diarrhoeal agents such as codeine or loperamide should be avoided if possible because they impair the clearance of the pathogen from the bowel.

Amoebiasis

Incidence
Occurs worldwide, but more commonly in the tropics.

Clinical features
In acute infection these include:
- Abdominal pain.
- Diarrhoea (often bloody).
- Nausea and vomiting.

Fulminant colitis and toxic dilatation can rarely occur.

Diagnosis and investigation
Investigations:
- Fresh stool samples are required for identification of amoebic cysts.
- Specific antibody can be measured in the serum.
- Sigmoidoscopy demonstrates ulceration of the colonic mucosa but it is not diagnostic.

Aetiology and pathogenesis
The disease is caused by *Entamoeba histolytica* which is digested in its cyst form via contaminated food or water, or direct person-to-person spread. Multiplication of the organism takes place in the colon, where they invade the colonic epithelium, causing ulceration. Not all who are infected will have clinical disease and some become asymptomatic cyst carriers.

Complications
Uncommon—perforation due to toxic dilatation can occur. Strictures can occur in chronic infection.

Hepatic abscesses are not uncommon (see Chapter 18).

Treatment
Metronidazole is the drug of choice. Education and advice regarding hygiene can help reduce person-to-person spread.

Cryptosporidiosis

Clinical features
Symptoms include:

- Watery diarrhoea.
- Fever.
- Abdominal pain.

Toxic dilatation and sclerosing cholangitis can be seen in patients with AIDS.

Diagnosis and investigation
Parasite can be identified by modified Ziehl–Nielsen stain of faeces or intestinal biopsy. Faecal oocysts should be quantified.

Aetiology and pathogenesis
The fungal parasite is found worldwide with its major reservoir in cattle, and is likely to be spread via contaminated water supplies.

Healthy individuals will have a self-limiting gastroenteritis and often the diagnosis is not confirmed. People who are immunocompromised tend to have a devastating illness with protracted episodes of diarrhoea.

The organism also causes sclerosing cholangitis in the immunocompromised patient.

Treatment
It may be self-limiting if the CD4 lymphocyte count is not too suppressed. Paromomycin has been shown to be effective. Good hygiene prevents spread of the infection.

Schistosomiasis
See also Chapter 18 and Fig. 18.28.

Clinical features
The main features are:
- Fever.
- Urticaria.
- Nausea.
- Vomiting.
- Bloody diarrhoea.

Diagnosis and investigation
Consider the following investigations:
- Specific antibodies can be detected by serology.
- Eggs can be isolated from stool, urine, or rectal biopsy.
- Sigmoidoscopy reveals mucosal ulceration which, as an isolated finding, is not diagnostic.

Aetiology and pathogenesis
Schistosoma mansoni predominantly affects the colon, causing erythema and ulceration of the

mucosa. A localized granulomatous reaction may be mistaken for colonic cancer. Progressive fibrosis leads to stricture formation but obstruction is rare.

Schistosoma japonicum affects the small intestine and proximal colon and epithelial dysplasia is seen with chronic infection which is now accepted to be a premalignant condition.

Complications
Periportal fibrosis and portal hypertension can ensue. Ectopic deposition of eggs elsewhere in the body (e.g. lung and brain).

Treatment
The drug of choice is Praziquantel, as it is effective against all human schistosomes, combining broad-spectrum activity with low toxicity.

Whipworm infection
Incidence
Found worldwide and prevalence can be as high as 90% in poor communities with poor hygiene.

Clinical features
Usually asymptomatic.

Heavy infestation causes bloody diarrhoea associated with weight loss, abdominal discomfort and anorexia. Involvement of appendix causes appendicitis.

Diagnosis and investigation
Stool examination for eggs.

Sigmoidoscopy—adult worms may be seen attached to the rectal mucosa.

Aetiology and pathogenesis
Caused by *Trichuris trichura*. Adult worms are more commonly found in the distal ileum and caecum. The whole colon may be affected in heavy infection.

The adult worm embeds itself in the colonic mucosa, causing damage and ulceration, leading to protein and blood loss in severe cases.

Treatment
The antihelmintic Mebendazole is the treatment of choice, but its use needs to be combined with hygienic measures to break the cycle of auto-infection. All family members should receive therapy.

Threadworm infection
Incidence
Occurs worldwide, but is more prevalent in temperate climates. Outbreaks are seen in institutional establishments and areas of overcrowded living conditions.

Clinical features
Pruritus ani is intense and usually nocturnal due to egg laying by the female worm.

Submucosal abscess is rare and due to secondary bacterial infection of the colonic mucosa.

Diagnosis and investigation
Adult worms may be seen directly leaving the anus. Clear adhesive tape can be applied to the peri-anal region to allow the identification of eggs microscopically.

Aetiology and pathogenesis
Caused by *Enterobius vermicularis* and commonly affects children. Adult worms reside in the colon and female worms migrate to the peri-anal region to lay their eggs. Superficial damage to the colonic mucosa is common during heavy infestations.

Autoinfection via scratching and poor hygiene aggravates the problem. Rarely, migration to the peritoneum and visceral organs occurs.

Treatment
Mebendazole given as two single doses, 2 weeks apart, is effective. Asymptomatic family members should also be treated.

- What drugs can be implicated in causing constipation?
- What are the contrasting features between ulcerative colitis and Crohn's disease?
- What are the clinical and laboratory features that would indicate a severe exacerbation of ulcerative colitis?
- How would you manage a patient presenting with an acute severe exacerbation of ulcerative colitis?
- What are the potential indications for surgery in ulcerative colitis?
- What is Dukes' classification of colonic cancer?
- What is the pathophysiology of Clostridium difficile infection and which antibiotics in particular are implicated?

18. Liver

Structure and function of the liver

The predominant pathological mechanisms affecting the liver are:
- Necrosis.
- Inflammation.
- Fibrosis.

The site at which these disease processes occur may produce different clinical syndromes, and the functions of the liver (Fig. 18.1) may be affected differentially:
- Centrilobular processes affect synthetic and metabolic functions and hepatocellular necrosis produces an enzyme rise predominantly of alanine transaminase (ALT) and aspartate transaminase (AST) (Fig. 18.2).
- Centrifugal or periportal processes have less effect on synthetic function but disproportionate effects on portal pressure and bile duct excretory function. Disease here tends to cause disproportionate increase in the 'biliary' enzymes alkaline phosphatase and gamma glutamyl transferase (Fig. 18.2).
- Alcoholic liver disease tends to have effects throughout all parts of the lobule and most progressive diseases ultimately will also involve both portal tracts and centrilobular areas.

Hyperbilirubinaemias

Unconjugated hyperbilirubinaemia
Gilbert's syndrome
Incidence and diagnosis
The most common congenital hyperbilirubinaemia affecting 2–5% of the population. It is:
- Usually detected incidentally on routine checks as an isolated, raised bilirubin.
- More commonly manifest in males.

The patient is often asymptomatic, and a positive family history of jaundice may be seen in 5–10% of cases. Serum bilirubin is usually less than 50 μmol/L

(normal <17). Intercurrent illness such as infection tends to elevate bilirubin levels.

Diagnosis can be made on the basis of an increase in unconjugated bilirubin following an overnight fast or during a mild illness. A genetic test is now available to confirm TATA box elongation in Gilbert's syndrome (see below).

Aetiology and pathogenesis
Aetiology of the syndrome involves a reduction in enzyme activity (UDP-glucuronosyl transferase or UGT-1), but many other factors can affect this, hence its variable presentation. UGT-1 is a cytoplasmic enzyme that conjugates bilirubin to allow it to be excreted in a soluble form. Recently, a mutation in the promoter region (TATA box) of the mRNA for this enzyme was described, which reduces the efficiency of transcription of this enzyme. The normal enzyme is present but is less efficient due to reduced synthesis. It is possible that Gilbert's syndrome represents an extreme end of a normal distribution.

Prognosis
This is excellent. It is important to reassure the patient that the condition is not serious and avoid any unnecessary investigations in the future. No treatment is required.

Crigler–Najjar syndrome
This is a more severe unconjugated hyperbilirubinaemia, again due to abnormalities of the UGT-1 enzyme (same as Gilbert's). Here, the mutations are in the translated region of DNA, not just the promoter region, so the enzyme may not be produced at all. Two types have been described, both of which are exceedingly rare conditions:
- Type I (autosomal recessive)—complete absence of glucuronosyl transferase.
- Type II (autosomal dominant)—decreased level of glucuronosyl transferase.

Type I deficiency: presents as neonatal jaundice due to unconjugated bilirubinaemia, usually fatal within the first year of life. Serum bilirubin can rise to 600–800 μmol/L. Death is from kernicterus, possibly due to an immature blood-brain barrier.

Functions of the liver	
Function	**Substrate examples**
Synthetic function	Albumin (half-life 20 days) Transferrin (half-life 3 days) Coagulation factors (all of them)
Storage	Glycogen, triglyceride, iron (ferritin), vitamin A
Metabolic homeostasis	Maintenance blood glucose (glycogenolysis and gluconeogenesis)
Metabolic activation and transformation	Vitamin D, lipoproteins
Metabolic deactivation and detoxification	Sex steroids, ammonia, drugs, alcohol
Excretion	Bilirubin

Fig. 18.1 Functions of the liver.

Type II deficiency—survival into adulthood is not uncommon. Serum bilirubin is usually less than 300 µmol/L. Kernicterus can be prevented by induction of the enzyme with phenobarbitone.

Liver biopsy is normal and transplantation is the only treatment for debilitated patients.

Conjugated hyperbilirubinaemia
Dubin–Johnson syndrome
Incidence and diagnosis
This is a rare and benign disorder that usually presents in adolescence. Plasma bilirubin is conjugated.

A bromsulphthalein (BSP) clearance test in Dubin–Johnson syndrome has a second recirculation peak at 90 minutes (see Chapter 24, liver function tests). Liver biopsy is stained black due to centrilobular melanin deposits.

Aetiology and pathogenesis
The condition is believed to be due to the failure to excrete conjugated bilirubin due to a defect in a transporter protein in the bile canaliculi. The inheritance is autosomal recessive.

Prognosis and treatment
No specific treatment is required and the prognosis is excellent.

Rotor syndrome
Also a benign and probably autosomal dominant condition of conjugated hyperbilirubinaemia. It can

be distinguished from Dubin–Johnson syndrome by a normal liver biopsy. Prognosis is also excellent for this syndrome.

Viral hepatitis

Traditionally, viruses with a predilection to cause hepatitis have come to be classified alphabetically. Currently, at least six different viruses are known to infect humans (A, B, C, D, E, and G). Other viruses such as cytomegalovirus (CMV), Epstein–Barr virus, yellow fever and herpes viruses can also infect the liver.

Hepatitis A
Incidence
This is the most common type of hepatitis worldwide, with the young most frequently afflicted. Epidemics are associated with overcrowding, poor hygiene and sanitation. Transmission is by the faecal–oral route or ingestion of contaminated water or shellfish.

Clinical features
In the prodromal phase:
- Symptoms mimic viral gastroenteritis (nausea, vomiting, diarrhoea, headache, mild fever, malaise and abdominal discomfort).
- A distaste for cigarettes said to be characteristic in young adults who normally smoke them.

The icteric phase occurs after 10–14 days (some patients remain anicteric) and resolves in 2–3 weeks:
- Mild symptoms such as malaise and fatigue may persist for months.
- Liver enlargement is common during the icteric phase; the spleen is palpable in approximately 10%.

Diagnosis and investigation
Diagnosis is usually made on clinical grounds. A definitive diagnosis can be made if there is a rising titre of anti-HAV immunoglobulin (Ig)M and/or demonstration of viral particles in stools by electron microscopy. Elevated anti-HAV IgG titre reflects previous exposure to hepatitis A and thus lifelong immunity. Transaminases are moderately elevated (500–1000 IU/L) but normalize rapidly (Fig. 18.3).

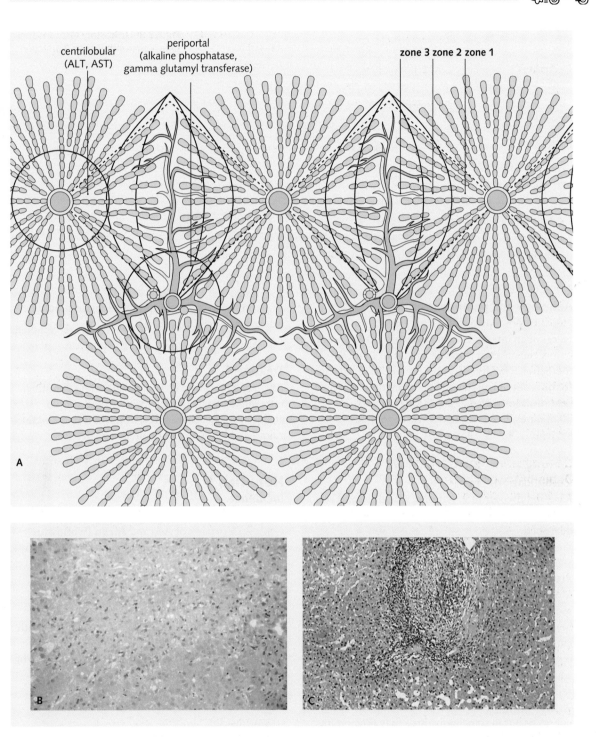

Fig. 18.2 (A) Hepatic lobular architecture showing functional zones and centrilobular or centripetal predilection for pathological processes. Different enzymes predominate in the different zones and their detection in serum may reflect liver damage in those zones. (B) Centrilobular necrosis with inflammation. (C) Inflammation centred on portal tract with early fibrosis.

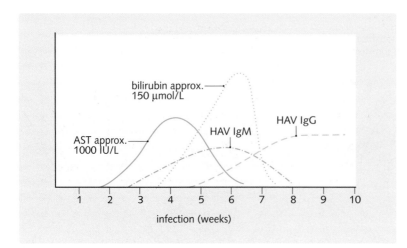

Fig. 18.3 Laboratory tests and their time course in hepatitis A infection.

Aetiology and pathogenesis
Hepatitis A is a pico-RNA-virus excreted in the faeces of an infected person approximately 2 weeks before the onset of jaundice and up to 1 week thereafter. The disease is most infectious just prior to the onset of jaundice. The RNA virus is relatively heat resistant withstanding 60°C for up to 30 minutes, hence it thrives in areas of poor hygiene.

Complications
Rare, but myocarditis, arthritis, vasculitis, and very occasionally, fulminant hepatic failure have been described.

Prognosis
Most patients recover completely without any sequelae; some have a self-limiting relapse of hepatitis. A few have a prolonged cholestatic jaundice (3–4 months) but in general the prognosis is excellent. Often, the course is more prolonged in adults or immunocompromised patients.

Hepatitis A infection does not have a carrier status. Progression to chronic viral disease does not occur but in some individuals may precipitate autoimmune liver disease. Previous infection confers lifetime immunity.

Aims and indication for treatment
Unless the patient is very unwell, hospital admission is unnecessary. Treatment otherwise is supportive.

Vaccination or hyperimmune globulin should be offered to people at high risk.

Treatment
Anti-emetics can be given for nausea and vomiting, intravenous fluids for dehydration, and simple analgesia for headaches. It is important to maintain caloric intake. Alcohol should be avoided.

Hepatitis B
Incidence
Symptomless infected carrier rate 0.1% in UK and USA, 20% in parts of Asia and Africa (worldwide prevalence of carriers estimated at 300–400 million).
Transmission:
- Contaminated blood products (incidence has fallen dramatically since the introduction of screening in UK, Europe, and USA in the late 1970s) and, subsequently, around the world with the WHO vaccination programme.
- Contaminated instrumentation (intravenous drug user, IVDU).
- Sexual intercourse with infected partner.
- Vertical transmission (most common mode worldwide).
- Viral particles have been isolated from insects such as mosquitoes.

Aetiology and pathogenesis
HBV is a DNA virus that replicates in the liver where the core antigen incorporates itself into the host

genome. The host's DNA polymerase then transcribes for the virus and may be the prime factor for the development of hepatocellular carcinoma.

Body fluid contact is essential for transmission. Infection in the birth canal during parturition is the most important mode worldwide, creating a large 'carrier state' reservoir of infection. In developed countries, promiscuous sexual practitioners and IVDUs form the largest reservoir of infection.

Hepatitis B syndromes may be acute, chronic, or the carrier state.

Clinical features

Features of acute hepatitis B include:
- Incubation time: 60–160 days (average 90 days).
- Non-specific prodromal symptoms: arthralgia, anorexia, abdominal discomfort.
- Jaundice, fever, and hepatomegaly are usual features.
- Urticarial or maculopapular rash may appear, together with a polyarthritis thought to be secondary to immune-mediated complexes.
- History of contact with contaminated source is usual (especially travellers to the Orient, drug addicts, accidental injury to health workers, etc.).

Features of chronic hepatitis B include:
- Most chronic carriers are asymptomatic.
- Majority discovered incidentally (e.g. blood donor screening, occupational health checks, routine liver function tests, etc.).
- Patients with chronic active hepatitis may present with features or complications of chronic liver disease, or cirrhosis: jaundice, ascites, portal hypertension, hepatic failure.
- Chronic hepatitis predisposes to cirrhosis of the liver and an increased risk of hepatocellular carcinoma, especially in males.

Investigation and diagnosis

Transaminases may be very high in the acute stage (1000–5000 IU/L) falling rapidly after the first week; chronic hepatitis produces only a mild elevation of ALT or AST.

Serology (Fig. 18.4): surface antigen (HBsAg) is the first serological marker to appear (6 weeks to

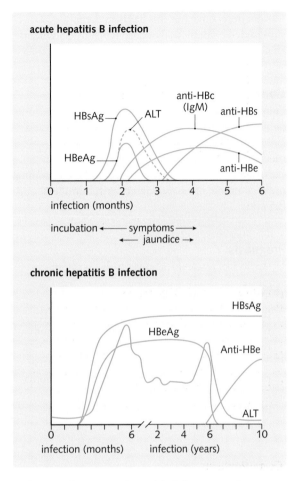

Fig. 18.4 Laboratory tests and their time course in hepatitis B infection. (Redrawn with permission from Kumar PJ, Clarke ML. Clinical Medicine, 3rd edn. London: Baillière Tindall; 1994.)

3 months); 'e' antigen (HBeAg) follows, reflecting viral replication, high infectivity, and more severe disease. This usually disappears before HBsAg, but its persistence correlates with HBV DNA in blood. HBsAg and HBeAg may be present in either acute or chronic HBV infection.

Anti-HBe antibodies appear from approximately 8 weeks after infection and their presence reflects low infectivity. Such seroconversion may occur spontaneously after several decades or with interferon. Anti-HBs antibodies appear late (>3 months) and confer lifelong immunity.

Antibodies to core antigen (HBcAg, IgM) were measured in the past when there was a window period where HBsAg disappeared and anti-HBsAg was not detectable but this has been largely superseded by detection of core DNA by polymerase chain reaction (PCR).

Complications

Fulminant hepatitis and death occurs in 1% of patients. Extra-hepatic complications: arteritis and glomerulonephritis may be immune-complex mediated. Cryoglobulinaemia may also occur. Variation in the viral genome (mutants) are becoming more common; often associated with fulminant hepatitis.

Prognosis

Up to 90% of acute infections resolve without sequelae:

- 5–10% of patients become chronic carriers (carrier rate is much higher following vertical transmission possibly due to immature immune response to the virus in the neonate).
- 5% develop chronic active hepatitis, which may progress to cirrhosis or hepatocellular carcinoma in cirrhotic patients, especially males (25% lifetime risk for hepatocellular carcinoma in cirrhotic males).

Aims of treatment

Acute infection: as in hepatitis A infection, symptomatic relief is all that is required with extra precautions taken when handling body fluids. Fulminant hepatitis carries a grave prognosis, requires intensive care and potentially liver transplantation. Chronic hepatitis can be treated with alpha-interferon to seroconvert from HBeAb negative to HBeAb positive. The success rate is variable, especially in cases of vertical transmission. Nucleoside analogues, which suppress viral replication, are an alternative treatment.

Vaccination is successful in preventing transmission. When combined with immunoglobulin at birth, this successfully prevents vertical transmission. Hyperimmune globulin or lamivudine, a nucleoside reverse transcriptase inhibitor, are used to prevent recurrence after transplantation.

Indication for treatment

Patients who are HBeAg positive and HBeAb negative have raised liver transaminases and evidence

Poor prognostic factors in hepatitis B and C	
Hepatitis B	**Hepatitis C**
Possibly duration of infection; age >40 years	Age at acquisition: older fare worse
Any signs, e.g. spider naevi, ascites	Viral inoculation or load may have a role; genotype 1b seem to fare less well
Activity on liver biopsy, especially if cirrhotic	Bridging fibrosis or cirrhosis on liver biopsy
Males fare worse than females	Males fare worse than females
Concomitant disease	Possibly higher iron stores and alcohol intake cause synergistic damage
Development of hepatocellular carcinoma, especially in males	Development of hepatocellular carcinoma, especially in males

Fig. 18.5 Poor prognostic factors in hepatitis B and C.

of chronic active hepatitis on liver biopsy and should be offered interferon treatment (Fig. 18.5).

Treatment plan

Subcutaneous injection of interferon alpha (5–10 mega units three times weekly) are used. Dose and duration of treatment are dependent on the patient's tolerance of side effects (an influenza-like syndrome and headaches). However, its use is also limited by a response rate of less than 50% and relapse occurs frequently. If there is no sign of improvement after a few months of therapy, then it tends to be discontinued. Interferon alpha should not be given to those who are immunosuppressed or patients with decompensated liver disease. Lamivudine has now been licensed for the treatment of chronic hepatitis B and other nucleoside analogues are emerging as effective treatment options.

All pregnant hepatitis B virus mothers should plan for vaccination of newborn at parturition. Vaccination should also be offered to other people at risk, such as IVDUs, health care personnel, and travellers to high-risk areas.

Hepatitis C
Incidence

Previously known as non-A, non-B hepatitis and now thought to be responsible for up to 90% of such cases. The hepatitis C virus was identified in 1988 and routine screening of blood products has been available only since 1991.

Transmission:
- Contaminated blood products.
- Contaminated instrumentation (IVDU).
- Sexual, vertical, or breast milk transmission is uncommon (less than 5%).

Clinical features
Features include:
- Clinical jaundice occurs in less than 20% of patients.
- Fatigue and malaise are common.
- Extra-hepatic manifestations such as arthritis, cryoglobulinaemia, and aplastic anaemia are rare.

A minority of patients with cirrhosis may have its attendant potential complications of portal hypertension, hepatic failure, or hepatoma.

Diagnosis
Most commonly, patients are referred for investigation of abnormal liver enzymes found incidentally or are referred by the blood transfusion service when they are discovered to be antibody positive:
- Transaminases are usually only slightly elevated (ALT 50–150 IU/L).
- Bilirubin and synthetic functions are usually normal.
- Ferritin may be elevated.
- Antibodies to hepatitis C are found in the serum using enzyme-linked immunosorbent assay or radioimmunoassay kits.
- Viral RNA is detectable by reverse transcription-polymerase chain reaction (RT-PCR); a positive result confirms current viraemia.
- Liver histology can demonstrate a spectrum of change, from fatty infiltration through lobular hepatitis to cirrhosis. These changes correlate poorly to liver enzyme derangement.

Aetiology and pathogenesis
Hepatitis C is a single-stranded RNA virus with several immunogenic subtypes, hence allowing epidemiological studies to establish modes of transmission.

Complications and prognosis
- 70% develop chronic indolent hepatitis of varying severity.
- 20% progress to cirrhosis.

Advanced age at infection, male gender, and high viral load predict a more rapid progression (Fig. 18.5). Progression is also much more rapid in the presence of coinfection with HIV. Fulminant hepatitis is a rare but fatal complication.

Aims of treatment
To reduce the level of viral replication in the liver and thus liver damage and cirrhosis. Interferon alpha can produce a viral remission in about 20% of cases. Recent evidence suggests that polyethylene glycol-conjugated 'pegylated' Interferon achieves a higher response. Pegylation prolongs the half-life of the interferon in the blood. Combination with Ribavirin (an antiviral drug that inhibits a wide range of DNA and RNA viruses) approximately doubles the response of interferon.

Indications for treatment
Most criteria are based on severity of inflammation and presence of fibrosis on liver biopsy. Hepatitis C virus antibody positivity and RT-PCR positive are prerequisites. There is some evidence that selection by certain criteria improves response rate (e.g. young age or low body weight, females, low iron indices). The National Institute for Clinical Excellence (NICE) recommends that the combination of interferon alpha (IFN-α) and ribavirin should be used for those with moderate to severe hepatitis C (preferably determined on histological grounds), including those who have previously responded to IFN alpha alone and then relapsed.

Treatment plan
The patient should be counselled regarding modes of transmission and advised against excess alcohol consumption, which appears to accelerate progression of the disease.

Alpha-interferon monotherapy (3–6 mega units for 3–6 months) achieves a biochemical response (normalization of ALT) in approximately two-thirds of patients but a clearance of virus detectable by RT-PCR in less than 50%. Treatment is continued for

6–12 months in PCR responders, but response is sustained in only about half of those treated. Ideally, combination therapy with ribavirin should be employed (where indicated) as the response rate is approximately double that of interferon alone. Combination therapy should be continued for 6 months; longer courses are sometimes given depending on viral genotype and clearance of circulating viral RNA. Currently, there is no vaccine for hepatitis C.

Hepatitis D
Incidence
Also known as the delta virus, it is an incomplete RNA particle which is unable to replicate by itself. It occurs as a coinfection with the hepatitis B virus and is particularly seen in IV drug abusers, but can affect any patient with hepatitis B.

Diagnosis
Coinfection is indistinguishable from acute hepatitis B infection, but occasionally superinfection produces an active flare-up of hepatitis with a rise of liver transaminases. Clinical jaundice may not be obvious.

   Presence of IgM anti-delta virus with IgM anti-HBcAg confirms coinfection and IgM anti-delta is replaced by IgG anti-delta over 6–8 weeks. IgM anti-delta in presence of IgG anti-HBcAg indicates superinfection because IgM anti-HBcAg is replaced by IgG antibodies after the initial infection. Hepatitis D RNA can be measured in the serum and liver, and is seen in both acute and chronic infection.

Aetiology and pathogenesis
The incomplete RNA particle is enclosed within HBsAg, suggesting that it is unable to replicate by itself but is activated in the presence of hepatitis B infection.

Complications
Fulminant hepatitis is a serious complication and is more common after coinfection. Chronic infection with hepatitis D is usually the case in the form of cirrhosis.

Aims of treatment
Supportive for fulminant hepatitis. Reduction of viral replication with interferon to reduce the risk of developing cirrhosis.

Indications for treatment
Chronic active hepatitis as demonstrated on liver enzymes and biopsy.

Treatment plan
As for other chronic viral hepatitis with interferon alpha, where it can induce remission but as with hepatitis C infection, relapse is common on withdrawal of treatment.

Hepatitis E
In summary of hepatitis E:
- An RNA virus spread via the faecal–oral route.
- Predominantly seen in developing countries.
- Mortality rises from 1% to 20% in pregnant women; the reason is still at present unclear.
- Hepatitis E RNA can be detected in serum or stool by PCR.
- Treatment, as for hepatitis A, is purely symptomatic.
- There is no carrier state, and no progression to chronic active hepatitis.
- Improved sanitation and hygiene are essential for prevention and control.

A summary of hepatitis viruses is shown in Fig. 18.6.

Hepatitis G
Hepatitis G (also called GB-C) has recently been identified and has some sequence homology with hepatitis C. It has been found in about 2% of blood donors who have been screened, but there is no routine screening test available. It is thought not to cause acute or chronic hepatitis and its precise clinical relevance is still not clear.

Epstein–Barr virus (EBV) (infectious mononucleosis)
Incidence and diagnosis
A common disease of the young, although it can occur at any age.

   Fever, malaise, tonsillar, and glandular enlargement are typical; mild jaundice associated with abnormal liver function tests is common. Rash can occur, particularly if the patient is given ampicillin (this does not imply future ampicillin allergy).

Hepatitis viruses				
Type	Spread	Incubation	Prevention	Treatment
A	Faecal–oral	2–6 weeks	Immunoglobulin or vaccine	Not specific
B	Contaminated body fluid: vertical, blood, semen	2–6 months	Hepatitis B immunoglobulin or vaccine	Alpha-interferon Lamivudine
C	Contaminated blood	6–8 weeks	None available	Alpha-interferon Ribavirin
D	Contaminated blood Requires hepatitis B	Unknown	Prevention of hepatitis B	None
E	Faecal–oral	2–9 weeks	Improve hygiene	None

Fig. 18.6 Summary of hepatitis viruses.

Heterophile antibodies (Paul–Bunnell or Monospot) can be detected early and disappear after 3 months. They agglutinate sheep red blood cells but do not react with EBV or its antigens. False positive Monospot tests can occasionally occur in other viral illness, lymphomas, or SLE. A rise in specific IgM antibodies to EBV is diagnostic of infectious mononucleosis. In addition, atypical, reactive lymphocytes can be seen on a peripheral blood film.

Aetiology and pathogenesis
Usually transmitted via saliva ('kissing disease') with an incubation time of 4–5 weeks.

Large mononuclear cells are seen to infiltrate the portal tracts but liver architecture is preserved.

Complications and prognosis
Hepatitis due to EBV carries an excellent prognosis, with a majority of patients retaining normal liver function. Splenomegaly and haemolytic anaemia can also occur.

Cytomegalovirus (CMV)
Predominantly in immunosuppressed patients: causes a hepatitis occasionally with fatal consequences.
- CMV may be detected in urine but isolation and growth is slow.

- The most sensitive test is to detect CMV antigen in buffy coat of ethylenediaminetetracetic acid peripheral blood. PCR technology can also be employed.
- A rising IgM titre to CMV can also be seen to aid diagnosis of acute infection.
- Liver biopsy shows intracytoplasmic inclusion bodies and giant cells.

Other infections involving the liver

Toxoplasmosis
Rare in the UK. Clinical features in an adult are often indistinguishable from infectious mononucleosis caused by EBV (negative Monospot test).

A congenital form of the infection can occur if a mother is infected during pregnancy.

Clinical features
Most infections are asymptomatic. Lymphadenopathy associated with a febrile illness is the most common form of presentation.

Maculopapular rash, hepatosplenomegaly, and reactive lymphocytes may be seen together with a biochemical rise in serum transaminases with or without clinical hepatitis. Rarely, chorioretinitis, myocarditis or encephalitis can occur, but this is more commonly observed in the immunocompromised.

Diagnosis

Rising IgM titres are diagnostic (although unreliable if HIV positive). The organism can also be isolated by injecting tissues (e.g. bone marrow or cerebrospinal fluid, CSF, from the patient) into the peritoneum of mice and peritoneal fluid examined 7–10 days later.

Aetiology and pathogenesis

Caused by *Toxoplasma gondii*, an intracellular protozoan that requires an animal host, such as cats or sheep, in addition to the intermediate human host. Infection is caused by ingestion of cysts via food contaminated by faeces of animal host.

Treatment

No treatment is required in mild cases because it is a self-limiting disease in people with normal immune systems.

Pyrimethamine and sulfadiazine can be given for severe cases and the patient should be treated for up to 1 month. Spiramycin can be given as an alternative to pyrimethamine during pregnancy (due to its teratogenic effects).

Strict hygiene when animal handling is essential for prevention of the disease.

Leptospirosis

This zoonosis is caused by the Gram-negative organism Leptospira interrogans, of which there are more than 200 serotypes. It is often referred to as Weil's disease, but this eponym should be limited to those with severe disease manifesting as jaundice, haemorrhage and renal failure.

Clinical features

Acute systemic infection (i.e. fever, arthralgia, headache, anorexia).

Jaundice, hepatomegaly, renal failure, skin rash, and haemolytic anaemia occur in 10–15% of cases.

Diagnosis and investigations

The rise in liver transaminases may be small. Blood, CSF, and urine cultures can isolate the organism. A complement fixation test can be employed and specific rising titres of IgM antibody are diagnostic.

Aetiology and pathogenesis

Majority of cases are due to the serotype *Leptospira icterohaemorrhagiae*, excreted by rats in their urine. Other Leptospira species are found in the urine of cattle, dogs, and pigs.

They gain access via abrasions in the skin or mucous membrane, and those particularly at risk are sewer workers, pot holers, and people who participate in watersports.

Complications

Renal and hepatic failure is seen in severe cases. Meningitis and myocarditis occur rarely.

Prognosis

Mortality can be as high as 20%, especially in elderly people.

Treatment

Penicillin is an effective antibiotic. Alternatively, erythromycin and tetracycline can be used. Doxycycline is useful prophylaxis for high-risk groups.

Brucellosis
Incidence

Extremely rare in UK. More commonly found in countries where raw unpasteurized milk is consumed. Must be considered in people with prolonged fever of an unknown cause.

Clinical features

The symptoms of an acute infection are often non-specific and insidious:

- Fever.
- Arthralgia.
- Weight loss.
- Headache.
- Night sweats.

Hepatomegaly and lymphadenopathy are commonly seen.

In chronic infection, the symptoms may persist for several months with bouts of fever and splenomegaly. Chronic derangements of liver biochemistry may be seen.

Diagnosis and investigations

Investigations to consider:

- Blood cultures are positive during acute infections in approximately half of patients. Rising titres are diagnostic.
- Liver biopsy may reveal presence of granulomas, but these are non-specific for brucellosis.

Aetiology and pathogenesis

A zoonosis due to a coccobacillus largely spread by ingestion of unpasteurized milk. Three species are recognized: *Brucella abortus* (cattle), *Brucella melitensis* (goats and sheep) and *Brucella suis* (pigs).

The organism travels via the lymphatics and infect lymph nodes and reticuloendothelial systems. Hypersensitivity may account for the formation of granulomas.

Treatment

A prolonged course of tetracycline and rifampicin is given. Alternatively, co-trimoxazole can be used.

Metabolic and genetic liver disease

In general, the following conditions often progress to chronic liver disease, but are considered separately here.

Haemochromatosis
Incidence

An autosomal recessive disorder due to excess iron accumulation affecting approximately 0.5% of the Caucasian population, with a heterozygote frequency of up to 10%.

Clinical features

Features are dependent on gender, dietary intake, age, and associated toxins (e.g. alcohol) (Fig. 18.7). Men tend to present up to a decade earlier due to the protective mechanism of menstrual blood loss in women. In developing countries, iron deficiency and hookworm infestation can result in later manifestation of organ damage.

Patients may rarely present between the fourth and fifth decade with the classic triad of
- Skin pigmentation (melanin deposition).
- Diabetes mellitus ('bronze diabetes').
- Hepatomegaly if the iron deposition is severe.

Other common presentations include gonadal atrophy and loss of libido secondary to pituitary dysfunction, cardiac failure, arthritis in small joints of the hand and chondrocalcinosis in the knees.

Diagnosis and investigation

Investigations include:
- Serum iron—usually elevated with a low total iron binding capacity.

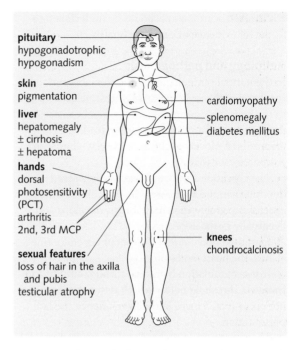

Fig. 18.7 Body map for haemochromatosis. (MCP, metacarpophalangeal joint; PCT, porphyria cutanea tarda.)

- Transferrin saturation—grossly elevated (often 100%; normal <50%) but levels can also be moderately raised in heterozygotes.
- Serum ferritin—usually grossly elevated (>1000 µg/L; normal <300 males, <200 females). Ferritin can also be elevated in rheumatoid or other inflammatory diseases or in alcoholic liver disease, as it is an acute-phase protein. This occasionally causes confusion (see below).
- Liver biopsy is the definitive diagnostic test and also provides an assessment of the extent of liver damage. Increased parenchymal iron deposition is also seen in alcoholic cirrhosis. Iron is demonstrated by Perl's potassium cyanide stain producing a Prussian Blue appearance if haemosiderin iron is present. Iron deposition is graded I–IV depending on degree and distribution. Grades III and IV are usually diagnostic of haemochromatosis. A hepatic iron index of >1.9 (mg iron per mg dry weight liver divided by the patient's age in years) is also diagnostic and is useful for differentiating genetic haemochromatosis from iron loading in alcoholic liver disease.
- Fasting blood glucose should be taken to exclude secondary diabetes mellitus.

131

- An electrocardiogram should be undertaken to detect evidence of cardiomyopathy.

Aetiology and pathogenesis

In the normal physiological state, iron absorption is regulated in the proximal small intestine according to the body's requirements. In haemochromatosis, the regulatory mechanism is faulty, leading to inappropriate levels of absorption even when iron stores are excessive.

The condition is characterized by increased deposition in the liver parenchymal cells in which extensive pigmentation and fibrosis develops and eventually cirrhosis occurs.

Increased iron content also occurs in endocrine glands, the heart, and skin.

Iron accumulation is gradual throughout life and there is a threshold below which tissue damage may not occur (e.g. 5 mg/g in the liver), hence the late presentation.

There is an association with HLA-A3, B14, and B7 groups. Recently, a mutation (C282Y) in a gene (HFE) has been identified on chromosome 6 and is responsible for almost all primary haemochromatosis.

Complications

If untreated, cirrhosis is a common end-point followed by liver failure, which may be accompanied by portal hypertension.

Up to one third of male patients who have cirrhosis may develop hepatocellular carcinoma (Fig. 18.8).

Treating patients reverses the tissue damage and improves the survival rate. However, the risk of malignant change may persist if cirrhosis is already present.

It is imperative to screen first degree relatives for the condition before the development of irreversible liver damage. This can be achieved by checking serum ferritin levels or by attempting to identify the culpable gene. Genetic testing is more useful in first degree relatives to predict risk even if ferritin is normal. Genetic testing for other subgroups has not been widely adopted because, although the condition tends to run 'true' in families, the phenotypic expression of the homozygous state in the wider population is variable (i.e. only a proportion of people homozygous for the mutation will develop iron overload). Biochemical testing with serum ferritin or transferrin saturation is more usually employed for screening the population.

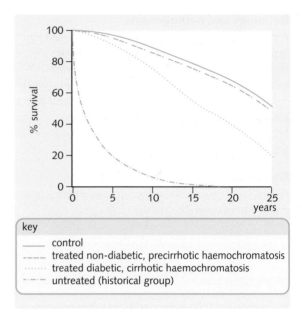

Fig. 18.8 Survival with iron overload depends on the development of complications. Even so, depletion of iron stores prolongs survival. Life expectancy is normal if treatment is started before the onset of end-organ damage.

Aims and indications for treatment

To reduce body iron stores (reflected by serum ferritin) to within normal levels and limit the progression of liver damage and other affected organs, in all patients who have a positive diagnosis of haemochromatosis.

Treatment plan

This should consist of:

- Venesection—a unit of blood (450 ml) contains approximately 250 mg iron. Weekly venesection is required for 6–12 months to remove the 20–40 g excess iron present. Regular removal of 2–3 units of blood per year thereafter maintains ferritin levels within normal limits.
- Chelating agents (e.g. desferrioxamine) can be used for patients who cannot tolerate venesection. Ascorbic acid supplements should be avoided by these patients as it enhances iron absorption.

Wilson's disease (hepatolenticular degeneration)
Incidence

A rare inborn error of copper metabolism affecting approximately 3 out of 100 000 people with pockets of higher prevalence in Northern India and Sicily.

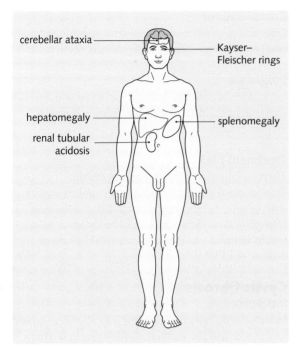

Fig. 18.9 Body map for Wilson's disease.

Clinical features
These include:
- Signs of chronic liver disease with neurological manifestation of basal ganglia damage (i.e. tremor, dysarthria, choreo-athetosis, and eventually dementia).
- Kayser–Fleischer copper brown ring in Descemet's membrane in the cornea (often requires slit lamp to see).
- Renal tubular damage giving rise to renal tubular acidosis and renal failure if severe.
- Haemolytic anaemia and osteoporosis in rare cases (Fig. 18.9).

Diagnosis and investigation
Serum copper and caeruloplasmin are usually low or normal. Urinary copper is grossly elevated in 24-hour collection (>10 times the normal range).

A definitive diagnosis depends on a liver biopsy and the amount of copper deposition, although elevated copper levels in the liver are found in chronic cholestasis.

Aetiology and pathogenesis
The condition is due to an autosomal recessive gene located on chromosome 13. There are at least 30 mutations described resulting in a faulty transporter protein (ATP7B) which excretes copper from the liver via the Golgi complex. Export of copper stimulates caeruloplasmin synthesis; hence, the explanation for its low levels in Wilson's disease.

Complications
These may include:
- Cirrhosis, with ensuing liver failure if left untreated.
- Neurological manifestations can be severe and disabling.
- Metabolic consequences of renal tubular acidosis and potentially renal failure.

Prognosis
Early diagnosis and treatment can lessen the risk of mortality and morbidity considerably but, once neurological features are established, these are often irreversible.

Aims and indications for treatment
All patients with Wilson's disease are treated in order to reduce copper deposition and to avoid life-threatening complications.

Treatment plan
Lifelong oral intake of penicillamine is an effective treatment, but serious side effects can occur, limiting its usage. Blood disorders including thrombocytopaenia, agranulocytosis and aplastic anaemia can occur. Proteinuria, associated with immune complex nephritis, occurs in up to a third of patients, but may resolve despite continuation of treatment. Full blood count and urine testing for blood and protein should be undertaken frequently, particularly after initiation of treatment. Urine copper levels should be monitored. All first degree relatives should be screened for early treatment.

Penicillamine and trientene (triethylamine) are copper chelating agents that have been shown to be effective. They increase urinary copper excretion, but do not completely 'decopper' the liver, instead causing the copper to be associated with metallothionein protein. Zinc treatment is also effective in reducing copper absorption and increasing metallothionein synthesis.

Alpha-1-antitrypsin deficiency
Incidence
Inherited as a rare autosomal recessive disorder. Alpha-1-antitrypsin is a protease inhibitor produced

Alpha-1-antitrypsin deficiency	
PiMM	Normal phenotype
PiMZ	Heterozygous for alpha-1-antitrypsin deficiency (variable type)
PiSZ	Heterozygous for alpha-1-antitrypsin deficiency
PiZZ	Homozygous for alpha-1-antitrypsin deficiency (severe type)

Fig. 18.10 Variants in alpha-1-antitrypsin deficiency. (Pi, protease inhibitor.)

in the liver that mediates various inflammatory processes.

Clinical features
These include:
- Late-onset liver cirrhosis (>50 years).
- Early-onset of pulmonary basal emphysema (5% of homozygotes by 40 years).

Diagnosis and investigations
Investigation of use:
- Low serum alpha-1-antitrypsin level (alpha-1 AT).
- Liver biopsy—changes of cirrhosis with periodic acid–Schiff positive staining globules within hepatocytes.
- Genotype—depending on the amino acid mutation various levels of severity of the disease can occur (i.e. ZZ have the worse prognosis) (Fig. 18.10).
- Chest radiograph and pulmonary function tests to identify evidence of emphysema.

Aetiology and pathogenesis
The gene responsible is located on chromsome 14. The variant of alpha-1 AT is characterized by position on a electrophoretic strip (i.e. M, medium; S, slow; and Z, very slow).
- Normal genotype is MM. S and Z variants are due to a single polypeptide mutation, resulting in reduced synthesis and secretion of normal alpha-1 AT. S produces approximately 60% of activity produced by M, and Z only 15%.
- Clinical phenotypes can be homozygous (e.g. ZZ) or compound heterozygous (e.g. MZ, MS, SZ).

Complications
Liver and respiratory failure due to cirrhosis and basal emphysema, respectively, usually occurs.

Prognosis
Up to 15% of patients with ZZ genotype will develop cirrhosis by the fifth decade and 5% will develop emphysema by the fourth decade.

Treatment plan
There are no specific treatments available. Treatments for chronic liver disease apply. Patients with hepatic failure should be considered for liver transplantation. Smoking should be stopped, as it results in up to a four-fold increase in the rate of decline of FEV1.

Cystic fibrosis
Incidence
More patients are now surviving into adolescence and adulthood, and the incidence of liver complications has risen. Up to 10% of patients may have established cirrhosis by their mid-20s.

Clinical features
Newborn infants may present with obstructive jaundice in the first few weeks of life due to the accumulation of viscous secretions in a similar fashion to meconium ileus. Recovery is usual within 6 months, but some will die of hepatic failure in infancy.

In those who survive, symptomatic liver disease can be seen up to 15% of adolescents.

Aetiology and pathogenesis
Thought to be due to obstruction of the biliary tree by mucus plugs, but the lesions can be patchy and can be missed on liver biopsy. Liver cirrhosis occurs in most cases in those with hepatic involvement.

Portal hypertension and splenomegaly may occur as a consequence of liver cirrhosis.

Prognosis
It is now recognized that the underlying liver disease is a significant prognostic factor for overall survival in cystic fibrosis. Patients with marked liver impairment have a worse outcome which may influence the timing of transplantation.

Treatment
Treatment of cirrhosis is the same regardless of the underlying aetiology. Patients who are suitable may

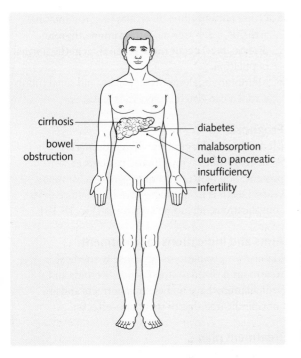

Fig. 18.11 Body map of extrarespiratory manifestations of cystic fibrosis.

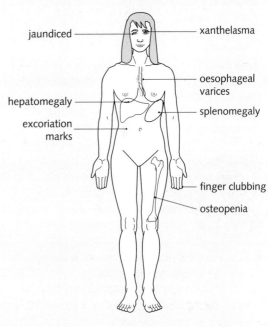

Fig. 18.12 Body map of primary biliary cirrhosis.

be considered for heart–lung–liver transplant which will significantly improve their outcome (Fig. 18.11).

Chronic liver disease

This section deals predominantly with chronic liver disease with an autoimmune basis. Other causes of chronic liver disease are discussed under each relevant section.

Primary biliary cirrhosis (PBC)
Incidence
Predominantly affects women with a female to male ratio of 10:1, presenting commonly between fourth and sixth decades.

Clinical features
These are:
- Pruritus, which often precedes jaundice; hepatosplenomegaly and signs of chronic liver disease are late features.
- Jaundice is cholestatic with dark urine and pale stools.

- Asymptomatic patients often present with an elevated level of alkaline phosphatase or with associated autoimmune disease.
- Xanthomas and other deposits of cholesterol may be seen.
- Metabolic bone disease may develop due to reduced absorption of fat soluble vitamin D (Fig. 18.12).

Diagnosis and investigation
Investigations to undertake:
- Liver tests—high levels of alkaline phosphatase initially, with derangement of other enzymes when cirrhosis occurs. Synthetic function, reflected by albumin and prothrombin time, is preserved until late in the course of the disease. A rising bilirubin heralds progression to the last stage of disease and is a useful prognostic indicator. Liver transplant is considered when the serum bilirubin reaches 100 µmol/L, although this is a fairly arbitrary figure.
- Autoantibodies—antimitochondrial antibodies (M$_2$ subtype) are detected in over 95% of cases. Lower titres of smooth muscle antibody and

antinuclear factor are often also present. IgM is generally raised.

- Elevated serum cholesterol is seen as a result of cholestasis.
- Liver biopsy—there is a characteristic picture of lymphocytic infiltration around the portal tract, together with plasma cells and occasionally granulomas, resulting in bile duct fibrosis, progressing to cirrhosis (see p. 142).

Consider the diagnosis of primary biliary cirrhosis if an elevated alkaline phosphatase (with or without gamma-glutamyl transferase) is seen in middle-aged or elderly women, with no discernible explanation, even if asymptomatic.

Aetiology and pathogenesis

The aetiology is unknown, but PBC is considered to be an autoimmune disease and is associated with other autoimmune phenomena such as hypothyroidism and sicca syndrome (xerostomia and xerophthalmia). Antimitochondrial antibodies (AMA) especially to M_2 antigen, are found in the majority of cases, but the level of titre does not correlate to the clinical or pathological picture; hence, it may play no part in the pathogenesis of the disease despite being a very specific marker.

The antigen appears to be the E_2 component of the pyruvate dehydrogenase enzyme complex on the inner mitochondrial membrane. It is unclear how this intracellular, seemingly inaccessible, antigen could be involved in the pathogenesis of PBC. It is thought that the antibodies may represent some form of cross reactivity with a bacterial antigen. Sensitized T-cells may account for the damage seen because patients with PBC have impaired cell-mediated responses and the reduction in T suppressor cells may allow cytotoxic T-cells to cause ductule damage.

High levels of IgM may be due to a defect in B cells to convert from secretion of IgM to IgG.

Complications

Complications include:
- Cirrhosis and hepatic failure eventually developing in most cases.

- Other autoimmune disorders (e.g. rheumatoid arthritis, scleroderma, autoimmune thyroid disease, etc.) occur more often than in the normal population.
- Membranous glomerulonephritis and renal tubular acidosis can also be associated features.

Prognosis

Median survival from time of symptoms is 8–12 years, but asymptomatic patients at presentation may not seem to progress for many years. Death is from progressive liver failure or its complications, including hepatoma (Fig. 18.13).

Aims and indications for treatment

Mainly symptomatic, as response to medical treatment is often disappointing. Steroids and penicillamine have no beneficial effects and are contraindicated due to their side-effects.

Treatment plan

Treatment should include the following:
- Ursodeoxycholic acid has been shown to benefit some patients with an improvement in biochemical and histology profiles. Ciclosporin, azathioprine, and colchicine have also been shown to have some effect but are not used routinely due to their side-effects.
- Pruritus is difficult to treat: colestyramine reduces bile salt absorption in the enterohepatic cycle and may be helpful.
- Fat-soluble vitamins (i.e. A, D, and K) are given to correct deficiencies.
- Liver transplant is indicated in severe disease.

Treatment of hyperlipidaemia is not usually required.

Primary sclerosing cholangitis (PSC)
Incidence

A rare condition in which over 60% of cases are associated with inflammatory bowel disease (patients may have no bowel symptoms and the diagnosis is made subsequently on histology or barium enema). Approximately 10% patients with ulcerative colitis may have overt or subtle evidence of PSC. More commonly presents in males (3:1).

Clinical features

These include:
- Symptoms referable to inflammatory bowel disease, particularly ulcerative colitis.

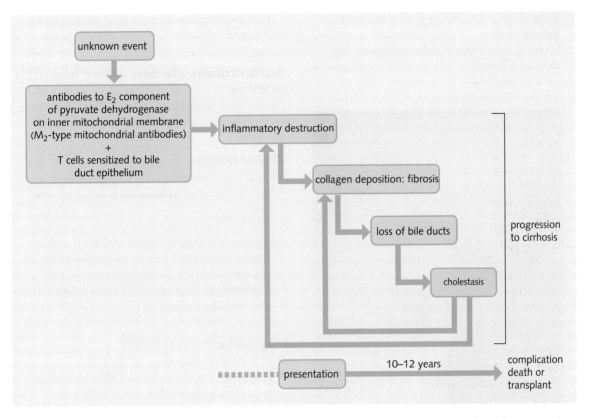

Fig. 18.13 Pathogenic mechanisms and progression in primary biliary cirrhosis.

- Abdominal pain and jaundice with or without pruritis.
- Cirrhosis and its complication in late stages.
- Asymptomatic.

Diagnosis and investigation
Investigations to consider include:
- Liver biochemistry—high alkaline phosphatase with or without hyperbilirubinaemia.
- Liver biopsy—a progressive fibrous obliterating cholangitis is seen. Polymorph infiltration of bile ducts is characteristic.
- Endoscopic retrograde cholangiopancreatography— a characteristic 'bead-like' appearance can be seen due to multiple strictures throughout bile ducts (Fig. 18.14).

Aetiology and pathogenesis
Putatively an autoimmune phenomenon, but the exact mechanism is unknown. Certain HLA types are associated with a worse outcome.

Some patients with AIDS appear to have a similar sclerosing cholangitis which may have an infective aetiology, possibly *Cryptosporidium* infection.

Complications
Are those of cirrhosis and liver failure in addition to those associated with inflammatory bowel disease.

Up to 30% patients may develop cholangiocarcinoma in the long term.

Prognosis
Often runs a benign course with an exception in a few cases where hepatic failure can be rapid.

Indications for treatment
These are:
- Ursodeoxycholic acid improves the biochemical profile and may ameliorate secondary bile salt damage. Otherwise, treatment is mainly symptomatic. Steroids and azathioprine are of limited use.

Liver

- Isolated strictures, if present, can be stented or balloon-dilated.
- Liver transplantation is indicated in late stage disease. A Roux loop biliary-enteric anastomosis is necessary because the patient's own bile duct is diseased.

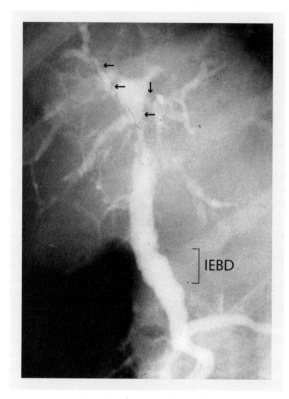

Fig. 18.14 Endoscopic retrograde cholangiopancreatography showing typical beading, irregular ducts in primary sclerosing cholangitis, and intra-hepatic strictures (arrows). (IEBD, irregular extra-hepatic bile duct.)

Autoimmune chronic active hepatitis
Incidence
Occurs more commonly in young women (<25 years) and occasionally in middle age (50–60 years).

Clinical features
The following modes of presentation are seen:
- Presents as an acute hepatitis in one quarter of cases.
- May be asymptomatic for years and present as chronic liver disease with or without jaundice.
- Features associated with an autoimmune disease (e.g. arthritis, rash, fever, malaise).
- Cirrhosis and its potential for complications in long-standing cases.

Diagnosis and investigation
Tests to consider include:
- Liver biochemistry—elevated bilirubin and ALT; increased globulins, particularly IgG; derangement of clotting factors and hypoalbuminaemia.
- Full blood count—normocytic normochromic anaemia, thrombocytopaenia, leucopaenia (changes also consistent with systemic lupus erythematosus).
- Liver biopsy—piecemeal necrosis of chronic active hepatitis.
- Autoantibodies—positive anti smooth muscle antibodies (present in 60%) (Fig. 18.15).

Interpretation of autoantibody tests in liver disease					
Antibody	Inference	ALT, AST elevation	Alk Phos, GGT elevation	Raised immunoglobulins	Diagnostic test
AMA	PBC	Slight	Moderate	Mainly IgM, some IgG	AMA-M$_2$ subtype, liver biopsy
SMA, ANF, LKM	AICAH	Moderate	Slight	Mainly IgG	Liver biopsy
pANCA	PSC	Slight	Moderate	Some IgG	ERCP

Fig. 18.15 Comparison of antibody profiles in autoimmune liver disease. (AICAH, autoimmune chronic active hepatitis; ALT, alanine transaminase; Alk Phos, alkaline phosphatase; AMA, antimitochondrial antibody; ANF, antinuclear antibody; AST, aspartate transaminase; GGT, gamma-glutamyl transferase; LKM, liver kidney microsomal antibody; pANCA, antineutrophil cytoplasmic antibody; PBC, primary biliary cirrhosis; PSC, primary sclerosing cholangitis; SMA, smooth muscle antibody.)

138

Aetiology and pathogenesis

Unknown cause. Thought to be immune-mediated because there are abnormalities in T suppressor cells which may result from autoantibody production against hepatocyte antigens. A polyclonal elevation of IgG suggests defects in humoral response.

Association with other autoimmune disease (e.g. pernicious anaemia, systemic lupus erythematosus, thyroid disease, etc.) suggests cell-mediated response to own tissues. Lupus erythematosus cells (LE) are found in a number of liver biopsies, hence the old term 'lupoid hepatitis' but this confusing term should be avoided.

A number of drugs (e.g. methyldopa, ketoconazole, isoniazid) may cause a chronic hepatitis similar to the autoimmune variety and in some cases are related to acetylation of the drug by the liver. Autosomal genes influences a person's acetylator status, with the 'rapid' allele being dominant to the 'slow' allele. Homozygotes for the 'slow' allele have lower levels of the enzyme N-acetyltransferase in the liver. 'Slow' acetylators are at an increased risk of developing chronic active hepatitis compared with 'fast' acetylators.

Complications

Cirrhosis and liver failure. Patients are also more likely to develop other organ-specific autoimmune diseases.

Prognosis

A pattern of remission and exacerbation for several years followed by cirrhosis is characteristic. Half will die within 5 years if no treatment is given, compared with a 90% survival rate with treatment.

Aims and indications for treatment

Early diagnosis and prompt treatment is paramount in order to lessen the risk of mortality and morbidity.

Treatment plan

Corticosteroids to induce biochemical and histological remission, with subsequent addition of azathioprine (an antiproliferative immunosuppressant) as a steroid-sparing agent is the adopted treatment strategy.

Sarcoidosis and liver

Sarcoidosis is a chronic, multisystem disease characterized by the presence of non-caseating granulomas which predominantly affect the lung, lymph nodes, and the skin, but the liver is also rarely affected. Cardiac, renal and neurological manifestations are also seen.

The underlying aetiology is unknown and the majority of cases present as an incidental finding of bilateral hilar lymphadenopathy.

It is a rare cause of hepatosplenomegaly, by producing portal hypertension either as a direct consequence of the granulomas compressing the portal venules or periportal scarring resulting in obstruction.

In cases of difficulty in diagnosing systemic sarcoidosis, a liver biopsy may be diagnostic especially in the presence of abnormal liver enzymes. Serum angiotensin-converting enzyme is often elevated, but not diagnostic, and more useful in monitoring disease activity. A Kveim skin test (still rarely performed by dermatologists) is positive.

Hepatic complications are those of portal hypertension with or without decompensated liver disease.

Treatment is with systemic steroids to induce remission of the disease. Methotrexate and azathioprine are sometimes used as steroid-sparing agents for protracted therapy or refractory disease, but the long-term benefit is currently unclear.

Alcoholic liver disease
Incidence and diagnosis

Approximately 1% of the population are psychologically or physically dependent upon alcohol:

- 20–30% of these develop alcoholic liver disease.
- Approximately 25% of liver cirrhosis is due to alcohol.

Current recommendations for safe alcohol consumption: 21 (male) and 14 (female) units per week.

- A unit of alcohol (approximately 10 g) represents a measure of spirit, a glass of wine, or half a pint of beer (see Fig. 21.3).
- An intake of 20 units (or more) per day is associated with a high risk of hepatocellular damage.

Clinical features

Diagnosis is made predominantly on clinical grounds, and the extent of liver damage can be determined by liver biopsy but does not always correlate well with deranged liver biochemistry.

Symptoms can often be vague, including nausea, vomiting, abdominal pain, and diarrhoea; and may be attributable to the effects of alcohol or alcohol withdrawal *per se*. More extensive hepatocellular damage may manifest from jaundice to hepatic failure.

Extra-hepatic manifestations include:
- Wernicke's and Korsakoff's syndromes.
- Proximal myopathy.
- Peripheral neuropathy (often painful).
- Cardiomyopathy, with cardiac failure and arrythmias.
- Gastritis and erosions.
- Porphyria cutanea tarda.
- Neglect and malnutrition.
- Psychosocial difficulties.

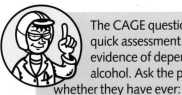

The CAGE questionnaire is a quick assessment for evidence of dependency on alcohol. Ask the patient whether they have ever:
- **C**ut down on alcohol for any reason.
- Become **A**ngry when people discuss their alcohol consumption.
- Felt **G**uilty because of their alcohol consumption.
- Needed an **E**ye opener early in the day to help them cope.

Pathogenesis

Three main types of liver damage are described:
- Fatty change.
- Alcoholic hepatitis.
- Fibrosis.

Fatty change

Ethanol is metabolized in the liver, which results in hepatic fatty acid synthesis and reduced fatty acid oxidation leading to accumulation and fatty destruction of the hepatic cells (Fig. 18.16). Similar changes can also be seen in obesity, diabetes, starvation, and pregnancy.

There is thought to be no permanent hepatocellular damage, hence fatty change resolves with abstinence from alcohol.

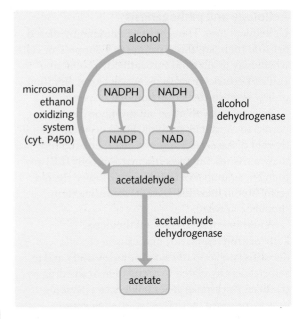

Fig. 18.16 Biochemical pathways for metabolism of alcohol. Alcohol under normal circumstances is converted to acetaldehyde by the action of alcohol dehydrogenase. In heavy drinkers, induction of the cytochrome P450 enzyme system occurs, hence increasing the metabolism of alcohol. Free radicals are a by-product of NADP and NAD production causing hepatocellular damage.

Alcoholic hepatitis

Infiltration with polymorphonuclear leucocytes and hyaline material (Mallory bodies) is typical. Fatty change often coexists with alcoholic hepatitis. Mallory bodies may also be seen in this form of chronic active hepatitis; they are not specific to alcoholic damage.

Fibrosis

Characterized by fibrosis with nodular regeneration which implies previous or continuing liver damage. A micronodular pattern progresses to macronodular in later stages.

Diagnosis and investigations

A background of chronic liver disease and a history of heavy alcohol consumption is highly indicative of alcoholic liver disease.

Other investigations may aid diagnosis:
- Full blood count—often reveals a macrocytosis (a sensitive indicator of heavy alcohol consumption). Iron-deficiency anaemia may be seen in cases of chronic gastrointestinal (GI) bleed due to varices or gastric or oesophageal erosion. Leucocytosis is

common. Thrombocytopaenia occurs as a result of the toxic effect of ethanol on megakaryocytes.

- Liver biochemistry: gamma glutamyl transferase is another indicator of heavy alcohol intake. In the presence of hepatitis, raised AST, ALT, bilirubin, and alkaline phosphatase will be seen. AST is usually only moderately raised at levels below 300 IU/L; ALT is usually less than half that value and it has been suggested that the AST:ALT ratio is a useful indicator of alcoholic liver disease when in excess of 2. Low albumin may suggest underlying cirrhosis and impaired synthetic function. Associated hyperlipidaemia with haemolytic anaemia can occasionally be seen (Zieve syndrome).
- Clotting screen—prolonged prothrombin time is typical of alcoholic hepatitis due to reduced production of clotting factors by the liver.
- Ultrasound will demonstrate fatty change and if there is macronodular cirrhosis may demonstrate an irregular margin with irregular intra-hepatic foci mimicking metastatic disease.
- Liver biopsy is the gold standard of diagnosis. Difficulty may arise due to deranged clotting and a transjugular liver biopsy may be necessary to reduce the bleeding risk. Features of fatty change and cirrhosis will be seen. End-stage cirrhosis seen on histology will not distinguish its underlying aetiology.

Complications
Liver failure and cirrhosis.

Prognosis
Dependent on abstinence. Patients without established cirrhosis have a 5-year survival of 60% if they continue drink alcohol, which rises to 90% if they discontinue. Cirrhotic patients who continue to drink alcohol have an even poorer prognosis with 5-year survival rate of 35%.

Treatment
Abstinence from alcohol is vital. Acute alcohol withdrawal (i.e. hallucinations, tremor, and fits, delirium tremens) should be treated with a decrementing regime of a benzodiazepine such as diazepam or chlordiazepoxide. Multivitamins, especially vitamin B complex, should be given in addition to high protein and calorie supplements except in cases of hepatic encephalopathy.

Treatment of cirrhosis is described separately.

Cirrhosis

Cirrhosis is the end-stage of any progressive liver disease.

Clinical features
Cirrhosis *per se* is usually asymptomatic. Symptoms arise due to either the underlying disease or when complications of cirrhosis ensue.

Abdominal examination may reveal:
- Hepatomegaly or splenomegaly (if portal hypertension is present).
- Ascites.
- Dilated umbilical veins (caput medusae; Fig. 18.17).

Stigmata of chronic liver disease in the skin include anaemia, jaundice, palmar erythema, Dupuytren's contracture, finger clubbing, leuconychia, pruritus, spider naevi, and xanthomas.

There may be endocrine features, such as loss of hair, testicular atrophy, parotid enlargement, gynaecomastia, amenorrhoea, and a loss of libido (Fig. 18.17).

Neurological features include drowsiness, confusion, flapping of hands, constructional apraxia, and fetor hepaticus (portosystemic encephalopathy).

Fluid retention may be apparent in the abdomen (ascites) or as peripheral oedema.

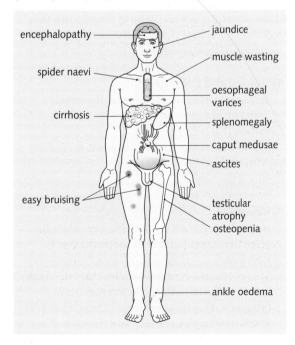

Fig. 18.17 Body map showing features of cirrhosis.

Investigations

Investigations to consider include the following:

- Liver biochemistry can be surprisingly normal but some abnormality will often be present with slightly raised transaminases and alkaline phosphatase. In severe cases, all liver enzymes will be abnormal. Low sodium and albumin are also seen. Hyperglycaemia can be evident if there is associated pancreatic insufficiency, and hypertriglyceridaemia is common.
- Full blood count may reveal anaemia due to variceal bleeding. Macrocytosis can be a direct effect of alcohol in addition to B_{12} or folate deficiency.
- Coagulopathy is a very sensitive indicator of liver dysfunction and is reflected in the prolonged prothrombin time.
- Alpha-fetoprotein is raised in hepatocellular carcinoma (although can be slightly elevated with cirrhosis—serial measurements are useful).
- Ultrasound provides information of liver size, fatty change, and fibrosis as well as hepatocellular carcinoma.
- Endoscopy identifies and allows treatment for varices.
- Liver biopsy may be indicated for patients in whom the underlying aetiology is unclear or to assess the severity of cirrhosis.

Other investigations are useful in establishing the underlying aetiology (e.g. hepatitis serology, ferritin, caeruloplasmin, autoantibodies).

Aetiology and pathogenesis

Cirrhosis of the liver is a result of cell necrosis followed by fibrosis and regeneration, hence nodule formation (Fig. 18.18).

The most common cause worldwide is chronic hepatitis B infection, whereas in the Western world, alcohol is the culprit.

Two types of cirrhosis have been described:

- Macronodular—regenerating nodules are generally larger and of a variable size. They are often due a result of chronic hepatitis B or C infection.
- Micronodular—contains nodules that are <3 mm in size, uniformly affects the liver, and is more often seen with ongoing alcohol abuse. However, a mixed picture can be seen and the underlying cause does not necessarily reflect the histological change.

A	Causes of cirrhosis
Alcohol excess	
Chronic viral hepatitis, especially B and C	
Genetic diseases, e.g. haemochromatosis, alpha-1-antitrypsin deficiency	
Chronic liver diseases, e.g. primary biliary cirrhosis, chronic active hepatitis	
Cryptogenic where no aetiology is apparent but the patient presents with complications	

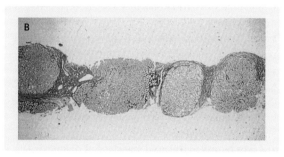

Fig. 18.18 (A) Common causes of cirrhosis. (B) Low power photomicrograph of needle liver biopsy showing fibrous nodular formation and established cirrhosis.

Complications

Portal hypertension

Portal vascular resistance is increased due to collagen deposition and fibrosis seen in liver cirrhosis and, hence formation of varices in the gastro-oesophageal junction (Fig. 18.20). In addition, sodium retention and vasoactive substances such as nitric oxide (due to accumulation of toxic metabolites) will increase plasma volume and splanchnic vasodilatation, respectively, and thus maintain portal hypertension.

Bleeding from the varices will result in haematemesis and melaena and can be precipitated by trauma (e.g. food bolus) or rising portal venous pressure (i.e. progressive liver cirrhosis).

Ascites

This is a result of fluid in the peritoneal cavity, and its pathogenesis involves several physiological processes.

Sodium and water retention occur as a result of activation of the renin–angiotensin system, secondary to arterial vasodilatation (caused by vasoactive substances such as nitric oxide.) Portal hypertension *per se* results in a transudative ascites due to increased hydrostatic pressure, hence further reduces intravascular volume and stimulates sodium and water retention via aldosterone (secondary hyperaldosteronism).

Ascites may be aggravated by a low plasma oncotic pressure resulting from hypoalbuminaenia, which occurs as a result of impaired synthetic hepatic function.

Spontaneous bacterial infection of ascites is a serious complication that carries a significant risk of mortality (50%). Common pathogens include *Escherichia coli*, *Klebsiella*, and other gut bacteria. Clinical deterioration (often non-specific), fever, and neutrophilia should raise the possibility of infected ascites. Aspiration of ascitic fluid should be performed for Gram stain and culture. Treatment with broad-spectrum antibiotics such as a third-generation cephalosporin (e.g. cefotaxime) should be employed.

Hepatic encephalopathy

Toxic metabolites that are usually detoxified by the liver accumulate in the bloodstream and pass through the blood–brain barrier to cause encephalopathy. Ammonia produced by the breakdown of proteins by intestinal bacteria appears to play a role in hepatic encephalopathy. Accumulation of false neurotransmitters is also important though poorly understood.

Clinically, the patient is confused, disorientated, has slurred speech, and in severe cases, convulsion and coma. Coarse flapping of hyperextended hands, hepatic fetor (sweet-smelling breath due to ketones), and constructional apraxia (unable to draw a five-pointed star) can also be seen.

Acute onset usually has a precipitating factor which can potentially be reversible (e.g. bleeding or infection).

Hepatorenal syndrome

Characterized by cirrhosis, jaundice, and renal failure.

It is thought to be due to a depletion in intravascular volume, activation of the renin–angiotensin system, and vasoconstriction of the renal afferent arterioles, hence reduced glomerular filtration.

Other mediators have also been implicated that are related to prostaglandin synthesis and the syndrome can be precipitated by the use of non-steroidal anti-inflammatory drugs (NSAIDs). More commonly, renal impairment occurs as a result of sepsis, diuretic use or excessive paracentesis causing intravascular volume depletion and renal hypoperfusion.

The renal abnormality is thought to be functional because transplanted kidneys from a donor patient with hepatorenal syndrome to a recipient will result in a normal functioning kidney. However, extreme cases will cause tubular necrosis and renal damage.

The patient should be treated for prerenal failure but the condition carries a very high mortality.

Hepatocellular carcinoma

Development of cirrhosis is an independent risk factor for hepatocellular carcinoma (see Liver tumours).

Prognosis

Grading of prognosis of cirrhosis is made on the Child's criteria (Fig. 18.19). Overall, there is a 50% survival in 5 years.

Modified Child classification			
Child's class	A	B	C
Serum bilirubin μmol/L	Normal	Up to twice normal	More than twice normal
Serum albumin g/L	Normal	30–35	Less than 30 g/L
Ascites	None	Minimal and responds to diuretics	Moderate or marked
Encephalopathy	None	None or mild irritability	Grades II, III, IV
Coagulopathy	None	Prothrombin time ≤4 s prolonged	PT ≥5 s prolonged

Fig. 18.19 Modified Child classification of cirrhosis based on functional capacity of the liver. Class C carries a poor prognosis.

Treatment

Generally consists of managing the complications that arise.

If ascites is present, spontaneous bacterial infection must be excluded and if found, appropriate therapy should be started.

A reduction in dietary sodium will allow the reabsorption of ascitic fluid back into the circulation.

Diuretic therapy is used to increase renal excretion of sodium and hence excess water. Hepatic dysfunction results in secondary hyperaldosteronism because of failure to break down aldosterone in the liver. Spironolactone, a specific aldosterone antagonist, is therefore the diuretic of choice. Further diuresis may be required and the use of loop diuretic such as furosemide (frusemide) is effective, but the patient is at risk of hyponatraemia, dehydration, and hypokalaemia. Paracentesis is often carried out for symptomatic relief (up to 20 L can be drained).

Hypovolaemia is problematic because ascites reaccumulates at the expense of circulating volume. This can be avoided by administration of salt-poor albumin or plasma expanders such as gelofusin.

Various shunts can be inserted for persistent ascites such that they drain peritoneal fluid into the internal jugular vein but infection and blockage of the shunts limits their use. Intra-hepatic shunts (TIPS, see below), have also been used but are controversial for this purpose.

For hepatic encephalopathy an underlying precipitating cause should be found and appropriate treatment instigated (i.e. correction of electrolyte imbalance, treatment of sepsis, etc.). Laxatives and enemas should be given to reduce ammonia load.

A low protein diet should be instituted in order to reduce nitrogenous waste which exacerbates encephalopathy.

Oesophageal and gastric varices

Incidence

Major complication of cirrhosis, whatever the underlying aetiology. Up to 70% of cirrhotic patients will develop varices and up to 40% of these will bleed.

Portal vein thrombosis causes non-cirrhotic portal hypertension.

Clinical features

Acute GI bleed in the form of melaena or haematemesis due to rupture of varices is the usual mode of presentation. Other features may include:

- Stigmata of chronic liver disease: palmar erythema, spider naevi, proximal myopathy or muscle wasting, pigmentation or jaundice, hypogonadism.
- Splenomegaly is usually present due to underlying portal hypertension.
- Features of liver failure (e.g. encephalopathy, ascites, jaundice, etc.).

Diagnosis and investigations

These include:

- Full blood count, biochemistry, clotting, etc., as for all patients with an acute GI bleed. A low platelet count may indicate hypersplenism due to portal hypertension. Prolonged prothrombin time is an indicator of diminished hepatic synthetic function.
- Urgent endoscopy is essential to confirm the diagnosis and differentiate variceal haemorrhage from other causes.
- Liver biopsy may be required, following recovery from the acute episode, if the aetiology of liver disease remains in doubt.
- Ultrasound and Doppler studies may be useful to diagnose hepatic or portal vein thrombosis.

Aetiology and pathogenesis

Due to presence of portal hypertension which can be:

- Presinusoidal.
- Sinusoidal.
- Postsinusoidal.

When portal pressures rises above 10–12 mmHg (normal = 5–8 mmHg), collateral communication with the systemic venous system occurs instead of blood flowing into hepatic vein. Portosystemic anastomoses occur at the gastro-oesophageal junction, ileocaecal junction, rectum, and anterior abdominal wall via the umbilical vein (Figs 18.20 and 21).

Presinusoidal

Blockage of the portal vein before its entry to the liver (e.g. portal vein thrombosis as a result of congenital venous abnormality, prothrombotic states or umbilical sepsis). Pancreatic disease is the most common cause in adults. A rare cause is schistosomiasis. Doppler studies usually identify the blockage.

Sinusoidal

The majority of cases are due to cirrhosis, where portal vascular resistance is increased due to distorted architecture and perivenular fibrosis. This

Fig. 18.20 Portal vasculature and sites of portal systemic anastomoses. Sites of portosystemic anastomoses are indicated by black circles. (A) Rectal varices or haemorrhoids. (B) Ileocaecal varices. (C) Umbilical varices (caput medusae). (D) Gastro-oesophageal varices. Varices at the gastro-oesophageal junction bleed most commonly only because they traverse the greatest pressure gradient between the negative pressure in the thorax and the positive pressure abdominal cavity.

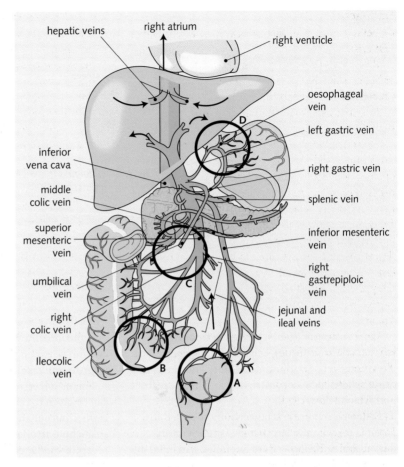

can also occur in congenital hepatic fibrosis and non-cirrhotic portal hypertension, where the histology shows mild portal tract fibrosis without cirrhosis.

Postsinusoidal

Budd–Chiari syndrome where there is occlusion of the hepatic veins as they exit the liver. The patient usually has a hypercoagulable state, underlying myeloproliferative disorder, or extrinsic occlusion by tumour or mass.

Portal hypertension develops if the condition becomes chronic. Other causes include constrictive pericarditis and right-sided cardiac failure.

Complications

Risk of developing encephalopathy is high with an acute variceal bleed.

Prognosis

Overall risk of recurrence after an acute episode is 80% over 2 years. Each variceal bleed carries a mortality risk of 15–40%.

Aims of treatment

Resuscitation, restoration of haemodynamic stability and arrest of variceal bleeding. Once this is successfully carried out, then preventive measures should be started.

Treatment

Resuscitation aims to replace depleted intravascular volume with plasma expanders and crystalloids initially, then blood once available (as with all major GI bleeds). Correction of coagulopathy with Vitamin K (takes 6–12 hours to work), fresh frozen plasma or cryoprecipitate should be undertaken if required.

Urgent endoscopy is required, during which sclerosant is injected in or around the varices to cause inflammatory obliteration (see Fig. 24.20). Alternatively, elastic band ligation of the varices at endoscopy produces thrombotic obliteration (Fig. 18.22). Repeat sclerotherapy or banding is usually needed to prevent further bleeds.

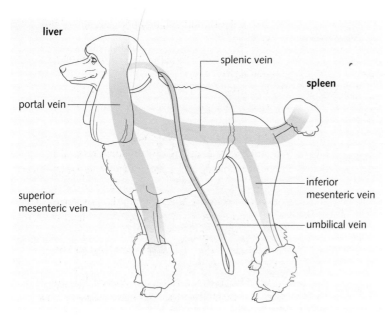

liver

portal vein

superior
mesenteric vein

splenic vein

spleen

inferior
mesenteric vein

umbilical vein

Fig. 18.21 Difficulty remembering the portal circulation? For portal, think poodle! (L, liver; S, spleen; PV, portal vein; SMV, superior mesenteric vein; Spl. V, splenic vein; IMV, inferior mesenteric vein; Umb. V, umbilical vein.)

Vasoconstrictor agents, such as octreotide (somatostatin analogue), can be administered intravenously as an adjuvant therapy. The aim is to cause splanchnic vasoconstriction and hence restrict portal blood flow.

Balloon tamponade is now mainly reserved for patients for whom sclerotherapy is temporarily unavailable or the procedure has failed. An inflatable tube is passed into the stomach and the balloon inflated with air. Traction on the balloon is maintained for 12 hours until the varices have collapsed. An alternative design of tube also has an oesophageal balloon. Prolonged inflation of the balloon is associated with mucosal ulceration and rupture of oesophagus. It also increases the risk of aspiration pneumonia.

Transjugular intra-hepatic portocaval shunt (TIPS) is a shunt formed between the systemic and portal venous system to treat varices (Fig. 18.23). A guide wire is passed under X-ray control via the internal jugular vein to the hepatic vein and passes into the liver. Contact is made through the liver substance with the portal venous circulation and a metal endoprosthesis is inserted to create the shunt. Encephalopathy occurs in up to 30% patients. Recurrence of varices can occur if the stent thromboses.

Surgery is rarely performed nowadays. Oesophageal transection can be done as an emergency with ligation of the vessels. Portosystemic shunts (mesocaval or splenorenal) can also be undertaken surgically but have a high incidence of

encephalopathy. Narrow gauge stents forming a conduit between the portal vein and vena cava can improve the results but have no advantage over TIPS.

A non-selective beta-blocker (e.g. propranolol) can be given to reduce portal pressure by reducing cardiac output and allowing vasoconstriction of splanchnic arteries by inhibiting the effects of β_2 receptor-mediated vasodilatation. This is the drug of choice in both primary prevention of variceal bleeding and in prevention of secondary haemorrhage following obliteration of varices. A long-acting nitrate such as isosorbide mononitrate can act as an adjuvant agent to beta-blockade in reducing portal pressure.

Tumours of the liver

The most common tumours are metastatic spread from another primary site (e.g. GI tract, breast, thyroid, and bronchus). Primary tumours of the liver are usually malignant.

Hepatocellular carcinoma
Incidence
One of the most common malignant diseases worldwide but rare in the Western world.

Clinical features
Include:
- Usually non-specific (i.e. weight loss, malaise, fever, right upper quadrant pain) and, in late

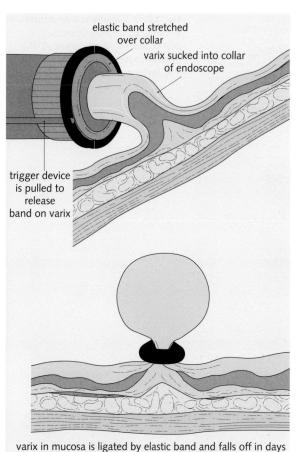

trigger device is pulled to release band on varix

elastic band stretched over collar

varix sucked into collar of endoscope

varix in mucosa is ligated by elastic band and falls off in days

Fig. 18.22 Strategy to control variceal haemorrhage by elastic band ligation.

stages, ascites (an exudate, that may be bloodstained).
- Cirrhotic patients who develop the above clinical features should have malignant change excluded.
- An enlarged irregular tender liver is more likely to be found in secondary metastasis or pre-existing cirrhosis than primary hepatocellular carcinoma.
- Metastases to lung and bone may produce pleural effusions and pathological fractures, respectively.

Diagnosis and investigations

Investigations to consider:
- Liver biochemistry—normal or mild abnormality of enzymes is usual in established, inactive cirrhosis. A rise in ALT or AST may be indicative of tumour necrosis. Elevated alkaline phosphatase may reflect bony metastases.
- Serum alpha-fetoprotein raised.

- Liver ultrasound will identify majority of liver tumours.
- Cytology of ascitic fluid may demonstrate malignant cells.
- Liver biopsy under ultrasound guidance is required for histological diagnosis.

Aetiology and pathogenesis

In areas where hepatitis B and hepatitis C are prevalent, over 90% of patients with hepatocellular carcinoma have positive serology and an equal number have pre-existing cirrhosis. The aetiology is presumed to be the integration of the virus into the host genome.

Most patients with cirrhosis, whatever the underlying cause, are at risk of developing hepatocellular carcinoma, but especially patients with hepatitis B and primary haemochromatosis. Development of a hepatoma occurs more commonly in males than females with cirrhosis.

Prognosis

Very poor—<5% survival at 6 months.

Treatment

Little response to radiotherapy or chemotherapy. Isolated lesions may be surgically resected.

Other tumours of the liver
Adenomas

Rare—associated with the oral contraceptive pill. Can present as an incidental finding or due to intra-hepatic bleeding. Surgical resection is only required if complications develop.

Haemangiomas

Most common benign tumour of the liver and usually found incidentally on ultrasound. No treatment is required. If diagnosis is in doubt, then angiography is required.

Focal nodular hyperplasia

As its name suggests this condition causes nodules in the liver, but hepatic function is normal. It is more common than hepatic adenoma but has no malignant potential. Its importance is that it can be mistaken for cirrhosis either on radiological imaging, or even on histology from a needle biopsy. It is usually asymptomatic and found incidentally, but is believed to be related to the oral contraceptive pill. In these circumstances, it is thought that about 50% become

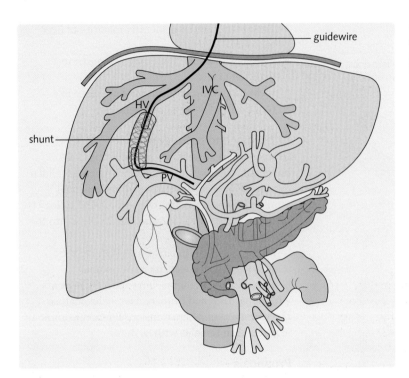

Fig. 18.23 Schematic representation of transjugular intra-hepatic portocaval shunt procedure. (IVC, inferior vena cava; HV, hepatic vein; PV, portal vein.)

symptomatic, usually with pain in the right upper quadrant. Symptomatic cases are treated by surgical resection.

Drugs and the liver

Many drugs are metabolized by liver enzymes and some are excreted in bile. Some drugs are fat-soluble and their bioavailability can be affected by bile salt micellar concentration in the intestine. Plasma proteins, especially albumin synthesized in the liver, affect the kinetics of many drugs. Hence liver dysfunction and disease can impair absorption, transport, metabolism, and excretion of several drugs (Fig. 18.24). Care must be taken when using most drugs in the presence of liver disease. Conversely, many drugs can cause deranged liver biochemistry or damage.

Drug toxicity to the liver
Incidence
Up to 10% of jaundice is drug induced and is mediated by different mechanisms.

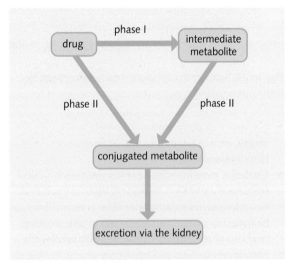

Fig. 18.24 Biochemical pathways of drug metabolism in the liver.

Aetiology and pathogenesis
Drug toxicity can be:
- Dose or duration related (e.g. azathioprine, methotrexate).
- Idiosyncratic (e.g. flucloxacillin, clavulanic acid).
- Due to overdose toxicity (e.g. paracetamol).

Fig. 18.25 Drugs known to cause disturbance in liver function.

Drugs affecting liver function	
Pattern of liver damage	**Drugs**
Hepatitis	Anti-tuberculous: rifampicin, isoniazid Anti-fungal: ketoconazole Anti-hypertensive: atenolol, verapamil Anaesthetics: halothane
Cholestasis	Anti-arrhythmics: amiodarone Anti-metabolite: methotrexate Allopurinol Anti-psychotics: chlorpromazine Antibiotics: erythromycin, clavulanic acid, flucloxacillin Immunosuppressives: ciclosporin A Contraceptives and anabolic steroids
Necrosis	Paracetamol, carbon tetrachloride

Three types of pathology are described (Fig. 18.25):

- Acute hepatitis typically occurs 2–3 weeks after starting the drug and normally resolves after cessation. In the case of halothane, repeated exposure sensitizes the patient and can cause fulminant hepatitis, suggesting an immunological cause. Clinically, this can mimic severe viral hepatitis.
- Cholestasis—bile stasis causes a functional obstruction, hence biochemically it produces jaundice with pale stools and dark urine usually after 4–6 weeks. The cause of bile stasis is unclear but inflammatory infiltration of bile ducts and interference with excretory transport proteins has been implicated. Anabolic steroids and oral contraceptives can cause profound cholestasis.
- Necrosis—mainly dose-dependent. Toxic metabolites are normally detoxified by the liver (e.g. conjugation by glutathione), and once the level of glutathione falls, toxic metabolites accumulate and liver necrosis follows. Concurrent ingestion of enzyme-inducing drugs (e.g. phenytoin, carbamazepine, an alcohol binge), severely ill patients, or starvation will render these individuals more susceptible to toxicity.

Clinical features

These can range from mild elevation of liver enzymes to acute fulminant hepatic failure:

- Jaundice is usually secondary to an acute hepatitis or cholestasis but rarely it can be due to haemolysis.
- In the majority of cases derangement of liver enzymes is found on routine examination before clinical jaundice develops.
- Nausea and vomiting or abdominal pain may occur.
- Pruritus, steatorrhoea, and dark urine if cholestasis occurs.

Diagnosis and investigation

Enquire carefully about the timing, chronology and duration of drug ingestion.

Liver enzymes can show an acute hepatitic picture (raised ALT or AST) or a cholestatic/obstructive picture (raised alkaline phosphatase and gamma glutamyl transpeptidase). Jaundice may be present in either type. It is important to establish whether there is clinical or laboratory evidence of hepatocellular dysfunction (encephalopathy, ascites, hypoalbuminaemia, coagulopathy, acidosis), or associated renal impairment.

Complications and prognosis

Fulminant hepatitis secondary to halothane-induced hepatitis has a mortality rate of up to 20%, but this is rare. Hepatic failure following acute liver necrosis most often and predictably follows paracetamol overdose.

Treatment

Withdrawal of the offending drug is usually sufficient to allow normalization of liver enzymes, within days to weeks. However in some cases, such as chlorpromazine-induced cholestatic hepatitis, it may take up to 12 months or longer before the liver biochemistry returns to normal.

Paracetamol toxicity

The analgesic paracetamol is commonly used for self-poisoning but this is a potentially treatable condition.

Poor prognostic factors for liver failure		
	Paracetamol	**Non-paracetamol**
Aetiology		Non-ABC hepatitis
		Drugs
Age		<10, >40 years
Encephalopathy	Present on day 2	Present
Serum creatinine	>300 µmol/L	>300 µmol/L
Prolonged prothrombin time	>100 s	>50 s
pH	<7.3	

Fig. 18.26 Factors associated with a poor prognosis in liver failure.

Occasionally, overdose of paracetamol can be accidental or there can be a pre-existing liver condition of which the patient was unaware. Unfortunately, delayed presentation can often be fatal. As this is such a common and important clinical scenario, it is worth describing in detail.

- Arterial gases—a low pH (<7.3) has a significantly poorer prognosis in patients presenting late (i.e. >24 hours) (Fig. 18.26).
- Blood glucose can be low and serial, measurements should be undertaken if there is evidence of hepatic failure.

Clinical features
Note that:
- Nausea and vomiting usually occur within the first 24 hours.
- Liver failure can be seen between 72 and 96 hours if left untreated. Acute renal failure can occur with or without liver failure (paracetamol can directly cause renal tubular necrosis).

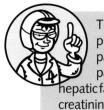

The three most prognostically influential parameters in the setting of paracetamol induced acute hepatic failure are: serum pH, creatinine and prothrombin time.

Diagnosis and investigation
Paracetamol levels are plotted on a chart (Prescott nomogram) and correlated to 'time post-ingestion' to establish the need for treatment. However, the exact timing may be difficult because the history from the patient is often unreliable. If there is doubt, it is safer to initiate treatment than to wait for, or rely upon, levels. Useful investigations include:
- Clotting screen—the prothrombin time is the most sensitive indication of hepatic damage.
- Liver biochemistry usually shows raised ALT and AST sometimes to very high levels (10000), but these do not correlate well with toxicity or give any prognostic information.
- Electrolytes are usually normal. Raised creatinine indicates significant renal damage and a level >300 µmol/L predicts a serious outcome.

Aetiology and pathogenesis
Paracetamol is converted to a toxic metabolite, *N*-acetyl-*p*-benzoquinonimine, which under normal circumstances is inactivated by conjugation with glutathione. In overdose, glutathione is depleted, hence there is a build up of toxic metabolite, thus hepatocellular necrosis (Fig. 18.27).

Patients with underlying liver impairment (e.g. chronic alcoholics or cirrhosis) or those concurrently taking an enzyme-inducing drug (e.g. phenytoin) are at greater risk of hepatocellular damage; hence, the threshold for treatment should be lowered. Those patients with HIV are also at higher risk, as they tend to have diminished stores of hepatic glutathione. There is a 'high risk' treatment line on the Prescott nomogram.

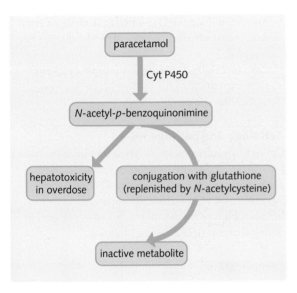

Fig. 18.27 Biochemical mechanism of paracetamol toxicity and prevention.

Complications

Fulminant hepatic failure is a serious and often fatal complication which is more often seen in those presenting later than 16 hours post-ingestion.

Treatment

N-acetylcysteine infusion is the treatment of choice, which replenishes hepatic glutathione by providing the sulphydryl group it requires. The decision of whether treatment is required is based on serum paracetamol levels taken 4 hours or more post-ingestion and the likelihood of severe hepatic damage is predicted. Oral methionine can be given as an alternative, but its absorption is unreliable, especially if the patient is vomiting.

Serum paracetamol levels are unreliable in patients who present later than 16 hours post-ingestion, hence if there is any doubt, treatment should be started and stopped when subsequent liver biochemistry and clotting are found to be normal.

Patients presenting within 1 hour of ingestion should be given activated charcoal, as this will reduce the absorption of the drug from the GI tract.

Patients at risk of severe liver damage or with fulminant hepatic failure should be referred to a specialist unit for expert care and possible liver transplantation.

Prognosis

Patients who recover from hepatocellular damage do not have any residual liver impairment and can be treated as normal.

Liver abscesses

Pyogenic abscess
Incidence

An uncommon complication of intra-abdominal sepsis (e.g. diverticulitis, appendicitis, perforated bowel, etc.), but it can occur sporadically without any overt sign of other sources of infection.

Clinical features

These include:
- Non-specific symptoms such as swinging fever, anorexia, weight loss, abdominal pain, malaise.
- Jaundice, tender hepatomegaly, and septicaemic shock in some cases.
- A reactive pleural effusion in the right lower lobe may be seen.

Diagnosis and investigation

Consider:
- Full blood count—normocytic normochromic anaemia with a neutrophilia.
- Liver biochemistry—raised alkaline phosphatase, raised bilirubin (if bile ducts are obstructed).
- Blood cultures—positive only in approximately one third of cases. Recent antibiotic therapy reduces this further.
- Chest radiograph—a raised right hemidiaphragm with or without pleural effusion may be seen.
- Liver ultrasound—cystic lesions (single or multiple) are seen and ultrasound-guided aspiration of pus with microscopy and culture aims to yield organism and its sensitivity.
- Further imaging (e.g. computed tomography scan of abdomen) may be required to identify primary source of infection.

Aetiology and pathogenesis

Escherichia coli is the most common pathogen isolated. Others include *Streptococcus faecalis* (enterococcus), *Streptococcus milleri*, *Proteus* sp., *Staphylococcus aureus*, and anaerobes.

Abdominal infection spread to the liver via the portovenous system is likely to be the most common

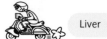

cause, but direct spread from biliary infection or perinephric abscess can also occur.

Complications and prognosis

Few or no complications will occur if the abscess is single and adequately treated. Rupture of the abscess can occur, producing bacterial peritonitis and consequently, a significant increase in mortality.

Multiple abscesses have a poorer outcome than unilocular, with a mortality rate of over 50% in some cases depending on the underlying cause.

Treatment

Treatment options include:
- Aspiration of the abscess under ultrasound control should be done as a therapeutic intervention as well as a diagnostic procedure.
- Surgical intervention may also be required if aspiration is unsuccessful or if multiple abscesses are unsuitable for aspiration.
- Broad-spectrum antibiotics are given immediately to cover Gram-positive, Gram-negative and anaerobic organisms, until sensitivity is known. A combination of benzylpenicillin, gentamicin and metronidazole is a reasonable initial regimen.

Amoebic abscess
Incidence

Occurs worldwide and it is endemic in the tropics and subtropics.

Clinical features

The main symptoms are:
- Diarrhoea as part of amoebic dysentry (but not always).
- Non-specific (e.g. malaise, anorexia, fever, abdominal pain).
- Tender hepatomegaly with or without right pleural effusion.

Rarely, clinical jaundice is seen.

Diagnosis and investigation

Investigations include:
- Liver biochemistry—may be normal or demonstrate an isolated, raised alkaline phosphatase.
- Blood cultures—usually negative.
- Microscopy of stool may demonstrate pus, red cells and trophozoites.

- Amoeba serology (IgG)—does not indicate current disease as it remains positive after the disease has resolved.
- Liver ultrasound—single or multiple cysts are seen: aspiration of the cyst yields an 'anchovy sauce'-like substance.

Aetiology and pathogenesis

Caused by *Entamoeba histolytica* that initially causes a diarrhoea illness with subsequent spread via the portovenous system into the liver. The initial bowel infection may not be clinically apparent. Inflammation of the portal tracts and development of single or multiple abscesses follows.

Complications

Rupture of the cyst causing peritonitis and secondary infection.

Prognosis

Good overall prognosis if treated adequately.

Treatment

Metronidazole is the antibiotic of choice, given for 2 weeks. Diloxanide may be required to eradicate intestinal amoebic cysts. Abscesses should be aspirated for diagnostic and therapeutic purposes.

Surgical drainage may be necessary in resistant cases or multiple large abscesses.

Parasitic infection of the liver

Hydatid disease
Incidence

Occurs worldwide, but more common where sheep and cattle farming are the main source of living. Rare in the UK, except for parts of Wales where there are large communities of sheep farmers.

Clinical features

These are:
- Asymptomatic.
- Right upper quadrant discomfort due to cystic enlargement and jaundice if obstruction of bile duct occurs.
- Rupture in the abdominal cavity may cause fever, abdominal pain, and peritonitis.
- Hepatomegaly due to cystic formation.

tract may cause haemoptysis and haematuria, respectively. Brain cyst may present as epilepsy due to its space-occupying effects.

Prognosis
If adequately treated, complete recovery is expected.

Treatment
Sterilization of the non-communicating cyst (e.g. by injection of formalin or oral albendazole—can also reduce the size of cysts), followed by surgical resection of the intact cyst. Fine needle aspiration is not routinely done due to risk of anaphylactic reaction to cyst contents.

Asymptomatic calcified cysts are usually left without treatment.

Prevention is by reducing carriage in domestic animal and improving hygiene.

Schistosomiasis
Incidence
Prevalent worldwide affecting over 200 million people mainly in the tropics.

Clinical features
The main features are:
- Acute inflammatory response at the site of penetration through skin by the cercariae ('swimmer's itch').
- Fever, myalgia, malaise, GI upset (i.e. vomiting and diarrhoea in the acute phase).
- Chronic infection produces hepatomegaly with or without portal hypertension.

Diagnosis and investigation
Investigations of use:
- Full blood count—eosinophilia.
- Liver function test—raised alkaline phosphatase.
- Immunological test—positive result is not necessarily indicative of current infection as IgG antibodies remain after the disease has resolved.
- Detection of ova in stool, liver, or rectal biopsy.

Aetiology and pathogenesis
Predominantly caused by *Schistosoma mansoni* (Africa and South America) and *Schistosoma japonicum* (China and SE Asia). Mode of infection is via swimming or bathing in contaminated water with its intermediate host as the snail.

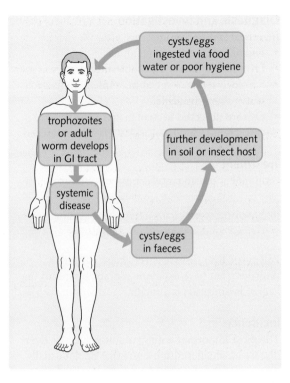

Fig. 18.28 Body map with parasitic life cycle.

Diagnosis and investigation
Investigations include:
- Full blood count—peripheral eosinophilia is typically seen.
- Haemagglutination test—positive for hydatid disease.
- Liver biochemistry —normal unless obstruction of bile duct occurs causing jaundice.
- Liver ultrasound—cystic lesion with or without daughter cysts.
- Plain abdominal X-ray—not routinely done but calcification of the cyst may be seen incidentally.

Aetiology and pathogenesis
Caused by ingestion of *Echinococcus granulosus*, which is a dog tapeworm, and its embryo via contaminated fruit and vegetables or direct ingestion due to poor hygiene (Fig. 18.28).

Within the duodenum, the embryos hatch, enter the portovenous system and systemic spread to lung, kidney, and brain can occur as well as to the liver.

Complications
Cyst rupture and secondary infection are the main complications. Rupture in the bronchus and renal

The infective form of the parasite, cercariae, penetrates the skin and migrates via the portovenous system into the liver. Here the parasite matures and eventually migrates along the portal and mesentric vein to produce a large amount of eggs, which leave the body by penetrating the intestinal wall to be excreted back into the river to complete its life cycle.

Granulomatous reaction to the trematode occurs in the liver producing a periportal fibrosis and hepatomegaly.

Complications

Portal hypertension and oesophageal varices occur in advanced cases, but cirrhosis is not usually seen.

Schistosoma japonicum produces a large number of eggs and systemic deposition of ova in lungs or brain can occur, producing epilepsy in the latter case. It also causes extensive chronic colitis and can cause premalignant changes in some cases.

Prognosis

Despite adequate treatment, fibrosis and risk of portal hypertension remains.

Aims and indications for treatment

The aim is to cause the trematode to vacate the portal and mesenteric vein and migrate to the liver or lung, where they are destroyed by the host's cell-mediated response. There may be difficulty in curative treatment, as the reinfection rate is high and it therefore may not be appropriate to attempt a cure.

Treatment

Praziquantel is an effective agent for all *Schistosoma* species. Abdominal pain and diarrhoea are common shortly after start of treatment.

Fascioliasis
Incidence

A zoonosis that infects sheep, cattle, and goats. Transmitted to humans via contaminated vegetables. Occurs worldwide, including UK.

Clinical features

These include:
- Fever, malaise, hepatomegaly, abdominal discomfort, weight loss.
- Urticarial reaction due to migration of parasite.
- Jaundice and cholangitis due to its presence in the biliary tract.

Diagnosis and investigation

Investigations to consider:
- Full blood count—eosinophilia.
- Liver biochemistry — a cholestatic picture is seen.
- Serological test— specific complement fixation test are now available.
- Ova are detected in stool in up to one third of cases, hence duodenal aspirate is often required.

Treatment

Bithionol or praziquantel are effective treatments.

Polycystic liver syndromes

Polycystic liver disease covers many different disorders that have in common cystic lesions of the liver. Classification is difficult.

Incidence

The most important entity is adult polycystic liver disease in which multiple cysts that do not usually communicate with the biliary tree develop in the liver. This condition is inherited as an autosomal dominant trait and its incidence is approximately $1:5000$ births. A related, but less common, condition is inherited as a recessive trait and often involves communication with the biliary tree.

Caroli's disease is a variant comprising cystic dilatation of the biliary tree.

Congenital hepatic fibrosis is often included under the umbrella classification as microcysts are common.

Polycystic liver disease is frequently associated with cyst formation elsewhere. Cysts are found in the kidney in 60% of cases and other viscera, especially the pancreas, in 5% of cases.

Clinical features

The clinical importance of these cysts (Fig. 18.29) is that they are often found incidentally during investigation for other problems and occasionally cause diagnostic confusion. Sometimes cysts present with pain, usually due to haemorrhage. Cysts related to the biliary tree or kidney can become infected.

Unless they are symptomatic in these respects, cysts of the liver or kidney do not usually present any problems. Cysts that communicate with the biliary tree are thought to have some malignant potential.

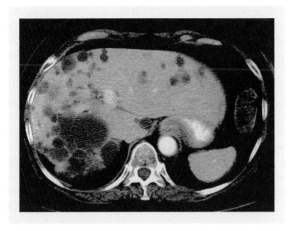

Treatment

As most cysts are asymptomatic, usually no treatment is indicated. Cysts causing haemorrhage or pain may require drainage, surgical fenestration or resection. Superadded bacterial infection should be treated empirically to cover Gram-negative organisms in particular. Cysts in the biliary tree occasionally require endoscopic drainage or resection.

Fig. 18.29 Computed tomography scan of abdomen showing multiple cysts of different sizes in the liver.

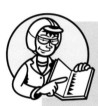

- Describe the functions of the liver under the subheadings of synthesis, storage, metabolic and excretory.
- What are the clinical manifestations of an acute viral hepatitis?
- Describe the sequence of serological markers and transaminases detected in the blood during acute hepatitis B infection (HBsAg, HBeAg, HBV DNA, ALT, Anti-HBe and anti-HBs antibodies).
- Name seven systemic manifestations of primary haemachromatosis in terms of end-organ damage.
- What are the clinical and biochemical parameters that comprise the modified Child classification of cirrhosis?
- How would you manage a patient presenting with paracetamol overdose? (include clinical assessment, investigations and initial treatment strategy)
- What are the factors associated with a poor prognosis in liver failure?
- Name some drugs known to cause disturbance in liver function.

155

19. Biliary Tract

Anatomy, physiology and function of the hepatobiliary system

Bile canaliculi between hepatocytes form ductules that merge into bile ducts in the portal tracts. These ultimately form the right and left hepatic ducts, which leave the respective lobes of the liver and join together to form the common hepatic duct at the porta hepatis. The cystic duct from the gallbladder inserts into the lower end of the common hepatic duct to form the common bile duct, which courses through the head of pancreas to emerge in the second part of the duodenum together with the pancreatic duct (Fig. 19.1).

Bile consists of:
- Water.
- Bile acids—these are synthesized from cholesterol, and act as a detergent for lipid stabilizers to form micelles with their hydrophilic and hydrophobic ends to enable absorption and digestion of fats.
- Cholesterol.
- Bilirubin—this is predominantly a by-product of the breakdown of red blood cells in Kupffer cells. Bilirubin is unconjugated and water insoluble. Conjugation occurs in the liver to allow excretion with bile in the small duodenum. Once in the terminal ileum, bacterial enzymes deconjugate the molecule and a small proportion of free bilirubin (water insoluble) is reduced to urobilinogen (water soluble) and excreted as stercobilinogen in the stool. The rest is reabsorbed in the terminal ileum and into the liver via enterohepatic circulation and further excretion in bile. Urobilinogen can also be excreted via the kidneys (Fig. 19.2).

Gallstones

It is important to distinguish between:
- Cholelithiasis, which refers to the presence of gallstones in the gall bladder, and
- Choledocholithiasis, which refers to the clinical scenario whereupon the gallstone passes into the cystic or common bile ducts.

Incidence

Gallstones can be found in approximately 30% of the population in the Western world in an age-related pattern (Fig. 19.3). Rare in Far East and Africa. Dietary factors may be influential.

Clinical features

Gallstones *per se* do not usually cause symptoms but more frequently, they are an incidental discovery during diagnostic imaging performed for another reason, or are identified at autopsy. Symptoms such as flatulence, dyspepsia, and fat intolerance are commonly attributed to underlying gallstones, but whether there is a true correlation between the two is still debatable.

About 15% of patients with gallstones will require cholecystectomy for symptoms which may be attributable. The following symptoms and signs may occur:
- Biliary colic and cholecystitis account for over 90% of clinical presentations of gallstone disease.
- Cholangitis may occur if bile is infected: features include fever, right upper quadrant pain, nausea and vomiting, and clinical jaundice is common.
- 'Murphy's sign'—elicited by placing two fingers on the right hypochondrium and asking the patient to breathe in. This results in pain and arrest of inspiration as the inflamed gallbladder moves below the costal margin. (It can only be regarded as 'positive' if the same manoeuvre in the left upper quadrant doesn't cause pain.) Localized rebound and guarding is characteristic of cholecystitis.

Diagnosis and investigation

A history of recurrent abdominal pain and jaundice with pale stools and dark urine, which subsequently resolves, may suggest an underlying diagnosis. Investigations to confirm diagnosis should include:

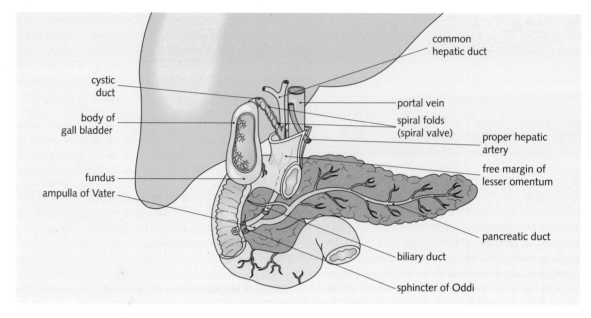

Fig. 19.1 Anatomy of the biliary tract and its relations.

- Full blood count—neutrophilia if acute cholecystitis is present. Biliary colic alone can exist without superimposed infection.
- Biochemistry—liver function tests may show features of obstructive jaundice (i.e. high bilirubin and alkaline phosphatase). Amylase should be checked to exclude acute pancreatitis, although may be modestly raised in biliary colic or cholecystitis.
- Abdominal X-ray—not routinely done because only 10% of gallstones are radio-opaque.
- Ultrasound is sensitive for the detection of gallstones, although they may not necessarily be the cause of clinical symptoms. Additional features such as gall bladder wall thickening, tenderness over visualized gall bladder, or sludge in gall bladder are more diagnostic.
- Radio-isotope scan shows the function of the gall bladder and will demonstrate any blockages in cystic or common bile duct by its delay in bile excretion.
- Endoscopic retrograde cholangiopancreatography (ERCP) will show blockage in the common bile duct which may not be seen ultrasound (Fig. 19.4).
- Endoluminal ultrasound or magnetic resonance cholangiography are useful alternatives to examine the bile duct without the risk of pancreatitis (Fig. 24.20).

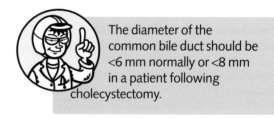

The diameter of the common bile duct should be <6 mm normally or <8 mm in a patient following cholecystectomy.

Aetiology and pathogenesis

Three main types of gallstones have been described:

- Mixed stones—constitute 70–90% of stones and predominantly contain cholesterol together with bile pigments and calcium. Multiple stones of different sizes are usually found, suggesting development in varying ages.
- Cholesterol stones account for up to 10% of stones, usually solitary, smooth, and pale in colour.
- Pigment stones, rare except in Asia, contain bile pigments (calcium bilirubinate) and are small and multiple. These are sometimes seen in patients with chronic haemolysis (e.g. hereditary spherocytosis, sickle cell disease, etc.) due to an increase in bile production.

The exact pathogenesis is unclear, although a high cholesterol intake and bile stasis have both been

Fig. 19.2 Bilirubin metabolism.

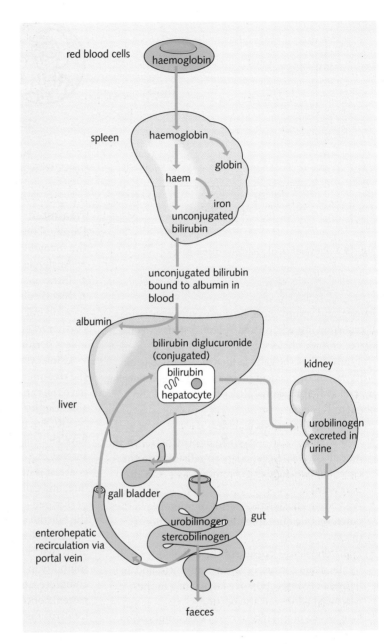

implicated. There is usually a nidus of organic material, often containing bacteria, where precipitation of calcium and cholesterol takes place. This is enhanced by biliary stasis either due to infection or biliary obstruction.

Patients with terminal ileal disease are at an increased risk of developing gallstones. As the terminal ileum is normally responsible for the resorption of bile salts, malfunction leads to a reduction of bile salts in the liver. Consequently, there is reduced micelle production and, hence, precipitation of cholesterol and formation of cholesterol stones.

Complications

In chronic cholecystitis, the gall bladder is shrunken and features of chronic inflammation are present. However, symptoms of intermittent abdominal pain,

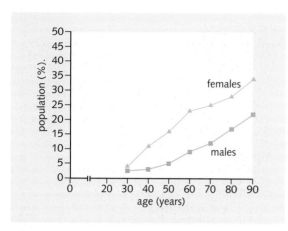

Fig. 19.3 Prevalence of gallstone disease.

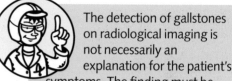

The detection of gallstones on radiological imaging is not necessarily an explanation for the patient's symptoms. The finding must be taken in context of the history, examination and laboratory investigations.

nausea, and vomiting can be due to other pathology. If recurrent, attacks of acute cholecystitis can give rise to chronic cholecystitis.

Empyema of the gall bladder means distension with pus, and the patient presents with a high, swinging pyrexia and septicaemia. Risk of perforation and peritonitis is high.

Other complications include:
- Acute pancreatitis—swelling or obstruction at the ampulla of Vater, secondary to gallstones in the common bile duct, is a common cause of acute pancreatitis.
- Ascending cholangitis—result of infection in the common bile duct spreading into intra-hepatic ducts.
- Gallstone ileus—erosion of the gall bladder wall by the stone can rarely cause peritonitis, and an ileus due to impaction of a large stone in the narrowed ileum can also occur.
- Carcinoma of gall bladder—a rare complication.

Prognosis
Definitive surgery is usually curative, but occasionally *in situ* stone formation can occur in the common bile duct, causing recurrent symptoms.

Aims and indication for treatment
Asymptomatic patients require no treatment. Symptomatic patients can be treated either medically or surgically. Approximately only 15% of patients have symptoms over a 15-year period.

Treatment
During acute episodes, if there are signs of infection, the following are required:
- Analgesia and anti-emetics.
- Intravenous fluids.
- Blood cultures, followed by broad-spectrum antibiotics.

Further intervention is not instituted at this stage unless perforation and generalized peritonitis occur.

Cholecystectomy, open or laparoscopic, is often the treatment of choice, but some patients may not have the cardiorespiratory fitness for a general anaesthetic.

ERCP is the treatment of choice for patients who have choledocholithiasis and are unsuitable for surgery. An endoscope is passed under sedation and contrast is injected to show any stones in the bile duct and gall bladder. A sphincterotomy is usually performed to allow passage of further stones once the bile duct is free of obstruction (Fig. 19.4).

Chenodeoxylate and ursodeoxycolic acid are bile acids that can be taken orally and increase cholesterol solubility in bile. Treatment takes up to 6 months to complete, and recurrence occurs in over 50% of patients once treatment is stopped. This dissolution treatment is rarely used.

Tumours of the biliary tract

Carcinoma of gall bladder
Incidence
Predominantly disease of elderly people (>60 years) but may also occur in younger people. There may be an association with pre-existing gallstones, suggesting chronic inflammation as a carcinogenic influence. Gall bladder cancer accounts for <1% of all adenocarcinomas.

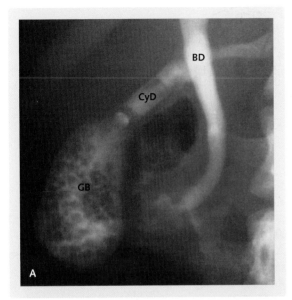

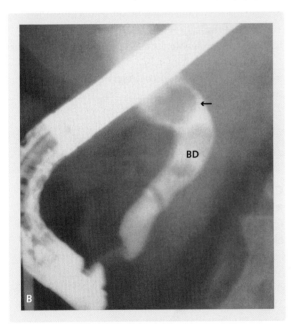

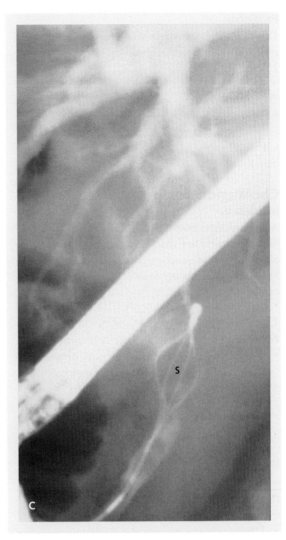

Fig. 19.4 Endoscopic retrograde cholangiopancreatography images. (A) There are multiple small stones in the gall bladder (GB), but the bile duct (BD) is clear. (B) A gallstone measuring 1 cm across can be seen in the middle of the common bile duct (arrow). (C) A gallstone (S) in the bile duct is being retrieved with the grasping basket following sphincterotomy. (CyD, cystic duct.)

Clinical features

Jaundice, right upper quadrant mass, in addition to general malaise and weight loss, are common features. A number of cases are found incidentally on routine cholecystectomy and confirmed on histology.

Diagnosis and investigations

Ultrasound is poor at detecting gall bladder carcinomas but will detect metastasis in the liver. The diagnosis is usually made at cholecystectomy for gallstone symptoms.

Prognosis

Due to its late presentation and early local metastasis, patients rarely survive for more than 1 year.

Treatment

Radical resection of the tumour may provide a cure, especially for patients only diagnosed incidentally. Chemotherapy and radiotherapy have unproven benefits.

Cholangiocarcinomas

Incidence

Adenocarcinomas of bile ducts associated with dense fibrous tissue. They can be intra-hepatic or extra-hepatic. They are uncommon tumours, accounting for only approximately 8–10% of primary liver tumours.

Clinical features

Features differ depending on the type of tumour:
- Extra-hepatic tumours present with progressive jaundice similar to sclerosing cholangitis.
- Intra-hepatic tumours tend to invade the liver parenchyma and present in a similar fashion to primary liver tumours, with jaundice being rare.

Clinical features such as weight loss, malaise, nausea, and vomiting may be evident.

Diagnosis and investigation

Investigations should include:
- Liver biochemistry indicates cholestatic jaundice with high alkaline phosphatase and bilirubin.
- Ultrasound shows dilated bile ducts if extra-hepatic lesions are present, or lesions within the liver parenchyma if intra-hepatic, but these features are not specific for cholangiocarcinoma, hence ERCP is required.
- ERCP—the dense fibrous tumour tends to grow along the duct system, with the appearance of a shouldered stricture.

Aetiology and pathogenesis

These are unknown, but in the Far East there is an association with infestation by the fluke *Clonorchis sinensis*. Up to 20% of patients who have chronic symptomatic primary sclerosing cholangitis develop cholangiocarcinoma.

Chronic inflammation or sepsis may therefore be important aetiological factors.

Prognosis

Poor, with survival rarely more than 6 months.

Treatment

Treatment options include:
- Radical resection of extra-hepatic tumours can offer a cure, but this is rare.
- Insertion of endoprostheses (stents) during ERCP (see Fig. 24.2) will provide symptomatic relief of jaundice and improve quality of life.

Radiotherapy and chemotherapy are unhelpful treatment modalities.

Ampullary tumours

An adenocarcinoma arising from the ampulla of Vater presents with obstructive jaundice which may be intermittent or progressive.

These tumours can be friable and bleed, presenting with melaena or anaemia with jaundice.

Diagnosis is made at ERCP and if made early, tumours are amenable to resection with a 60% 5-year survival.

Figure 19.5 shows the pattern of bile duct tumours.

Benign anatomical bile duct problems

Choledochal cyst and other anomalies

Congenital dilatations of the bile duct are known as choledochal cysts. The majority are asymptomatic but can produce jaundice and abdominal pain. Intra-hepatic cystic dilatations are known as Caroli's disease and can predispose to cholangitis. Treatment of symptoms initially is with antibiotics, but surgical reconstruction may be required.

Benign stricture of bile duct

A result of damage to bile ducts due to trauma or inflammation (gallstones, ascending cholangitis, or previous gall bladder surgery). Presents as progressive jaundice and can be mistaken for cholangiocarcinoma or sclerosing cholangitis.

Diagnosis is usually made by temporal association with trauma or surgery. Differentiation from tumours can be difficult if the trauma was a long time ago. Endoscopic brush cytology or histology may be helpful. Strictures occur in up to 15% patients

Fig. 19.5 Depiction of tumours involving the bile duct that may then present with jaundice. (A) Ampullary tumour. (B) Carcinoma of the head of the pancreas. (C) Carcinoma of the cystic duct or gallbladder. (D) Cholangiocarcinoma involving the hilum or below.

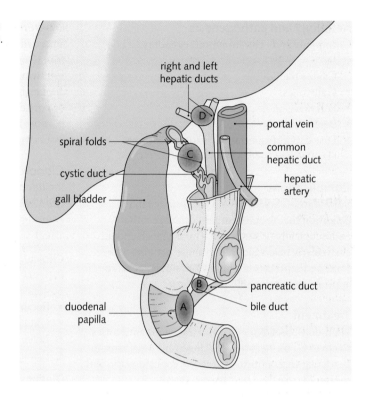

following liver transplantation. Localized strictures can be treated with stenting or reconstruction surgery.

Infections of the biliary tract

Under normal circumstances, bile within the biliary tree is sterile. The sphincter of Oddi, together with hydrochloric acid in the gastric juice, prevents bacteria ascending the tract.

Infection tends only to occur when the integrity of the bile duct sphincter function has been disrupted (e.g. after surgery or by inflammation caused by gallstones).

Cholangitis
Incidence
A potentially serious, but common complication of bile stasis secondary to gallstones, bile duct dilatation, or strictures.

Clinical features
In the majority of people the symptoms are:
- Fever.
- Jaundice.
- Right upper quadrant pain.

Septicaemic shock may be a feature in severe cases, especially in elderly people.

Diagnosis and investigation
Investigations to consider:
- Full blood count demonstrates a neutrophilia.
- Liver biochemistry reveals a cholestatic picture (i.e. raised alkaline phosphatase and bilirubin, mild increase in transaminases). As a sensitive marker of infection and inflammation, C-reactive protein is high.
- Blood cultures are positive in over 90% of cases on repeated cultures (usually the Gram-negative *Escherichia coli*).
- Ultrasound shows dilatation of bile ducts; liver abscesses can sometimes be seen.

Always consider the biliary tract as a potential site of infection when faced with a patient in whom the source of (Gram-negative) bacteraemia is not obvious.

Aetiology and pathogenesis

Commonly an *E. coli* infection secondary to bile stasis.

Causes include:

- Gallstones.
- Following cholecystectomy.
- Benign strictures.
- Post-ERCP (especially if a stent is inserted, because stents occlude with time).

Complications

Suppurative cholangitis is a potentially fatal condition that requires urgent drainage either endoscopically or surgically. The diagnosis should particularly be considered in those patients whose fever and septicaemic shock does not respond to appropriate intravenous antibiotics.

Treatment

High-dose, broad-spectrum intravenous antibiotics to cover Gram-negative and anaerobic organisms in particular (e.g. a third-generation cephalosporin and metronidazole).

Any underlying cause needs to be addressed once the infection has been adequately dealt with (e.g. removal of gallstones, blocked endoprosthesis, etc.).

Other infections of the biliary tract

These are rarely seen in the Western world and include *Opisthorchis* and *Clonorchis sinensis*, which are liver flukes that cause ascending cholangitis. There may be a predisposition to cholangiocarcinoma following such an infection. Patients with AIDS following HIV infection can develop sclerosing cholangitis, and it is possible that this could be due to opportunistic infection with *Cryptosporidium parvum* in the gastrointestinal tract, but its exact association is unclear.

Clonorchis and Opisthorchiasis

Incidence

Clonorchis sinensis and *Opisthorchis felineus* are common flukes found in the Far East that mainly affect animals such as dogs, cats, and pigs.

Clinical features

Patients may remain symptom-free but repeated and prolonged exposure will cause:

- Recurrent jaundice.
- Cholangitis.
- Liver abscess.
- Possibly cholangiocarcinoma.

Diagnosis and investigation

Microscopic examination of faeces or duodenal aspirate is required for diagnosis.

Treatment

Praziquantel is the treatment of choice.

- What are the main constituents of bile?
- Describe the sequence of bilirubin metabolism and excretion.
- What are the clinical manifestations of gallstone disease and what initial investigations would you perform?
- How would you manage a patient presenting with symptoms and signs suggestive of acute cholecystitis?
- What is Murphy's sign?
- Why are patients with terminal ileal disease at increased risk of developing gallstones?

20. Pancreas

Anatomy, physiology and function of the pancreas

The pancreas is a retroperitoneal structure that extends from the second part of the duodenum to the spleen (Fig. 20.1). The pancreatic duct, together with the common bile duct, enter the duodenum at the ampulla of Vater.

The pancreas has two distinct functions, exocrine and endocrine:

- Exocrine secretions include lipase, amylase, and proteases which are responsible for digestion of fat, carbohydrate, and protein, respectively. The enzymatic secretion is influenced by gut hormones, such as cholecystokinin, which are released when fatty acids and amino acids enter the duodenum.
- Endocrine secretions are insulin, glucagon, and somatostatin; hormones that are primarily involved in the regulation of glucose storage and use.

Acute pancreatitis

Incidence
A relatively common condition affecting approximately 1% of the general population.

Clinical features
These include:

- Severe epigastric pain that typically radiates to the back; sitting forward is sometimes said to provide some relief.
- Nausea and vomiting are invariably present.
- Tenderness and guarding, depending on severity.
- Tachycardia, tachypnoea, fever and shock may be manifest in severe cases.
- Abdominal wall discoloration, i.e. bruising around the umbilicus (Cullen's sign) or over flanks (Grey–Turner's sign) is rare. This reflects retroperitoneal haemorrhage that is likely to be due to a coagulopathy as a result of disseminated intravascular coagulation (DIC).

Beware of tachypnoea in a patient with acute pancreatitis; this may be a reflection of severe metabolic acidosis or a manifestation of ARDS.

Diagnosis and investigation
Investigations should be as those for an acute abdomen, as other conditions may mimic clinical signs and symptoms of acute pancreatitis.

In particular, consider the following tests:

- Serum amylase—>1000 units is usually diagnostic. A lipase assay, although less readily available, has a longer half-life and a greater specificity.
- Biochemistry—poor prognosis associated with high glucose, high urea, low calcium, and low albumin (Fig. 20.2).
- High white cell count and evidence of DIC suggested by low platelets, high prothrombin time and activated partial thromboplastin time, low fibrinogen and elevated D-Dimers.
- Arterial gases—hypoxia with metabolic acidosis in severe cases.
- Chest radiograph may demonstrate a reactive pleural effusion or bilateral infiltrates suggestive of adult respiratory distress syndrome (ARDS).
- The reported abdominal x-ray findings in acute pancreatitis are unreliable and not usually of diagnostic help.
- Ultrasound/computed tomography (CT) scans are not routinely done, except if there is diagnostic uncertainty. Swollen pancreas, ascites, and gallstones can be seen. Despite its unreliability in diagnostic terms ultrasound is recommended initially in all patients with acute pancreatitis. An early diagnosis of gallstones in a severe case may prompt the need for endoscopic retrograde cholangiopancreatography (ERCP) to be undertaken.

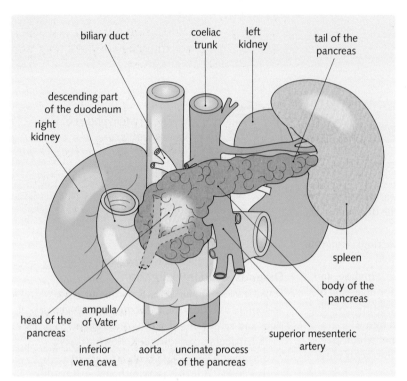

Fig. 20.1 The pancreas and its relations.

Poor prognostic criteria in pancreatitis	
Age	>55 years
White blood cell count	>15 x 10 9/L
Blood glucose	>10 mmol/L
Urea	>16 mmol/L
Albumin	<30 g/L
Calcium	<2 mmol/L
AST	>100 IU/L
LDH	>600 IU/L
PaO$_2$	<8 kPa

Three or more of these factors indicates a poor prognosis (Glasgow scoring system)

Fig. 20.2 Prognostic criteria of severity in pancreatitis.

Modest elevations in serum amylase levels (usually <1000) can be seen in a range of intra-abdominal conditions, such as acute cholecystitis, mesenteric infarction, perforated peptic ulcer.

Aetiology and pathogenesis

Exact mechanism is unclear, but is thought to be due to autodigestion by proteolytic enzymes in the pancreas, leading to self-perpetuating pancreatic inflammation with oedema in mild cases and haemorrhagic necrosis in severe cases.

The reflux of bile in the pancreatic duct may contribute to pathogenesis of acute pancreatitis in cases of pre-existing gallstones.

The causes of acute pancreatitis are listed in Fig. 20.3.

Causes of pancreatitis
Alcohol
Gallstones
Drugs, e.g. azathioprine, corticosteroids
Infections, e.g. mumps, coxsackie
Metabolic, e.g. hypercalcaemia, hyperlipidaemia
Iatrogenic, e.g. post-ERCP, postsurgical
Trauma
Scorpion bite

Fig. 20.3 Causes of pancreatitis.

Complications

Usually associated with a higher mortality, particularly if organ failure ensues.

Early:

- ARDS is a rare but severe complication of acute pancreatitis which requires artificial ventilation.
- Metabolic abnormalities such as hypocalcaemia and hyperglycaemia are commonly seen.
- Disseminated intravascular coagulation is often a life-threatening complication.
- Acute renal failure.
- Paralytic ileus is commonly seen.

Later:

- Pseudocysts can occur in up to half of patients seen with severe acute pancreatitis. Often no treatment is required because they are usually small and resolve spontaneously. A pseudocyst is a collection of pancreatic fluid in the lesser sac and has no epithelial lining.
- Pancreatic abscesses are due to infection of pancreatic pseudocysts or cysts within the pancreas following acute infection.
- Chronic pancreatitis occurs following repeated attacks of acute pancreatitis, especially secondary to alcohol.

Prognosis

A multifactor scoring system such as the modified Glasgow scoring system can be used to assess prognosis (Fig 20.2). The greater number of factors, the poorer the prognosis. The mortality rate reaches up to 60% in patients with severe pancreatitis and bad prognostic factors. However, in mild cases, mortality is low (<1%). Other scoring systems such as APACHE II can be applied, and levels of C-reactive protein have an independent prognostic value; see UK guidelines for the management of Acute Pancreatitis: Gut 1998; 42 (suppl 2).

Aims of treatment

This is to reduce the amount of proteolytic enzymes produced and hence autodigestion, which is achieved by 'resting' the bowel.

Treatment

Conservative management includes:

- Inspired oxygen to correct hypoxia.
- Restoration of haemodynamic stability with intravenous colloid, crystalloid and blood if required.
- Strict fluid balance monitoring; a urinary catheter is usually required.
- Correction of electrolyte imbalance: insulin may be required for hyperglycaemia.
- A nasogastric tube should be inserted, particularly if vomiting, and the patient should be 'nil by mouth'.
- Intravenous antibiotics should be reserved for proven bacteraemia or abscess formation.
- A central venous line may be indicated in severe cases, particularly if there is haemodynamic instability or a history of cardiac disease.
- Blood products such as fresh frozen plasma, cyroprecipitate and platelets may be indicated if there is bleeding with DIC.

In severe cases with systemic complications such as DIC, ARDS and renal failure, an intensive care setting is often required.

Surgery may be indicated to remove necrotic pancreatic tissue. Pseudocysts and abcesses can often be drained under radiological guidance.

Chronic pancreatitis

Clinical features

These include:

- Chronic epigastric/upper abdominal pain, usually radiating to back. Intermittent severe pain can be precipitated by heavy alcohol consumption, similar to that in acute pancreatitis.
- Steatorrhoea and malabsorption occurs due to reduction in pancreatic enzyme activity.
- Weight loss may be a prominent feature.
- Secondary diabetes mellitus due to destruction of Islet cells.
- Less common presentations include obstructive jaundice and cholangitis.

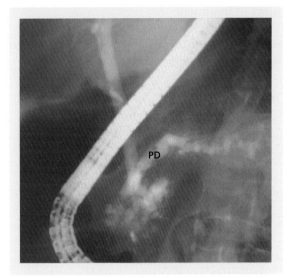

Fig. 20.4 Endoscopic retrograde cholangiopancreatography signs of chronic pancreatitis. The pancreatic duct (PD) is dilated and grossly distorted with ectatic side branches.

Diagnosis and investigation

Investigations should include:
- Serum amylase—not usually raised unless an acute attack is present on background of chronic disease (and can be normal even with an acute attack).
- Biochemistry—can show high serum glucose due to underlying diabetes.
- Deranged liver biochemistry often reflects high alcohol consumption.
- Abdominal X-ray—may reveal the characteristic appearance of pancreatic calcification.
- Abdominal CT—may demonstrate pancreatic swelling or pseudocyst formation.
- ERCP—demonstrates distorted and irregular pancreatic ducts indicative of fibrosis (Fig. 20.4).

Aetiology and pathogenesis

The majority of cases are due to high consumption of alcohol. Early changes are due to protein deposition along the pancreatic ducts which lead to duct dilatation. This is followed by acinar atrophy and fibrosis around pancreatic ducts. Calcification of protein plugs occurs.

Damage to the pancreas is long term, but cessation of alcohol intake may prevent further damage.

Rarer, but important, causes include cystic fibrosis, haemochromatosis and hyperparathyroidism.

Complications

Unfortunately, complications of chronic pancreatitis are common and include:
- Pain—a significant complication for many patients of whom some become dependent on opiates for pain relief.
- Malabsorption—due to reduced secretion of pancreatic lipases causing steatorrhoea and fat-soluble vitamin deficiencies.
- Diabetes—often requires insulin treatment as pancreatic function declines.
- Pseudocysts —these are commonly found on ultrasound and cause pain.
- Jaundice—rare, but can occur with ascending cholangitis.
- Portal hypertension occurs occasionally when the portal or splenic vein becomes thrombosed.

Prognosis

Depends on whether the patient is abstaining from alcohol, and in the majority of cases, complete abstinence is rare.

In some patients, there are continuing intermittent attacks of acute pancreatitis on a background of chronic pancreatitis. This is known as chronic relapsing pancreatitis.

Treatment

Stop drinking alcohol!

Other treatment options include:
- Pain control usually in some form of opiates with its problem of addiction.
- Pancreatic enzyme supplements (lipase) are given to improve fat absorption and fat-soluble vitamins.
- Oral hypoglycaemic agents or insulin may be required.
- Surgery, if required, involves removal of pancreatic duct stones with partial pancreatectomy and drainage of ducts into the small bowel. Occasionally, a total pancreatectomy is done. Good result from surgery is variable.
- Coeliac ganglion blockade can provide permanent pain relief, but has no effect on continuing inflammation.

Pseudocysts

Incidence
Seen following an attack of moderate to severe acute pancreatitis in over 50% of cases. True cysts are those occurring within the pancreas and pseudocysts are those without an epithelial lining, consisting of a collection containing inflammatory fluid and pancreatic enzyme within the lesser sac. They are far more common than true cysts.

Multiple small cysts can also be seen in the pancreas with polycystic disease involving the kidney and liver. This is inherited as an autosomal dominant condition, and the pathology is quite different to that following acute pancreatitis and a more detailed text should be consulted.

Clinical features
Main features are:
- Abdominal pain—particularly if the pseudocyst is large, together with nausea and vomiting mimicking unresolved acute pancreatitis.
- An epigastric mass may be palpable (the cyst will make the aorta more palpable and occasionally is mistaken for an aortic aneurysm).
- Ascites—these can occur due to rupture of the cyst within the peritoneal cavity. Ascitic fluid will have a high concentration of amylase.

Diagnosis and investigation
Persistence or recurrence of symptoms following an episode of acute pancreatitis should alert one to the suspicion of pseudocyst formation (Fig. 20.5).

Ultrasound is the investigation of choice, and small cysts are frequently seen in asymptomatic patients.

Aetiology and pathogenesis
Thought to be due to inflammatory exudate produced by the inflamed pancreas collected in the lesser sac. High levels of pancreatic enzyme found in the fluid may indicate extensive damage to the pancreas, causing secretions to leak out. They are more commonly found in severe and chronic pancreatitis.

Complications
Pancreatic abscess is due to infection of the cyst, which can occur spontaneously or as a consequence of repeated aspiration.

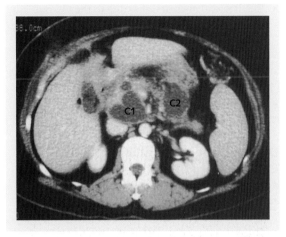

Fig. 20.5 Computed tomography scan of pancreatic pseudocyst. A heart-shaped cyst (C1) is seen in the head of the pancreas and a second cyst (C2) is seen near the tail.

Prognosis
Dependent on underlying pathology. Prognosis is poor if pseudocyst is secondary to alcohol-induced chronic pancreatitis, whereas it is excellent if the pancreatitis is due to a treatable cause (e.g. gallstones).

Treatment
No treatment is required for small asymptomatic pseudocysts, as they usually resolve spontaneously.
Therapeutic manoeuvres include:
- Aspiration of cyst—usually carried out under ultrasound guidance and may need to be repeated.
- Surgery if persistent; the cyst can be 'marsupialized' such that fluid will drain into the stomach.

Cystic fibrosis

Incidence
Affects 1 in 2500 live births.

Clinical features
These include:
- Recurrent chest infections—usually the presenting feature in childhood.
- Pancreatic insufficiency leading to diabetes, steatorrhoea, and failure to thrive despite a good appetite.

- Small bowel obstruction—due to the viscous secretions. Neonates may present with meconium ileus.
- Infertility—females are more likely to conceive. Males are invariably infertile. Delayed puberty is seen in most patients.
- Liver cirrhosis seen in patients who survive into adulthood.

Diagnosis and investigation
Consider the following:
- Sweat test reveals a high sodium concentration.
- Genetic analysis for the recessive gene and the identification of cystic fibrosis protein.
- Pancreatic function tests (e.g. PABA test) (see p. 198).
- CXR may demonstrate bronchiectatic changes; spirometry and sputum culture should also be performed.

Aetiology and pathogenesis
Due to a gene mutation on the long arm of chromosome 7, resulting in an abnormality of a transmembrane protein known as cystic fibrosis transmembrane conductance regulator, which results in production of thick viscous secretions (high in salt, low in water) due to reduced chloride transport.

Complications
The main complications include malabsorption, especially of fat-soluble vitamins, and bronchiectasis and pneumothorax, which are common. Infertility and liver disease occur in adults. Death is usually due to respiratory failure.

Prognosis
The median survival is 30 years, with many affected adults in active employment. Persistent respiratory colonization with *Pseudomonas* conveys a poorer prognosis.

Treatment
Treatment of chest infections includes intensive physiotherapy and appropriate antibiotic therapy. A recombinant nebulized DNAse aids in reducing sputum viscosity. Also:
- Enzyme supplements (capsules containing trypsin and lipases, which break down in the duodenum delivering the enzyme).
- Immunizations.
- Vitamin supplements and high calorie intake.

- Gene therapy has been attempted but early results are disappointing so far.
- Lung transplant is considered in some patients.

Carcinoma of pancreas

Incidence
Increases with increasing age and most patients are over 60 years. It is the fourth most common cancer in the UK. More common in males than females.

Clinical features
Signs and symptoms include:
- Weight loss can be dramatic.
- Persistent abdominal pain is a common feature usually radiating through to the back and tends to be relieved by sitting forward.
- Jaundice is usually the presenting feature of carcinoma affecting the head of pancreas. Jaundice is obstructive and progressive and is characteristically painless in the early stages.
- Diabetes is thought to be due to insulin resistance, caused by hormones secreted by pancreatic beta cells rather than its destruction.
- Thrombophlebitis migrans is a skin manifestation due to a paraneoplastic phenomenon.
- Ascites occurs in the late stages with hepatomegaly due to liver metastases.

Figure 20.6 shows the sites at which pancreatic tumours occur.

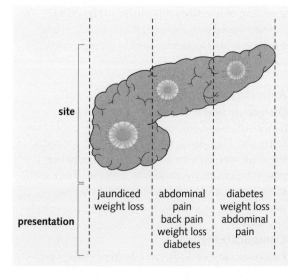

Fig. 20.6 Anatomical sites for pancreatic tumours.

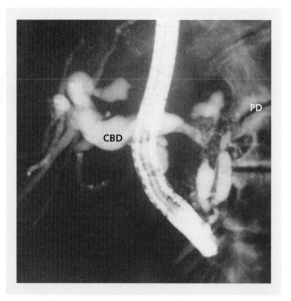

Fig. 20.7 Endoscopic retrograde cholangiopancreatography showing 'double duct stricture' (arrows) in pancreatic carcinoma. (CBD, common bile duct; PD, pancreatic duct.) Note incidental scoliosis and vertebral collapse.

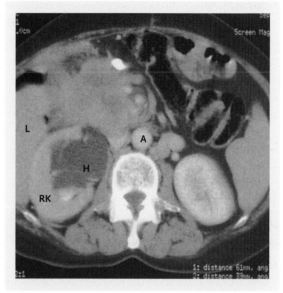

Fig. 20.8 Computed tomography scan of pancreatic tumour (arrows) obstructing the right ureter and causing hydronephrosis (H). (A, aorta; L, liver; RK, right kidney.)

Courvoisier's sign—in the case of painless obstructive jaundice, a palpable gall bladder suggests cancer because a dilated gall bladder is not found with gallstone disease as the stones induce a fibrotic reaction in the gall bladder which then shrinks down.

Diagnosis and investigation

Investigations may include:
- ERCP, as part of an investigation for obstructive jaundice, will usually be diagnostic especially of periampullary tumours (Fig. 20.7).
- CT of the abdomen will diagnose most pancreatic tumours, and it is ideally confirmed by biopsy. It will also demonstrate nodal spread at the porta hepatis (Fig. 20.8).
- Ultrasound is less sensitive at detecting pancreatic tumours, especially those along the body or the tail of pancreas.

Aetiology and pathogenesis

The aetiology is unknown but smoking and high alcohol consumption have been implicated. The role of chronic pancreatitis as a risk factor is uncertain as familial chronic pancreatitis is associated with a significantly increased risk of cancer.

Almost all tumours are due to adenocarcinoma arising from the duct epithelium and around 70% are in the head of the pancreas. The tumours have usually already metastasized to local lymph nodes and the liver by the time of presentation.

Prognosis

Very poor due to its late presentation. The 5-year survival is <5%.

Aims of treatment

This is mainly for palliation because curative treatment is unlikely to be successful due to the nature of the disease.

Treatment

Options include:
- Radical surgical resection provides the only possible chance of a cure, but it is seldom carried out, as most patients are unsuitable for surgery and it carries a high mortality rate. A by-pass operation

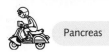

for the relief of jaundice can be performed where the common bile duct is anastomosed to the small bowel as a palliative measure.

- Stent insertion can be achieved endoscopically where a stent is inserted into the narrowed part of the common bile duct to allow free drainage of bile (see Fig. 24.20).
- Analgesia in the form of opiates are indicated, as dependence is not an issue.
- Coeliac axis block may be useful for patients with pain that is not controlled by conventional analgesia.

Endocrine tumours

Incidence
These are rare tumours in the pancreas and can occur with tumours of the pituitary and parathyroid to form a syndrome of multiple endocrine neoplasia (MEN).

Clinical features
Depends on the cell type and the hormone produced.

Gastrinomas (Zollinger–Ellison syndrome)
These arise from the G-cells of the pancreas and they secrete gastrin and present as peptic ulceration which is often large and multiple. Perforation and gastrointestinal haemorrhage is common and diagnosis should be considered in young patients presenting with recurrent peptic ulcer disease.

Diarrhoea due to excess acid production is also common (low pH).

Insulinomas (Islet cell tumours)
Produce insulin and present as episodes of fasting hypoglycaemia (i.e. early morning or late afternoons).

Presentation is often bizarre, hence diagnosis may not be made for years and the patient learns to live with the symptoms, as glucose abolishes the attacks.

Vipomas
This is a rare pancreatic tumour in which vasoactive intestinal peptide is produced causing severe secretory diarrhoea, leading to dehydration by stimulating adenyl cyclase to produce intestinal secretions.

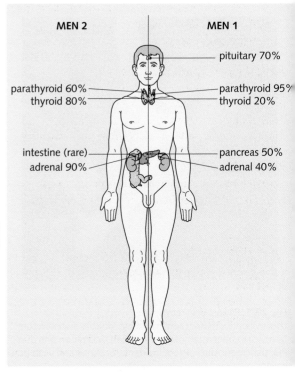

Fig. 20.9 Depiction of multiple endocrine neoplasia I and multiple endocrine neoplasia 2.

Glucagonomas
Tumour of alpha cells that produce glucagon in patients with diabetes mellitus. A characteristic rash (necrolytic migratory erythema) has also been described.

Somatostatinomas
Somatostatin is an inhibitory hormone that produces a reduction in the secretion of insulin, pancreatic enzyme, and bicarbonate, hence produces the clinical syndrome of diabetes mellitus, steatorrhoea, and hypochlorhydria.

Weight loss is also a common feature.

Diagnosis and investigation
This again is dependent on the type of tumour involved and the clinical presentation:

- A CT scan will identify the majority of endocrine tumours in the pancreas.
- Hormone assays—measurement of the specific type of hormone produced will often give the diagnosis. Selective venous sampling from the pancreas will also help to locate the tumour. In cases

of insulinoma, measurement is usually made during a 24–48-hour fast when symptoms of hypoglycaemia appear.

Aetiology and pathogenesis
The tumours arise from the APUD cells (amine precursor uptake and decarboxylation), hence their hormonal secretory nature. The MEN type 2 syndrome has an autosomal dominant inheritance.

Prognosis
Gastrinomas are often malignant, hence carry a worse prognosis than insulinoma, which is benign.

Overall prognosis will depend on associated MEN syndrome and other tumours involved.

Treatment
Surgical resection of the tumour is required.

Identification of other possible tumours associated with MEN syndrome may be required, and screening of relatives in those with MEN type 2 syndrome (Fig. 20.9).

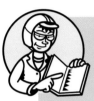

- Describe the functions of the pancreas.
- How would you manage a patient in the first few hours following an episode of acute pancreatitis?
- What are the factors indicating a poor outcome in the context of acute pancreatitis?
- What are the systemic complications of acute pancreatitis?
- What investigations would you undertake in the investigation of suspected chronic pancreatitis?
- What is Courvoisier's 'law'?
- What is the genetic abnormality described in cystic fibrosis?

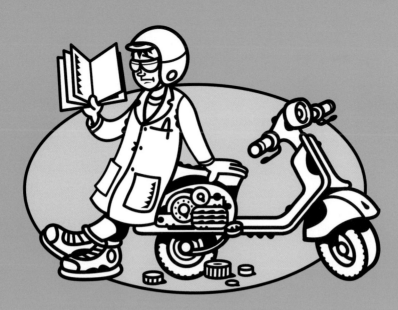

HISTORY, EXAMINATION, AND COMMON INVESTIGATIONS

21. Taking a History

Preliminaries
Introduce yourself, be polite, listen carefully, and look interested, even if you have been up all night!

Give patients the time and the opportunity to tell you what you need to know and put them at their ease as many symptoms are embarrassing.

Maintain eye contact (even if patients do not) and watch carefully for clues on how ill they look. Are they agitated, distressed, or in pain? Is there a discernible tremor or involuntary movement? Is there evidence of significant weight loss (cachexia)? Do they have a pale, pigmented, or jaundiced complexion?

Look around the bedside for clues (e.g. inhalers, oxygen, a walking stick or frame, cards from family and friends, sputum pots, reading material and glasses, special food preparations, etc.).

The purpose of taking a history is to arrive at a differential diagnosis. Some information is background and may not be immediately obvious or useful, but can often be vital later on.

The standard structure of a history

It is important to maintain a structured approach to your history taking, particularly in the early stages of your career. You are less likely to omit relevant questions if your history is structured. It is preferable to commit the format to memory, and acquire the relevant information in conversational form, so that constant reference to notes is avoided during the interaction.

Description of the patient
This should include brief demographic details, including the patient's age, sex, ethnic origins, and occupation. It should allow others who have not met the patient to picture him or her in their mind.

Presenting complaint
What prompted the patient to seek help? This will usually be a specific or particular symptom, but may be difficult to identify immediately. Your task is to focus on the symptoms and crystallize them into problems that can be addressed.

Note down the sites of pain (Fig. 21.1).

History of presenting complaint
This is a complete description of the problem that brought the patient to see you, including:
- How and when the symptoms started.
- The speed of onset—was it rapid, or slow and insidious?
- The pattern of symptoms, their duration and frequency—are they continuous or intermittent? How often do they appear?
- If the symptoms include pain, you should describe it comprehensively! Relevant features are onset, site, severity, character (sharp, crushing, gnawing, etc.), radiation, frequency, periodicity, associated features, precipitating and relieving factors, relationship to meals, posture, and alcohol.
- Why has the patient decided to consult the doctor at this juncture? What is different?
- Find out the extent of any deficit. Is there any loss of function, anything specific the patient cannot do or any impact on their lifestyle?
- Is there anything else the patient thinks may be relevant, however trivial?

Past medical history
Has the patient had any medical or surgical contact in the past? Ask specifically about operations, previous transfusions, drugs, especially antibiotics, allergies, and previous investigations.

Obstetric and menstrual history should also be recorded.

Drug history
Ask about all drugs, including contraceptive pills and over-the-counter medicines, as well as medicines that have been prescribed.

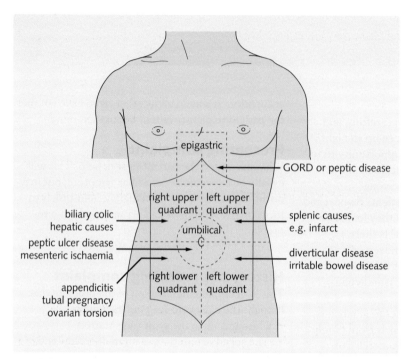

Fig. 21.1 Sites of pain and possible significance.

epigastric

GORD or peptic disease

right upper quadrant | left upper quadrant

biliary colic hepatic causes

umbilical

splenic causes, e.g. infarct

peptic ulcer disease mesenteric ischaemia

diverticular disease irritable bowel disease

right lower quadrant | left lower quadrant

appendicitis tubal pregnancy ovarian torsion

Non-steroidal anti-inflammatory drugs are commonly taken as over-the-counter medicines and can cause ulcers.

It may be necessary to contact family members or the General Practitioner to establish an accurate list of the patient's current prescribed therapy.

It is common for patient to profess to having a drug allergy, when in fact an adverse side-effect has occurred (e.g. diarrhoea after taking penicillin), or dyspepsia with aspirin. It is important to establish whether they are truly allergic to a particular drug, as you may be denying them the best treatment. However, you must not prescribe anything they say they are allergic to, unless you are confident they are not!

Family history

Ask about the cause, and age, of death of close relatives, especially parents and siblings. Practise drawing quick sketches of family trees (Fig. 21.2). Is there a specific family history pertinent to the suspected diagnosis?

Social history

The purpose of this assessment is to see the patient in the context of their environment and gain some

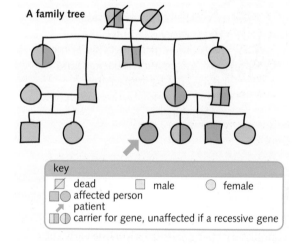

A family tree

key
- ▨ dead
- ■ male
- ○ female
- ■○ affected person
- ↗ patient
- ▥◑ carrier for gene, unaffected if a recessive gene

Fig. 21.2 Example of Mendelian recessive inheritence depicted in a family tree. Arrow indicates the propositus, or individual who brought the pedigree to notice.

idea of how the illness affects this particular patient, what support the patient has and whether he or she can reduce any health risks.

It should include information about the patient's
- Marital status.
- Children and other dependants.

Fig. 21.3 Alcohol measures and recommended limits. Try to work out the units of alcohol for yourself. One unit of alcohol is in fact 8 g, but when working out measures it is rounded up to 10 g to simplify the calculations.

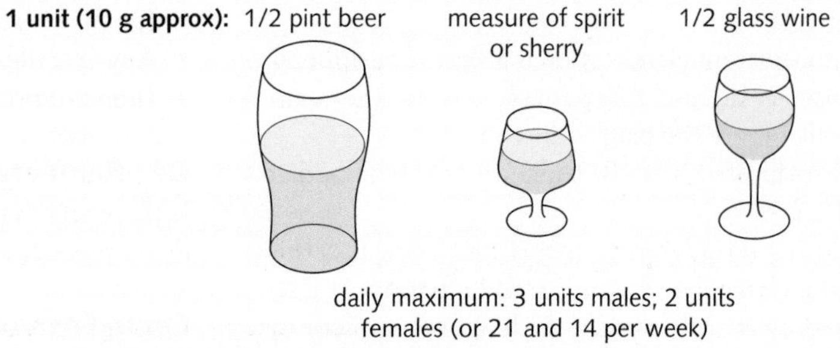

1 unit (10 g approx): 1/2 pint beer   measure of spirit or sherry   1/2 glass wine

daily maximum: 3 units males; 2 units females (or 21 and 14 per week)

- beer contains approximately 5% alcohol (i.e. 5 g/100 ml), i.e. 250 ml or 1/2 pint is 1 unit
- wine is usually about 12% alcohol: 750 ml standard bottle is 9 units, 1 unit per 1/2 glass
- spirits are often 40% alcohol: 25 ml measure is 1 unit

- Occupational history (including previous occupations)—this is especially relevant regarding exposure to toxins, musculoskeletal disorders, and psychiatry.
- Hobbies that may result in exposure to toxins or other risk.
- Accommodation: put yourself in the patient's position. Will he or she be able to cope at home? Are there stairs, lifts, bath, shower, etc.?
- Diet—is it adequate? High cholesterol? Vegetarian?
- Exercise—does he or she take any? Is it appropriate?

Is there any risk behaviour?
Consider the following:
- Ask about alcohol—record as units per day or week (Fig. 21.3).
- Ask about smoking—this is best described in terms of the number of 'pack-years', whereby 20 cigarettes smoked each day for 1 year is termed '1 pack year'. (40 cigarettes a day for three years would equate to 'six pack years'.)
- Be tactful but thorough in asking about illicit or recreational drug use.
- Industrial toxins are important in claims for compensation (e.g. asbestos).
- A history of travel to certain regions of the world may be relevant.
- In addition to occupation or hobby, exposure to animals can be important.
- Sexual practice or orientation may be important for some conditions.

Review of symptoms (functional enquiry)
The purpose of this review is to go through the organ systems logically and ensure nothing is forgotten. In addition, it often gives information into the cause or effect of the presenting complaint.

This can be very brief and some of the important questions to ask are listed. If the patient has any of these problems, clearly it is important to take a relevant extended history.

Gastrointestinal tract
Ask about:
- Abdominal pain.
- Indigestion.
- Nausea and vomiting.
- Heartburn.
- Dysphagia.
- Haematemesis and melaena.
- Jaundice.
- Abdominal swelling.
- Change of bowel habit.
- Diarrhoea.
- Rectal bleeding or pain.
- Weight loss.

(For a full discussion of these symptoms, refer to Part I.)

Cardiovascular system
Ask about chest pain:
- Related to exertion or posture.
- Relieved by rest.

- Are there any palpitations or postural syncopal attacks?
- Intermittent claudication is a sign of peripheral vascular disease. Ask patients how far they can walk before the pain comes on.
- Breathlessness can be a manifestation of cardiac disease.
- Orthopnoea refers to the patient being breathless when lying flat. This is due to increased hydrostatic pressure in the lungs consequent upon left ventricular dysfunction. It is usually measured in terms of the number of pillows required for sleeping. However, it is important to clarify why the patient uses several pillows—it may just be for a bad back!
- Paroxysmal nocturnal dyspnoea—the patient wakes up from the lying down position gasping for air for reasons similar to those for orthopnoea.

Respiratory system

Any chest pain? Is it 'pleuritic' or related to phases of respiration? Has there been any wheeze, cough, or haemoptysis? If there is sputum, enquire about colour, nature, and amount.

Endocrine and reproductive system

Has there been:
- Any polyuria or polydipsia (indicative of diabetes, hypercalcaemia)?
- Any heat or cold intolerance with mood change and/or weight change (suggestive of thyroid disease)?

- Any fatigue with pigmentation and dizzy spells (possibly Addison's disease)?
- Any erectile/fertility (male) or menstrual/fertility (female) problems?

Genitourinary tract

Is there any dysuria, nocturia, hesitancy, dribbling or incontinence, urethral discharge?

Central nervous system

Is there history of specific symptoms, such as:
- Headache?
- Speech or visual disturbance?
- Dizzy spells?
- Fits or blackouts?
- Loss of power or sensation in any area?

Joints

Has there been pain or swelling in any joint, or any back pain?

Skin

Is there a skin rash, itchiness (pruritus), or lumps or bumps?

Try to formulate an impression or differential diagnosis based on the history before proceeding to examination. You may be able to anticipate abnormal physical signs.

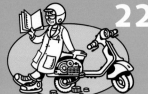

22. Examination of the Patient

The purpose of the clinical examination is to find evidence in support of or against the differential diagnosis you are considering after taking the history. It should be thorough enough so as not to miss other possibilities that you had not considered and to consider causes and effects of each putative diagnosis.

Examination preliminaries

The main purpose of a general inspection is to determine how ill the patient is. Bear this in mind as you introduce yourself and take a history; if the patient is very ill, do not waste valuable time asking questions that can wait until later.

During the examination:

- Look at the patient's facial expression: is he or she comfortable, in obvious distress, looking furtive, receptive, hostile?
- Assess the patient's body posture and mobility, and his or her weight and size.
- Consider whether he or she is appropriately dressed and behaving appropriately in the circumstances.

Many diseases and conditions do not have a direct effect on the gut. However, always remember that the patient may be receiving medication for a pre-existing condition, and this may affect the dose of drug you are intending to give for his or her gastrointestinal (GI) condition (e.g. the patient may already be receiving enzyme-inducing drugs for another condition). Current medication may even be producing the gut symptoms (e.g. diarrhoea caused by antibiotic therapy).

The following examination primer is orientated for GI disorders and is not comprehensive. You should read the relevant system in Crash Course for other disorders.

Face

The face can be a mine of information. Some 'facies' are pathognomonic of certain conditions (e.g. dystrophia myotonica, Graves' disease, and acromegaly), and have a peculiar habit of appearing in clinical examinations. Here, we concentrate on the facial signs of GI disease.

General inspection

Ask yourself the following questions:

- Are there any signs of mania or psychosis (possibly related to steroids, systemic lupus erythematosus, Wilson's disease, porphyria)?
- Is the patient agitated and not just anxious to see you (possible sign of hyperthyroidism, alcohol withdrawal)?
- Is the general appearance unkempt or neglected (e.g. due to alcohol or depression)?
- Is there excessive skin hair (hypertrichosis can occur with excess steroids, ciclosporin, or minoxidil)?
- What is the skin's colour and its relevance (Fig. 22.1)?

Are there specific skin lesions suggestive of a particular disorder (Fig. 22.2), such as:

- Dermatitis herpetiformis (coeliac).
- Psoriasis (colitis, sometimes liver disease).
- Eczema (atopy).
- Telangiectasia (CREST—calcinosis cutis, Raynaud's phenomenon, oesophageal stricture or dysmotility, scleroderma, telangiectasia).
- Spider naevi (liver disease).
- Erythema nodosum (inflammatory bowel disease, tuberculosis).
- Pyoderma gangrenosum (ulcerative colitis).

Specific examination

Examine the face specifically for particular signs indicative of disease (Fig. 22.3).

181

Pigmentation of the skin and its significance in gastroenterology	
Colour	**Possible significance**
Yellow	Jaundice, carotenaemia
Grey	Haemochromatosis
Brown	Addison's
Dusky	Primary biliary cirrhosis, renal failure
Blue	Cyanosis (cardiac, respiratory)
Red	Plethora, carcinoid flush
Blotchy	Vitiligo

Fig. 22.1 Pigmentation of the skin and its significance in gastroenterology.

Hands

Examine the hands for particular signs indicative of GI-related disease (Figs 22.4 and 22.5).

Take the pulse, blood pressure, and feel the palms for temperature.

Find out whether there is:
- Any tremor: is it coarse or fine? Does it disappear with voluntary intent?
- A flap indicative of liver failure or CO_2 retention.

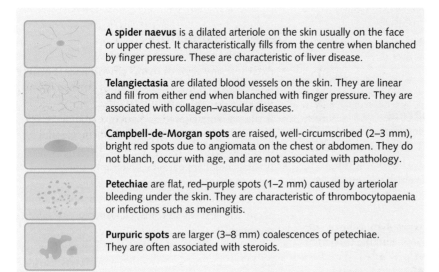

A spider naevus is a dilated arteriole on the skin usually on the face or upper chest. It characteristically fills from the centre when blanched by finger pressure. These are characteristic of liver disease.

Telangiectasia are dilated blood vessels on the skin. They are linear and fill from either end when blanched with finger pressure. They are associated with collagen–vascular diseases.

Campbell-de-Morgan spots are raised, well-circumscribed (2–3 mm), bright red spots due to angiomata on the chest or abdomen. They do not blanch, occur with age, and are not associated with pathology.

Petechiae are flat, red–purple spots (1–2 mm) caused by arteriolar bleeding under the skin. They are characteristic of thrombocytopaenia or infections such as meningitis.

Purpuric spots are larger (3–8 mm) coalescences of petechiae. They are often associated with steroids.

Fig. 22.2 Definitions of common skin lesions found in gastrointestinal examination.

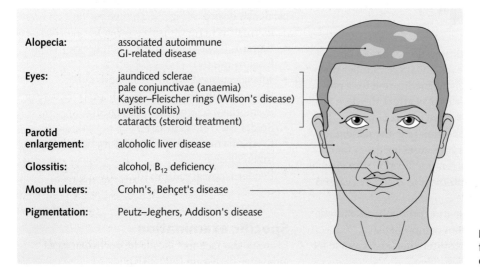

Alopecia:	associated autoimmune GI-related disease
Eyes:	jaundiced sclerae pale conjunctivae (anaemia) Kayser–Fleischer rings (Wilson's disease) uveitis (colitis) cataracts (steroid treatment)
Parotid enlargement:	alcoholic liver disease
Glossitis:	alcohol, B_{12} deficiency
Mouth ulcers:	Crohn's, Behçet's disease
Pigmentation:	Peutz–Jeghers, Addison's disease

Fig. 22.3 Specific facial features of disease.

Fig. 22.4 Clinical signs in the hands indicative of disease.

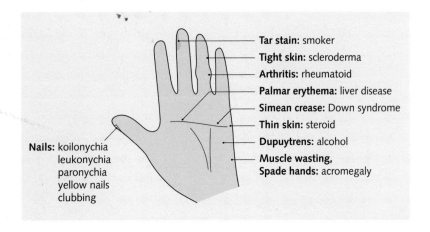

Tar stain: smoker
Tight skin: scleroderma
Arthritis: rheumatoid
Palmar erythema: liver disease
Simean crease: Down syndrome
Thin skin: steroid
Dupuytrens: alcohol
Muscle wasting,
Spade hands: acromegaly

Nails: koilonychia
leukonychia
paronychia
yellow nails
clubbing

Causes of clubbing of the nails		
GI causes	**Cardiac causes**	**Respiratory causes**
cirrhosis coeliac disease Crohn's disease ulcerative colitis	bacterial endocarditis congenital cyanotic heart disease atrial myxoma	fibrosing alveolitis suppurative disease (bronchiectasis, empyema) mesothelioma bronchial carcinoma

Fig. 22.5 Causes of clubbing of the nails.

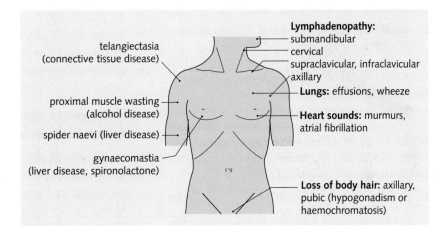

Lymphadenopathy:
submandibular
cervical
supraclavicular, infraclavicular
axillary
Lungs: effusions, wheeze
Heart sounds: murmurs,
atrial fibrillation

telangiectasia
(connective tissue disease)

proximal muscle wasting
(alcohol disease)

spider naevi (liver disease)

gynaecomastia
(liver disease, spironolactone)

Loss of body hair: axillary,
pubic (hypogonadism or
haemochromatosis)

Fig. 22.6 Signs relating to gastrointestinal pathology to be sought in upper torso.

Neck, thorax, and upper limbs

Examine the neck and upper chest together looking for signs of:
• Liver disease.
• Portal hypertension.
• Cardiac failure (Jugular venous pressure).

• Metastatic disease.
• Systemic disease (e.g. endocrine) that may produce GI symptoms (Fig. 22.6).

Inspect and palpate the neck, supra- and infraclavicular fossae, and axillae for lymph nodes indicative of metastatic disease or lymphoma.

183

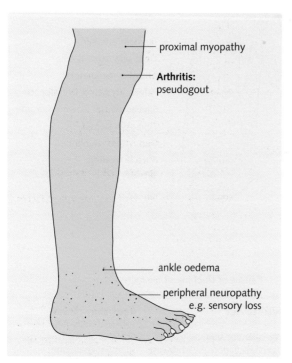

Fig. 22.7 Signs of gastrointestinal disease in the legs.

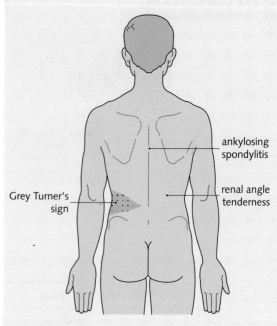

Fig. 22.8 Examine the back for signs of intra-abdominal pathology.

Lower limb

Proximal myopathy may be a sign of generalized debility or due to biochemical pathology (e.g. alcoholism, diabetes or hyperthyroidism). Steroids used for chronic inflammatory disease such as colitis may produce proximal muscle weakness.

A patient with arthritis may be taking medication that can cause GI problems (e.g. non-steroidal anti-inflammatory drugs cause gastritis and gastric erosions). Conversely, the arthritis may be an extra-intestinal manifestation of GI pathology (e.g. arthritis of colitis or chondrocalcinosis associated with haemochromatosis).

Ankle oedema can be due to hypoalbuminaemia from liver cirrhosis or chronic diarrhoea (e.g. coeliac disease).

Fig. 22.7 shows a summary of the signs of GI disease in the legs.

Back

Do not forget to examine the patient's back (Fig. 22.8):

- Are there structural bone problems such as ankylosing spondylitis (associated with colitis) or kyphoscoliosis?
- Tender renal angles from pyelonephritis may be an explanation for abdominal pain. Haemorrhagic pancreatitis may manifest as haematoma in the flanks or back (Grey–Turner's sign).

Abdominal examination

Warm your hands before you start or you may produce reflex guarding. Stand at the end of the bed and inspect the abdomen. Ask the patient to lift their head up from the pillow. This simple manoeuvre involves the abdominal wall muscles and can provide useful information: it may accentuate or reveal abdominal masses, organomegaly or asymmetry; and a patient with peritonitis will not be able to do it! Inspect for:

- Asymmetry
- Lumps and bumps
- Pulsation
- Peristalsis
- Scars
- Distension

Fig. 22.9 Examination of the abdomen—expected normal findings.

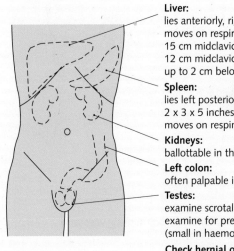

Liver:
lies anteriorly, right upper quadrant
moves on respiration
15 cm midclavicular line (male)
12 cm midclavicular line (female)
up to 2 cm below costal margin is common

Spleen:
lies left posteriorly, normally impalpable
2 x 3 x 5 inches, 7 ozs, under ribs 9–11
moves on respiration

Kidneys:
ballottable in thin people, listen for renal bruits

Left colon:
often palpable in left iliac fossa, can indent faeces

Testes:
examine scrotal sac
examine for presence and size
(small in haemochromatosis)

Check hernial orifices:
umbilical, inguinal, femoral, scrotal

Now move on to palpation. Position yourself at an appropriate level to the abdomen but maintain a steady posture. Adopting a kneeling position is often best, but make sure you check the floor surface first! During palpation it is helpful to form a visual map in your mind of normal intra-abdominal anatomy. Some abdominal organs may be just palpable in thin, normal subjects. Be systematic in your approach, palpating each contiguous area in turn.

Use superficial palpation initially to detect tenderness or guarding. Your hand should simply rest on the abdominal surface, and employ a gentle flexing action at the metacarpal-phalangeal joints. Follow with deep palpation, using a similar technique, to detect organomegaly and masses. Do not hurt the patient, watch their face! If you detect a mass, you need to be able to provide an accurate description. Note its position, size, shape, upper and lower borders, whether it is ballotable. Is it tender, hard, smooth or irregular? To determine whether it is pulsatile, lay your hand still for several seconds. Does it move with respiration?

Following systematic superficial and deep palpation of the abdomen, specifically seek evidence of hepatomegaly or splenomegaly. Begin palpation in the right iliac fossa, as both these organs can enlarge to this extent. Use the lateral border of your hand/forefinger and palpate in a parallel fashion, toward the right or left upper quadrant for the liver and spleen respectively. For each palpation, the patient should inspire and exhale as you press. You may feel the edge of the enlarged organ 'meet' your hand during inspiration. Now attempt to 'ballot' the kidneys. For each kidney in turn, slide one hand under the loin area whilst firmly pressing over the kidney with your other hand. The hand underneath should attempt to 'bounce' the kidney upward, whilst the other hand should remain still, and attempt to feel any abnormality.

Percussion is useful to confirm enlargement of liver, spleen, or distended bladder if present. This is performed in the usual way and a dull note signifies a solid viscera or fluid collection beneath. Always percuss beyond both the upper and lower borders of the mass; remember that the liver can be 'pushed down' by hyperinflated lungs and appear enlarged, unless the upper border is determined by percussion. Percussion is also discriminatory if the abdomen is distended, to differentiate fluid (dull) from air (tympanitic).

You must know how to check for:
• Shifting dullness (dull percussion note becomes resonant when you roll the patient and gravity shifts the fluid).
• A fluid thrill (this can transmit 'tapping' from one side of the abdomen to the other).

Listen for bowel sounds and bruits. Accentuated auscultation (listening with stethoscope over solid structure while lightly scratching over organ edge) can also be used to confirm liver or spleen enlargement.

Check inguinal, scrotal, and umbilical hernial orifices, particularly in the scenario of intestinal obstruction.

Expected normal findings on examination of the abdomen are shown in Fig. 22.9.

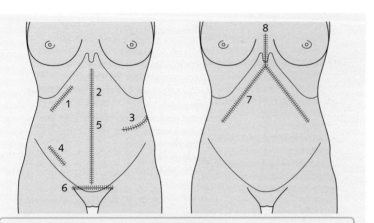

Fig. 22.10 Illustration of common abdominal surgical scars and their possible significance.

1. Kocher's incision commonly for cholecystectomy
2. Upper midline incision commonly for peptic ulcer surgery: vagotomy, pyloroplasty, oversewn DU, gastrectomy
3. Lateral loin scar often for nephrectomy
4. Short scar in right iliac fossa for appendicectomy
5. Lower midline scar for colonic resection, laparotomy, caesarean section
6. Pfannensteil's incision for caesarian section
7. 'Rooftop' scar common for pancreatectomy or liver resection
8. 'Mercedes' scar is an upper extension of 'rooftop' to enable access to the IVC required in liver resection or transplantation

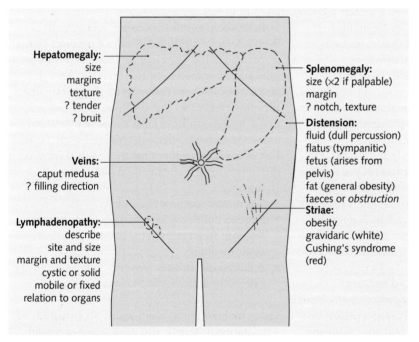

Fig. 22.11 Characterization of abnormal abdominal findings.

The abnormal abdomen

Inspect the abdomen for scars—you need to be aware of their possible significance as, occasionally, the patient is not (Fig. 22.10). Any abnormality detected should be characterized carefully; establish whether an organ is involved and evaluate the nature of the mass. Does it move with respiration?

Masses or organomegaly in particular should be measured (cm) and commented on as in Fig. 22.11. Causes of common abdominal masses are listed in Fig. 22.12.

Fig. 22.12 Causes of common abdominal masses. (CML, chronic myeloid leukaemia; CMV, cytomegalovirus; EBV, Epstein–Barr virus; PA, pernicious anaemia; PBC, primary biliary cirrhosis; TB, tuberculosis).

Causes of abdominal masses		
Right iliac fossa mass	**Hepatomegaly**	**Splenomegaly**
Appendix abscess	Cirrhosis (PBC)	Portal hypertension
Ectopic pregnancy	Metastases/neoplasia	Myelofibrosis or CML
Crohn's mass	Hepatitis	Lymphoma
Ileocaecal TB	Alcoholic liver disease	CMV or EBV
Ovarian tumour/tubal	Congestion	mononucleosis
pregnancy	(Budd–Chiari)	Anaemia: sickle cell, PA
Carcinoma caecum	Storage disorders	Storage: Gaucher's
Carcinoid tumour	Riedel's lobe	
Amoebic abscess		

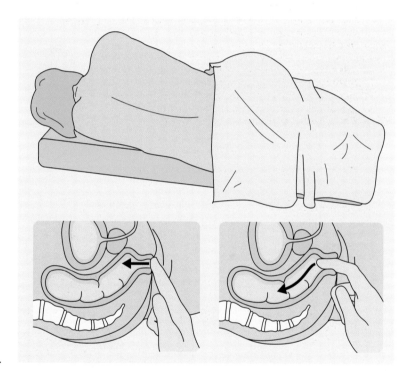

Fig. 22.13 Rectal examination technique: press gently on the anal margin with the pulp of your forefinger and gently rotate inwards.

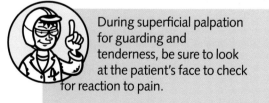

During superficial palpation for guarding and tenderness, be sure to look at the patient's face to check for reaction to pain.

Rectal examination

This is a very important part of GI examination, but must be carried out properly or is not worth doing. Clearly, there are sensitive issues of modesty and cultural code of which you need to be aware. Examination of a patient without consent may constitute an assault, and the more intimate examinations can be an area where failure to communicate your intention can produce difficulties.

Preparation:
- Make sure the patient understands what you want to do and why (consent).
- Have a chaperone or assistant present (same sex as patient if possible).
- Position patient in left lateral fetal position (bottom over edge of couch).
- Use xylocaine or KY jelly on gloved hand.

Rectal examination technique

Inspect the anus for:

- Excoriation (pruritus ani).
- Tags (associated with colitis).
- External haemorrhoids.
- Fistulae (associated with Crohn's disease).

Press gently on the anal orifice with the pulp of your index fingertip and flex the finger through anal canal (Fig. 22.13). Gauge the sphincter tone: if necessary ask patient to squeeze.

Rotate your finger to feel the prostate or uterus anteriorly, the rectal mucosa all around, and assess the consistency of any stool present.

Look at the glove stain for blood or mucus.

Ancillary examinations are often available in clinic to help with diagnosis. These include:

- The guaiac test (Haemoccult) to examine the faecal stain for blood.
- Proctoscopy to examine the anal canal for fissures (painful) or haemorrhoids.
- Rigid or flexible sigmoidoscopy to inspect the rectal mucosa and take a biopsy.

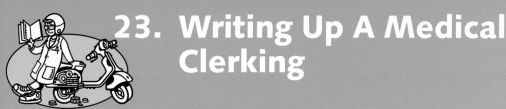

23. Writing Up A Medical Clerking

Purpose

The purpose of recording a history and examination in notes is to remind yourself and convey to others what the patient's problems were at the time. Notes must be legible, timed or dated, and signed in order to be used by other professionals. Do not use abbreviations unless they are so well recognized as to be easily understood.

 Be sure to remember 'PDNUA'—please do not use abbreviations!

Structure

Your history and notes will be much easier to follow if they are structured. Follow the same structure used in the history section of the sample medical clerking (see. pp 189–190). This is conventional and has the advantage that your colleagues will know where to look for specific information.

Illustration

This can be very useful to document images or to convey very precisely the site of pain. Take care if you are using illustrations that, where they convey quantitative rather than qualitative data, they are clear (e.g. audible murmur 2/6, diminished muscle power 3/4). Examples are given in Figs 23.1–23.4.

Formulating a differential diagnosis

It is important that you convey your impression at the time of taking a history. The clinical picture may change later, but valuable clues can be gained by recording early impressions.

Investigation

If you are ordering investigations, these should be listed and dated so that it is clear when they were ordered. It is also very useful, if a list of investigations is required, that a summary of results is put alongside the list as they come through.

Continuity

Clinical situations are rarely static. For subsequent entries, it is useful to state briefly the purpose or context of your review (e.g. called to see because complaining of chest pain).

If the clinical notes are extended because the patient has a long or complex history, a frequent update or summary is very useful to keep everyone focused on the problems. Some clinicians find it useful to keep a problem list which is updated daily. The important element throughout is clarity of thought and intent.

Sample medical clerking

An example of a medical clerking is shown overleaf. It highlights some of the points discussed earlier in this chapter.

Hospital No: X349182
BROWN, Jane
23/4/79
20/6/04 18.00   (26) Clerical worker   Referred by GP – seen in A & E
                          ♀

PC   Lower abdominal pain

> 1. Presenting complaint should be brief, but it is helpful to mention relevant background information.

HPC   6 month history
            Left iliac fossa
            Intermittent, every few days
            Relief with bowels opening
            Associated with: diarrhoea,
            semi-formed x 4/day
            Intermittently constipated
            No vomiting
            no weight loss / PR blood or mucus
            Appetite good

> 2. Mention only the relevant negatives. In this case it is important to mention the absence of weight loss and rectal bleeding.

PHHX   Appendectomy 1998
            NO asthma/diabetes/epilepsy

SYSTEMS review
            General: fatigue lately
            No sweats/itching
            sleeps well
     CVS: no chest pain/palpitations/oedema
     RS: no dyspnoea/wheeze/cough/sputum
     GIU: LMP 3 weeks ago
            Regular cycle
            No urinary symptoms
            Joints: No aches/swelling

DH   Combined oral contraceptive pill: 5 years
            No over the counter or herbal medicine

> 3. Always clarify an up-to-date drug history, with doses if applicable. Determine the nature of any drug allergies.

Allergies   penicillin → itchy red rash

DIET   Low residue
            Irregular meals
            High caffeine intake

Fam Hx   Father died aged   SHx   Lives with boyfriend
         42 years (IHD)   Non-smoker
         Mother well, siblings well   Alcohol 10 units /week (at weekends)
         No family hx of colonic disease No recreational drug use
                                         No regular sport activity

O/E   Looks well
Overweight
No evidence jaundice/anaemia/cyanosis
No lymphadenopathy or goitre
Clinically euthyroid
P 80/minute + regular BP 120/62
JVP normal
HS I + II + O
Chest resonant + clear throughout

> 4. Record your initial observations – they are important. 'Alert & chatty' or 'Distressed & looks unwell' tell you a lot about the patient.

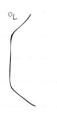

°L   °S

No peripheral oedema
No herniae
PR + sigmoidoscopy to 15cm
Normal mucosa
'Pellet' stool

Tender
but not
marked
+ no guarding

> 5. Always use diagrams to clarify your examination findings.

CNS   Grossly intact. GCS 15 PERLA
Alert and responsive.

> 6. If there is no abnormality of the CNS, simply include a one-line summary.

Imp   △ Irritable bowel syndrome

Plan   Explanation, reassurance and advice
Review in outpatients to reinforce
+ plan to discharge at 3 month followup
Blood tests: FBC (to exclude anaemia),
CRP/ESR (to look for evidence of infection
or inflammation)
Further investigation not indicated
at this stage

> 7. Always include a management plan – even when you are still a student. It might not be right but you need to start training yourself to think like a doctor.

FOX 752

> 8. Sign your notes, including printed surname and bleep number.

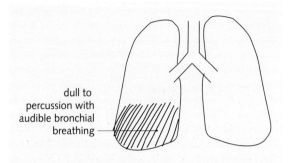

Fig. 23.1 Sample illustration of chest examination: usually the trachea and lung fields are drawn. In the example shown, an area of dullness to percussion, with audible bronchial breathing, in the lower right zone is shown.

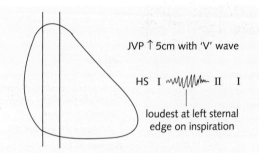

Fig. 23.2 Sample illustration of cardiac examination, showing how a murmur may be represented. In this example, a crescendo–diminuendo murmur was heard in systole (between the first and second heart sounds) and was best heard at the left sternal edge.

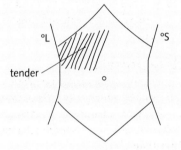

Fig. 23.3 Sample illustration of abdominal examination. In this example, there was an area of tenderness in the right upper quadrant. The degree symbol is often used to denote absence or negative findings (e.g. °L and °S indicate no hepatosplenomegaly found).

	Right arm	**Left arm**
Tone	↑	normal
Power	3/5	normal
Reflexes	++	+
Co-ordination	N/A (weak)	normal
Sensation	normal	normal

Fig. 23.4 Sample illustration of neurological examination findings. Reflexes are often represented as present (+), brisk (++) or absent (–). The MRC (Medical Research Council) scoring system for power should be used. Comments regarding type and distribution of sensory loss are made.

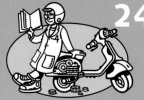

24. Common Investigations

Investigations are used to confirm, reinforce or refute a differential diagnosis. You ought to be able to justify any test you order on clinical grounds. Brief notes follow to aid interpretation of tests in gastrointestinal (GI) disease.

> Be careful not to rely upon investigations to make a diagnosis. They should be used appositely and discriminately to aid the diagnosis achieved following the history and examination.

Routine haematology

A full blood count (FBC) tends to be performed routinely on every patient and can provide vital information if interpreted correctly (Fig. 24.1).

A blood film can be very valuable if anaemia is present:

- Red cells can appear small (microcytosis), with variation of size (anisocytosis), and shape (poiklocytosis), in iron-deficiency anaemia.
- Red cells are large (macrocytic) with vitamin B_{12} deficiency.

Reticulocytes may be raised following recent blood loss and can account for a spurious macrocytosis on an automated FBC result. Target cells (ringed red blood cells) are common in liver disease. Be wary of a combined deficiency of B_{12}/folate and iron, resulting in both microcytes and macrocytes. This can appear as a normocytic anaemia.

A high platelet count (thrombocytosis) may be seen in cases of chronic blood loss or inflammatory disease.

Other haematological investigations can be helpful in GI disease:

- Vitamin B_{12}—if low, consider gastric or ileal resection, or disease (e.g. pernicious anaemia, Crohn's disease), blind loop syndrome, bacterial overgrowth, malabsorption. Disruption of liver architecture can lead to high levels (e.g. fibrolamellar hepatoma—rare) or hepatic abscess.
- Schilling test: replacing deficient intrinsic factor allows radiolabelled vitamin B_{12} to be absorbed (e.g. gastrectomy, pernicious anaemia: positive test), but has no effect if absorptive (ileal) mucosa is absent or diseased (e.g. ileal resection, Crohn's disease, tuberculosis: negative test) (Fig. 24.2).
- Folate can be low with any chronic debilitating state, malabsorption, excess alcohol, and certain drugs (e.g. sulphonamides, colestyramine, anticonvulsants). It can be elevated in small intestinal bacterial overgrowth.
- Erythrocyte sedimentation rate (ESR)—non-specifically raised in inflammatory and malignant diseases. Limited usefulness, and rises with advancing age.

C-reactive protein

C-reactive protein is an acute-phase protein, rising within 6 hours of an infective or inflammatory insult, correlating well with inflammatory activity in some diseases (e.g. in Crohn's). It is more reliable, specific and sensitive than ESR.

Biochemistry

Urea and electrolytes are requested routinely for the majority of patients. Sodium is commonly slightly low in many sick patients due to the syndrome of inappropriate anti-diuretic hormone secretion. Some inference about GI pathology can be made from routine biochemistry (Fig. 24.3).

Amylase

Amylase:

- Should be at least moderately raised (500 IU/L) in acute pancreatitis.
- Is usually normal in chronic pancreatitis.
- Is commonly raised without pain following endoscopic retrograde cholangiopancreatography (ERCP).
- Is raised non-specifically in many causes of abdominal pain, e.g. perforated viscus, ruptured ectopic pregnancy, cholecystitis.

Routine haematology tests		
Parameter	**Level**	**Inference**
HB	Low	?Dietary iron deficiency, malabsorption, or blood loss (achlorhydria, gastrectomy, coeliac disease)
WCC	Low High	Viral infection (e.g. hepatitis) Bacterial infection, colonic inflammation, alcoholic hepatitis, steroids
Platelets	Low High	Portal hypertension and hypersplenism Inflammatory disease (e.g. Crohn's) or chronic GI blood loss
MCV	Low High	Iron deficiency Reticulocytosis (recent bleed), macrocytosis (B_{12} deficiency or alcoholic liver)

Fig. 24.1 Routine haematology tests in gastrointestinal disease.

Arterial blood gases

Patients who are ill from any cause (e.g. sepsis, liver/renal failure, pancreatitis) develop metabolic acidosis, often with compensatory respiratory alkalosis (hyperventilation). Following a paracetamol overdose, pH is a particularly useful prognostic measurement (along with the serum creatinine and prothrombin time).

Glucose

Diabetes mellitus can present in a spectrum of guises, including weight loss. Glucose measurement is often forgotten.

Calcium

Hypercalcaemia can lead to constipation and low levels can be seen in malabsorption and vitamin D deficiency.

Alcohol

Alcohol measurement can be useful in specific circumstances, such as determining occult causes of coma or abnormal liver enzymes in patients presenting acutely.

Endocrine and metabolic

Thyroid function

Thyroid disease does not usually cause GI problems, but may accentuate symptoms such as diarrhoea (hyperthyroidism) or constipation (hypothyroidism) from other causes. Hyperthyroidism needs to be excluded as a cause of weight loss (in children, it can cause weight gain!).

Catecholamine levels

A 24-hour urinary collection for free catecholamines (adrenaline (epinephrine), noradrenaline (norepinephrine) and dopamine) is used to diagnose catecholamine excess secondary to tumours of the adrenal medulla. These may present with GI symptoms of weight loss, nausea, vomiting, and altered bowel habit. Associated features are flushing and cardiovascular dysfunction (arrhythmias and episodic hypertension). Note that some hospitals still measure urinary vanillylmandelic acid as a surrogate of catecholamine excess.

Cortisol

An absent or impaired cortisol response following administration of an analogue of adrenocorticotrophic hormone is useful to diagnose Addison's disease. This can present with nausea, vomiting, weight loss, diarrhoea or postural dizziness. Acute adrenal failure may present as severe abdominal pain, mimicking an acute abdomen.

Gut hormone profile
Serum gastrin

Serum gastrin is raised slightly in patients with *Helicobacter pylori* infection, peptic ulcer disease, or in patients on long-term treatment with proton pump inhibitors. It is markedly raised in gastrinomas. These APUD (amine precursor uptake and decarboxylation) tumours arise most commonly in the pancreas, but also in the mucosa of the duodenum or antrum. They present with peptic ulcers, diarrhoea, and weight loss.

Fig. 24.2 Schematic representation of Schilling test: An intramuscular dose of B₁₂ is first administered to saturate the cell receptors. Radiolabelled vitamin B₁₂ is then given orally and absorption is assessed by its appearance in the urine. Dietary vitamin B₁₂ combines with intrinsic factor (IF) secreted by the stomach and can then be absorbed in the terminal ileum. Lack of IF causes pernicious anaemia and can be identified by the Schilling test. A positive test (correction of B₁₂ malabsorption with IF) indicates a gastric cause. A negative test may indicate terminal ileal disease.

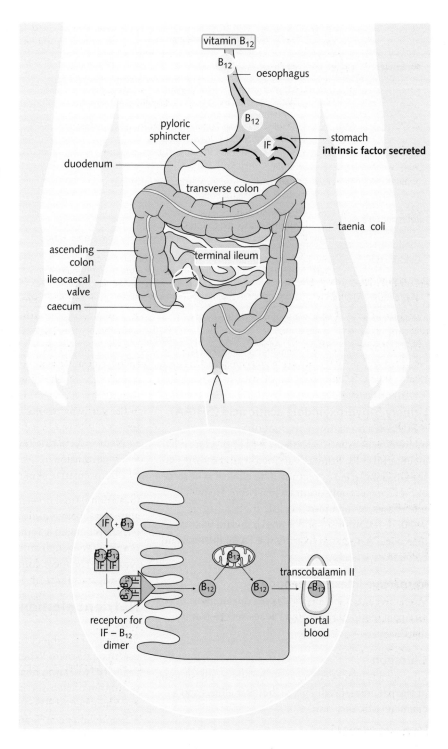

Routine biochemistry		
Parameter	Level	GI significance
Urea	Low High	Malabsorption or liver disease Slightly (up to 14 mmol/L): dehydration (nausea, vomiting, Addison's) Moderate (up to 20 mmol/L): profound dehydration, GI bleed (protein load) Severe (more than 20 mmol/L): renal failure, hepatorenal syndrome
Sodium (Na)	Low	Common in diarrhoea, vomiting, alcoholic liver disease, diuretics
Potassium (K)	Low High	Common in diarrhoea, vomiting, alcoholic liver disease, loop diuretics Possible renal failure, diuretics especially spirononlactone
Calcium (Ca)	Low High	Correct for albumin, common in coeliac disease Associated with malignant disease, hyperparathyroidism
Magnesium (Mg)	Low	Commonly in malnutrition, malabsorption, alcoholic diseases
Creatinine	High	Renal failure (all causes)
Glucose	High	Hyperglycaemia can cause abdominal pain, dehydration and acidosis Acute and chronic pancreatis can lead to high glucose in serum

Fig. 24.3 Routine biochemistry and its significance in gastrointestinal disease.

Urinary 5-hydroxyindole acetic acid (5HIAA)

5-HIAA is a breakdown product of 5-hydroxytryptamine (serotonin, 5-HT) produced by argentaffin cells. Primary carcinoid tumours arise in the small intestine or rectum. The clinical syndrome of 5-HT excess only occurs when there are liver metastases, as 'first pass' hepatic metabolism is avoided. It comprises abdominal pain and watery diarrhoea. Associated features are facial flushing and respiratory wheeze.

Vasoactive intestinal peptide

Vasoactive intestinal peptide is produced in excess by rare pancreatic tumours and causes severe watery diarrhoea.

Glucagon

Glucagon is produced in excess by alpha cell tumours of the pancreas, producing diabetes mellitus and a characteristic skin rash.

Somatostatinomas

Somatostatinomas produce diarrhoea and weight loss with diabetes mellitus.

Porphyrins

These are intermediate metabolites in the haem biosynthetic pathway. Enzyme absence or deficiency in the pathway results in their accumulation leading to:

- Neuropsychiatric disorder.
- Hypertension.
- Photosensitive skin rashes.

Gastrointestinal presentation is common with abdominal pain, vomiting, and constipation. Excess porphobilinogen is found in urine. Red blood cell porphobilinogen deaminase and aminolaevulinic acid synthase, the most common enzyme deficiencies, can be measured (Fig. 24.4).

Nutrient elements

Iron

Serum iron is subject to too much fluctuation to be useful on its own. When compared with its binding capacity (total iron binding capacity), the percentage saturation of transferrin can be derived:

- Values below 20% are considered iron deficient.
- Values above 50% are probably iron overloaded.

(see Chapter 11)

Ferritin

Ferritin reflects body iron stores in adults and is a useful tool for investigating iron overload. However, as an acute-phase protein, it is elevated in any cause of inflammation. It can therefore be misleadingly normal or high, in rheumatoid arthritis or in alcoholic hepatitis, in which it may be difficult to differentiate from haemochromatosis.

Caeruloplasmin

A plasma protein that binds copper, caeruloplasmin is reduced in most cases of Wilson's disease, but this is not sufficient to make a diagnosis. Serum copper should also be elevated and 24-hour urinary copper excretion increased.

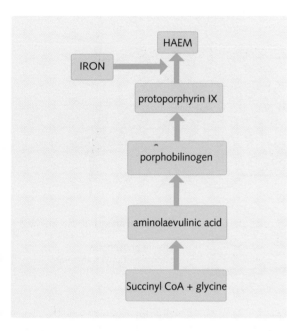

Fig. 24.4 Haem biosynthetic pathway.

Zinc

Zinc is low in alcoholic liver disease; its deficiency can cause an enteropathy as well as skin rashes.

Liver enzymes and liver function tests

Liver enzymes

Elevated liver enzymes in serum signify hepatic injury of some kind, but give no information about liver function. For this, routine measurement of metabolites made or excreted by the liver are very useful, e.g. bilirubin, albumin, coagulant factors. Dynamic function tests are also available, although rarely used.

Use Figs 24.5 and 24.6 to help you to work out how to interpret liver enzyme levels.

The pattern of elevation may give some clue about the disease process. This is easiest to understand by reference to the hepatic lobule in Fig. 24.6:

- A predominant or disproportionate rise in alkaline phosphatase and gamma glutamyl transferase indicates biliary tract pathology such as obstruction or biliary cirrhosis.
- A predominant rise in transaminases usually indicates a parenchymal process such as hepatitis.

Elevation of liver enzymes	
Liver enzymes	**Significance**
AST (aspartate transaminase)	Very high (thousands) in acute hepatitis or necrosis Moderate (approx. 500) in chronic active inflammatory disease Mild (<300) in portal tract damage, focal hepatitis Also present in muscle (raised in myocardial infarction)
ALT (alanine transaminase)	As for AST, but more specific to liver In alcoholic hepatitis usually less than AST by ratio of 2
Alkaline phosphatase	Highest in cholestatic syndromes (portal tract disease or bile duct obstruction). Remember other sources: bones (especially young), placenta (females), intestine (rare)
Gamma glutamyl transferase	Very labile enzyme, often mildly elevated Highest levels in portal tract disease and alcoholics

Fig. 24.5 Elevation of liver enzymes and their significance.

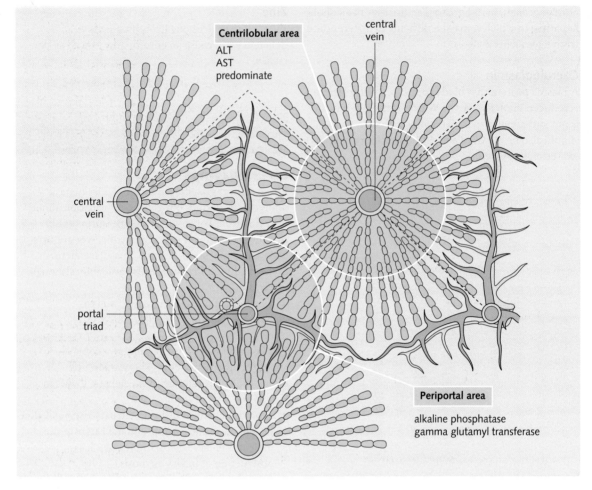

Fig. 24.6 Liver enzymes predominate in different areas of the liver lobule and their relative proportions in serum give a clue about the pathological process in the liver. (ALT, alanine transaminase; AST, aspartate transaminase.)

Tests of liver function
Standard blood tests
Prothrombin time is a sensitive test of hepatic synthetic function because it reflects interaction of all the clotting factors made by the liver (II, VII, IX and X). It is sometimes expressed as international normalized ratio (INR) against a control, although this should be reserved for patients on warfarin therapy.

In cholestatic syndromes, prothrombin time may also be abnormal because absent bile reduces absorption of vitamin K from the intestine. In this situation, the INR will correct with parenteral vitamin K but not in parenchymal liver disease. Be aware that parenteral vitamin K will take at least

6 hours to become effective. Albumin depletes rapidly in chronic debilitating or inflammatory conditions. It is made in the liver (half-life = 20 days) and is low in chronic liver disease and malabsorption. It can also fall in the acute setting, such as severe sepsis or an acute inflammatory condition.

Bilirubin in serum can be conjugated or unconjugated:
- Unconjugated elevation (clinically referred to as acholuric jaundice) occurs in haemolytic disorders or with deficiencies of conjugation enzyme (e.g. Gilbert's disease, Rotor syndrome).
- Conjugated hyperbilirubinaemia indicates cholestasis or loss of hepatocyte function.

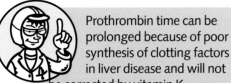 Prothrombin time can be prolonged because of poor synthesis of clotting factors in liver disease and will not be corrected by vitamin K. Alternatively it may be prolonged due to a lack of vitamin K absorption because of biliary obstruction. In this instance parenteral vitamin K can be expected to correct the prothrombin time.

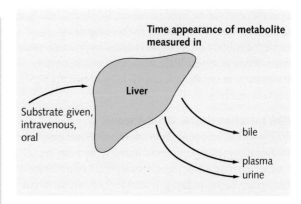

Fig. 24.7 Principle of dynamic liver function tests: a known amount of substrate is given and its metabolite(s) measured at set time points in plasma or urine. Metabolism is a function of hepatic functional mass and blood flow.

Causes of jaundice include (see Chapter 12):
- Hepatitis (viral and alcoholic).
- Drugs (e.g. phenothiazines, anticonvulsants, some antibiotics such as clavulanic acid and flucloxacillin).
- Poisons (e.g. carbon tetrachloride, CCl_4).
- Chronic liver diseases such as primary biliary cirrhosis (PBC) or primary sclerosing cholangitis (PSC).
- Extra-hepatic bile duct obstruction (gallstones and benign or malignant bile duct strictures).

It is often forgotten that gluconeogenesis and glycogenolysis (the mechanisms for the homoeostasis of blood glucose levels) take place in the liver.

Profound hypoglycaemia can occur in some acute liver diseases (e.g. fulminant hepatic failure, Reye syndrome) and occasionally with alcoholic binges. Glucose tolerance is impaired in chronic liver diseases.

Immunoglobulins are commonly elevated in chronic liver disease, but not usually in obstructive jaundice or in drug-induced cholestasis.

The mechanisms of elevation are poorly understood, however:
- In cirrhosis, this may involve antigens from the gut bypassing the liver and producing an antibody response predominantly of the immunoglobulin IgG and IgM class.
- In alcoholic liver disease, a decline in Kupffer cell activity may explain the rise in IgA because of reduced clearance.
- High IgG is usually associated with chronic active hepatitis and IgM with primary biliary cirrhosis.

Dynamic and metabolic liver tests

These are based on the principle that certain substances are either metabolized or excreted by the liver and their products can be measured after administration as a bolus (Fig. 24.7).

They are mainly useful as research tools and for evaluating response to new treatments. Some of the more commonly used tests are described briefly below.

Bromosulphthalein (BSP) excretion

This organic anion is rapidly taken up by the liver and bound by Y and Z proteins before being excreted. This test can detect subtle changes in hepatic dysfunction in mild disease, but is not now much used clinically. Changes in serum albumin and hepatic blood flow affect the result. Delayed excretion is pathognomonic of Dubin–Johnson syndrome.

Indocyanin green

This is another organic anion which is more avidly bound to plasma protein and more actively extracted by the liver. It is safer, easier to measure and less susceptible to variability than BSP, but less useful in detecting subtle changes in function. It reflects hepatic blood flow very well and is mostly employed for this purpose. Normal in Dubin–Johnson syndrome.

Bile acids

Bile acids more specifically reflect excretory hepatic function than serum bilirubin. They are sensitive and specific, and can be used to detect subtle dysfunction or differentiate liver disease from congenital hyperbilirubinaemias or haemolysis. In practice their measurement offers little advantage over enzyme estimation in combination with measurements of protein and bilirubin.

IDA excretion (HIDA, DISIDA scans)

Imino-iodoacetic acid (IDA) derivatives are taken up by hepatocytes and excreted in bile. They can be tagged with a radioactive isotope (^{99}Tc) to evaluate excretory function and gall bladder concentration of bile. They can be useful in difficult cases of intra-hepatic bile duct stasis.

Metabolic challenge tests

These rely on functional hepatic mass to produce or excrete a metabolite.

Antipyrine clearance, aminopyrine breath test, and caffeine or lidocaine (lignocaine) clearance have been used to investigate and test microsomal function. They correlate well with hepatic dysfunction but offer little advantage over measurement of prothrombin time, serum albumin, or the Child–Pugh score.

Galactose tolerance test

Galactose is rapidly phosphorylated in hepatocytes and eliminated. After an infusion or bolus, the rate of elimination can detect subclinical cirrhosis and distinguish parenchymal from obstructive liver disease. It offers no clinical advantage over orthodox tests.

Liver biopsy

Ultimately, for a detailed assessment of liver pathology a liver biopsy will often be required.

The usual indications are to help in diagnosis or to assess the severity of inflammation and fibrosis in established disease to guide treatment and prognosis.

The procedure is undertaken under ultrasound guidance usually with a slicing or suction needle percutaneously under local anaesthetic. A Menghini hollow, wide-bore needle inserted into the liver with suction via a syringe may be used as an alternative.

Sub-costal or shoulder tip pain (diaphragmatic referred pain) is common. More serious complications include bile leak or haemorrhage. Perforation of a viscus is rare (mortality 1:1000).

If coagulation is abnormal (a 4-second prolongation of prothrombin time) or there is significant thrombocytopenia (80 000), a biopsy can be obtained with a long flexible needle via the jugular and hepatic veins or by laparoscopy under direct vision. The standard vital stains used are haematoxylin and eosin and reticulin to demonstrate fibrosis.

Tests of pancreatic and gastric function

These tests are now rarely used and for the majority, the sensitivity and specificity is too poor to be relied upon.

Pentagastrin

The gastric acid output is measured preceding and following the administration of pentagastrin (a synthetic gastrin analogue).

- High basal output results from high gastrin levels (now known to be due to *Helicobacter* infection) or very high levels in Zollinger–Ellison syndrome.
- A low maximal output response indicates atrophic gastritis or achlorhydria.

Lundh test

Following a fatty meal, duodenal content is aspirated and assayed for trypsin and lipase. The levels are low in chronic pancreatitis. Variations of this test are also undertaken with secretin or cholecystokinin provocation.

Para-aminobenzoic acid (PABA)

Para-aminobenzoic acid (PABA) is a peptide hydrolysed by chymotrypsin causing release of free PABA which is excreted in the urine. A less than expected amount of PABA in the urine following an oral load is diagnostic of pancreatic insufficiency.

Fat malabsorption

Fat malabsorption can be determined by detecting a high proportion of unabsorbed fat following a test meal (3-day faecal fat collection) or detecting a lower than expected amount of $^{14}CO_2$ in exhaled air following an oral dose of ^{14}C-labelled triglyceride (e.g. ^{14}C trioleine). To confirm that this result is due to pancreatic insufficiency, this is often compared and expressed as a ratio to $^{14}CO_2$ following an oral dose of fatty acid (e.g. ^{14}C oleic acid).

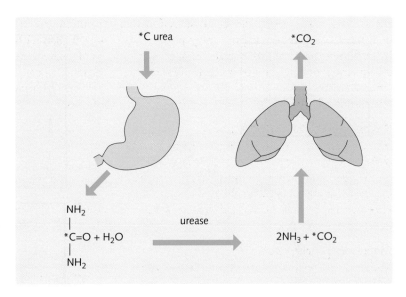

Fig. 24.8 Schematic representation of the biochemical basis of gut breath tests. The example shown is the urea breath test in which ^{13}C or ^{14}C urea is given orally. If urease is present in the stomach (on the cell membrane of *H. pylori*), the urea is split into ammonia and radiolabelled CO_2 which can be detected in the exhaled breath. *C indicates that C is radiolabelled.

Pancreolauryl test

Fluorescein-conjugated dilaurate is hydrolysed by pancreatic esterase; the released fluorescein is absorbed and detectable in urine. False positives may occur if bacterial esterases are present.

Breath tests

The general principle of these tests is that a substrate is metabolized when the relevant enzyme is present in the gut lumen, resulting in release of CO_2 or hydrogen which are absorbed by diffusion and exhaled in the breath. Normally, breath hydrogen is undetectable, so elevation is consistent with bacterial hydrolysis. To detect CO_2 by this process, either ^{13}C or ^{14}C is used in the substrate (Fig. 24.8).

Lactulose

Lactulose is hydrolysed by bacterial enzymes causing the release of hydrogen. Once bacteria in the oral cavity are neutralized with an antiseptic mouthwash, an early rise will indicate bacteria in the proximal small intestine beyond the acid stomach. A late rise, due to bacteria resident in the colon, is normal.

Lactose

Lactose is cleaved by disaccharidase, allowing its constituent sugars to be absorbed. Failure to detect a rise of plasma glucose following an oral load of lactose indicates disaccharidase deficiency, which can be congenital or secondary to any small bowel disorder. Avoidance of dairy produce usually alleviates the associated diarrhoea.

D-Xylose

D-xylose is a synthetic sugar absorbed, like all sugars, from the proximal small intestine. Measurement of serum xylose following an oral load has been used as a test for malabsorption but is too sensitive and non-specific to be clinically useful.

Urea

Urea labelled with ^{13}C or ^{14}C and given orally is cleaved to ammonia and radiolabelled CO_2, which is detectable in exhaled breath if urease is present in the stomach. This enzyme is present on the coat of *Helicobacter pylori* and the test identifies patients with current gastric infection.

Glycholic acid

Glycholic acid is a bile salt which can be conjugated to ^{14}C glycine. Bacteria, if present in the small intestine, deconjugate the bile salt and the glycine is metabolized, releasing $^{14}CO_2$ which is absorbed and exhaled in expiration.

Motility physiology

Oesophageal manometry

This is undertaken for the investigation of non-cardiac chest pain if oesophageal dysmotility is suspected, or in the assessment of gastro-oesophageal reflux disease or non-mechanical dysphagia.

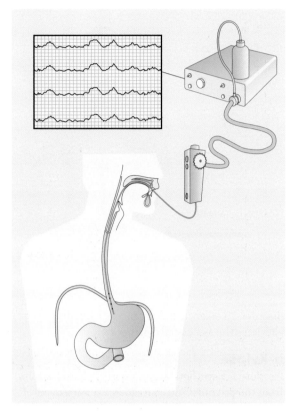

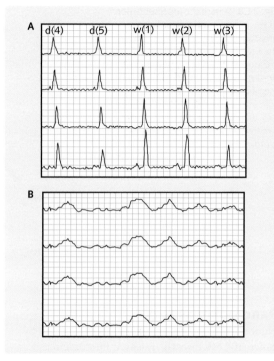

Fig. 24.10 (A) Oesophageal motility showing normal peristalsis and (B) from a patient with achalasia where the peristalsis is uncoordinated The lower sphincter also fails to relax in achalasia (not shown in this tracing).

Fig. 24.9 Measurement of oesophageal motility. A probe is passed nasogastrically with several transducers at 1 cm intervals. These pick up sequential pressure waves as the peristaltic swallow travels down the oesophagus. This is represented by the waveforms shown in Fig. 24.10.

A tube with either solid-state or water-pressure transducers at intervals along its length is passed nasogastrically and peristaltic swallow waves are recorded (Figs 24.9 and 24.10).
- Uncoordinated peristalsis with failure of the lower oesophageal sphincter to relax is diagnostic of achalasia.
- High pressure waves (nutcracker oesophagus) may indicate oesophageal spasm.
- Diffuse hypomotility is common in scleroderma.

Ambulatory oesophagogastric pH

This is often undertaken in combination with manometry in the assessment and management of reflux disease. The patient wears the tube attached to a small solid-state recorder for 24 hours and the result is then analysed by a computer (Figs 24.11 and 24.12).

The transducer is placed 5 cm above the gastro-oesophageal junction where the pH is normally above 4, and detects reflux of acid when the pH drops below 4. Results are expressed as the number of reflux episodes and the proportion of time that oesophageal pH is below 4 (normally <5%).

Anorectal manometry

This is undertaken for the investigation of faecal incontinence or chronic constipation. A narrow tube with pressure transducers is passed across the anus and measures resting tone and squeeze–relaxation activity. An inflatable balloon device attached to a pressure gauge is used to assess rectal pressures. The patient can be instructed by a biofeedback mechanism to improve anal sphincter tone and defecation technique.

Serological tests

A large variety of tests are based on the interaction of antibodies with antigen in radioimmunoassay kits and

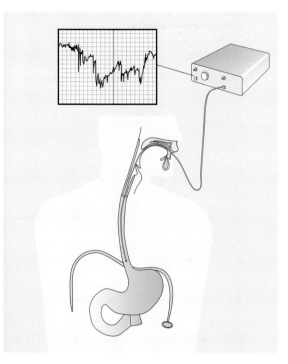

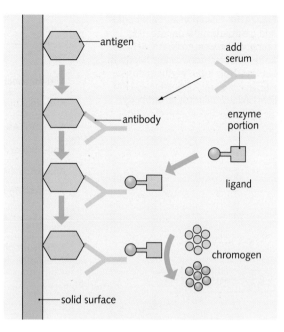

Fig. 24.11 Method for assessing oesophageal pH: a nasogastric tube with a probe sensitive to hydrogen ions is placed 5 cm above the gastro-oesophageal junction. pH here should be greater than 4. Dips below this identify episodes of gastro-oesophageal acid reflux. This is represented by the waveforms shown in Fig. 24.12.

Fig. 24.13 The principles of enzyme-linked immunosorbent assay (ELISA). A solid surface is labelled with antigen (the solid phase). The patient's serum is added and if the specific antibody is present, it is held by the antigen and can be detected by a labelled antibody sandwich technique with a colouring agent.

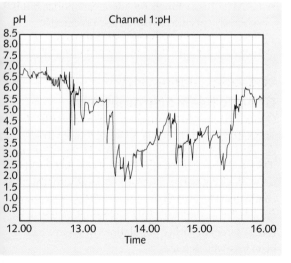

Fig. 24.12 Example of 24-hour pH recording from a patient with significant acid reflux. pH dipping below 4 indicates acid reflux from the stomach.

enzyme-linked immunosorbent assay kits (Fig. 24.13). Their principal use is to screen for infection, tumours, or immunoinflammatory disease when those conditions are suspected by the clinical presentation or the results of other tests.

These are useful confirmatory tests, but are much less useful and often confusing if used as screening tests. Here, they are classified according to their clinical implications in GI pathology.

Markers of autoimmune disease

Antibodies to various nuclear components are found in a number of diseases (Fig. 24.14), but also in up to 20% of the normal population.

More specific antibodies to double-stranded DNA are found in 50% of patients with systemic lupus erythematosus, and speckled pattern anti-nuclear factor in mixed connective tissue disease.

- Smooth muscle antibodies are found in 60% of cases or autoimmune chronic active hepatitis. Anti-liver–kidney microsomal antibodies are found in a subgroup of these patients with a more protracted course of disease.

203

Fig. 24.14 Common autoantibodies and gastrointestinal disease. (PBC, primary biliary cirrhosis; AICAH, autoimmune chronic active hepatitis; SLE, systemic lupus erythematosis; ALT, alanine aminotransferase; LKM, liver–kidney microsomal antibody.)

Common autoantibodies		
Test	Significance	Application
Anti-mitochondrial Ab	PBC	When biliary enzymes raised
Anti-smooth muscle Ab	AICAH	When ALT raised
Anti-LKM Ab	AICAH	When ALT raised
Anti-nuclear Ab	CAH	When ALT raised
Anti-dsDNA Ab	SLE	Abnormal LFTs
Anti-endomysial Ab	Coeliac	In chronic diarrhoea/ malabsorption
Anti-gliaden Ab	Coeliac	In chronic diarrhoea/ malabsorption
Anti-neutrophil cytoplasmic Ab	Ulcerative colitis	In blood diarrhoea

- Gastric parietal cell antibodies are found in 90% of patients with pernicious anaemia.
- Rheumatoid factor (IgM class autoantibody against own IgG) is found in 70% of patients with rheumatoid-like arthritis and is the determining factor for seropositivity which tends to run a more severe course.
- Anit-neutrophil cytoplasmic antibody (ANCA) antibodies are found in a variety of connective tissue diseases, but the p-ANCA variety is found more commonly (in 70% of cases) in primary sclerosing cholangitis.
- Endomysial antibody is the most reliable marker for coeliac disease as long as the correct antigen is used in the laboratory. In this situation, it is found in up to 90% of cases and is specific enough to have clinical value.
- Alphagliaden antibody was initially thought to be a good marker of coeliac disease, but is only present in about 50–70% of cases.

Markers of infection
These are shown in Fig. 24.15.

Markers for tumours
It is important to note that these are not diagnostic tests, and are often more useful for monitoring disease following treatment.

Examples of markers for tumours may include:
- Alpha-fetoprotein is a marker for hepatocellular carcinoma. It can be mildly elevated in chronic liver diseases. Higher levels are found in the third trimester of pregnancy.
- Carcinoembryonic antigen levels are high with colonic tumours or metastatic disease. It can be raised non-specifically in inflammatory colonic disease. It is usually used as serial measurements following colonic resection.
- CA19.9 is a marker for adenocarcinoma, but is relatively specific for pancreatic carcinoma.
- CA125 is a marker also for adenocarcinoma, but is relatively specific for ovarian carcinoma.
- CAM17.1 is a marker for adenocarcinoma, but is relatively specific for pancreatic carcinoma.

Genetic markers

Genetic haemochromatosis
Genetic haemochromatosis has been formerly associated with HLA type A3 and B7 in up to 70% of patients. More recently, a mutation (C282Y) in the 'HFE gene' on chromosome 6 has been described and is present in more than 90% of patients with this condition (Fig. 24.16). It is currently used to screen families where an index case has been identified: its role in screening other populations or groups has been less-well defined.

Wilson's disease
A variety of genes associated with this condition have been localized to chromosome 13. There is no specific screening test as no single mutation can

Markers of infection

Test	Significance	Application/comment
Hepatitis A IgM	Indicates acute or recent infection	Use for acute presentation of hepatitis
HBsAG (surface antigen)	Indicates current or chronic infection or the carrier state. Becomes negative after the virus has been cleared	Used to screen in acute hepatitis and blood donors
Anti-HBs	Indicates immunity to hepatitis B virus	May appear in this situation or following vaccination
HBcIgM (core antigen)	Indicates recent infection	
HBeAg (envelope antigen)	Indicates current infection and correlates with viral replication and serum levels of hepatitis B virus DNA	Used to confirm infection if HBsAg positive
Anti-HBe	Indicates that immune response has been successful against viral replication	Infectivity is low, virus dormant or cleared
HCV-Ab	Indicates current or past infection with hepatitis C virus	Screening tests are undertaken with an ELISA kit and these are confirmed by RIBA assays. Blood products have been screened only since 1991
HCV PCR	RNA can be detected by PCR or the b-DNA (branched DNA) assay	PCR positivity indicates active viral infection
CMV	Antibody kits are available to determine past or current infection	Is endemic in many countries and does not usually pose problems except in the immunocompromised host, e.g. after transplantation
EBV	This is tested by an immunoprecipitation test formerly called the Paul–Bunnell or monospot test	Is the cause of infectious mononucleosis
Helicobacter pylori	An antibody test indicating past or current infection with the organism	Should be considered in the investigation of patients with dyspepsia. Its clinical use is limited, as it cannot discriminate past from current infection
Leptospira		Should be considered as a cause of jaundice or headache in patients whose occupation takes them into contact with rodent infested areas
Brucella		Should be considered in patients, particularly farmers, with pyrexia of unknown origin, or granulomatous liver disease
Entamoeba histolytica		CFT should be considered in patients returning from Africa or Asia with pyrexia, diarrhoea, or pain in the right upper quadrant
Hydatid		Should be considered in any patient with pain in the right upper quadrant, pyrexia of unknown origin, or unexplained liver abscess, who may have been in contact with animals, particularly sheep
Clonorchis		Is endemic in parts of Asia and the fluke worm ends up in the bile duct, sometimes causing obstruction with cast formation. This should be considered in patients with obstructive jaundice from endemic areas
HIV		Indicates exposure to HIV
Toxocara		This protozoan infection is uncommon, but should be suspected in patients with obscure liver disease who are in contact with animals, particularly cats and dogs
Toxoplasma		This protozoan infection is uncommon, but should be suspected in patients with obscure liver disease who are in contact with animals

Fig. 24.15 Markers of infection.

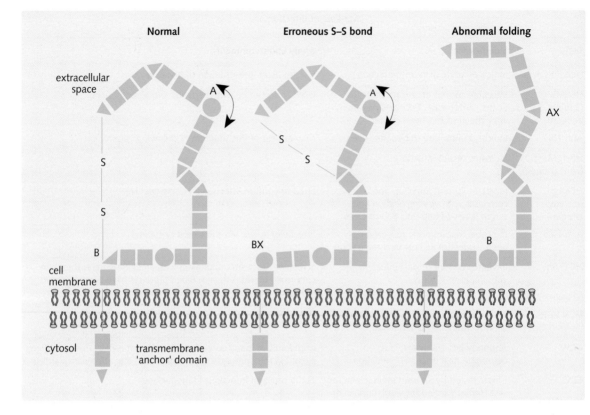

Fig. 24.16 Schematic drawing showing how protein conformational structure and function can change with a single amino acid substitution at sites A or B. Amino acid substitution in turn is due to a single nucleotide substitution or mutation in its coding DNA. Some amino acids allow more flexible conformation (e.g. A) and if substituted will not allow conformational change (AX). Cysteine residues in particular (e.g. B) allow -S–S- bonds to stabilize conformations and can affect ligand binding. If substituted this can also affect conformational possibilities (BX).

explain all cases. The genetic defect is in an ATP protein which exports copper to the Golgi complex, where it stimulates production of and is bound to caeruloplasmin. Hence, the absence of ATPB7 protein is associated with low caeruloplasmin levels.

Cystic fibrosis
The gene responsible for this is a chloride transporter and a marker is available (Δ508).

Alpha-1-antitrypsin
A number of genotypes and corresponding phenotypes exists for alpha-1-antitrypsin. The varieties associated with liver disease included PIZZ and PIMZ (Fig. 18.10).

Gilbert's disease
This is possibly the commonest reason for raised serum bilirubin in younger patients and can affect up to 5% of the male population (genetic predisposition is even more common). It is due to an inefficient transcription of the uridine glucuronosyl transferase enzyme (UGT-1) because of a slightly longer promoter region (TATA box) on the gene. A simple genetic test is available and used to confirm suspected cases.

Imaging

Endoscopy
The principle of endoscopy is shown in Fig. 24.17.

Upper GI endoscopy
Upper GI endoscopy is useful:
- For the investigation of dyspepsia.
- To identify the cause of bleeding or blood loss in patients who present acutely or with iron-deficiency anaemia.

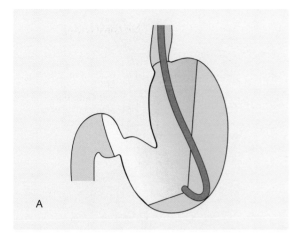

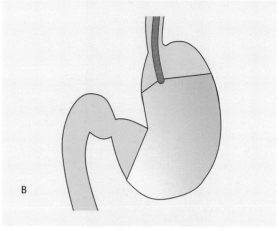

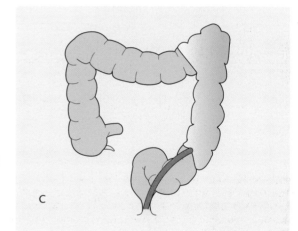

Fig. 24.17 Principle of endoscopy: a flexible tube is passed into the GI lumen and relays video images to the operator. The endoscope can be manoeuvred to see all areas. Specially designed instruments can be used to undertake techniques (e.g. forceps biopsy, polypectomy) through channels in the endoscope.

Endoluminal biopsy

This is now commonly undertaken endoscopically, during which 2–5 mm pinch biopsies are obtained by forceps.

- In the oesophagus, stomach, and colon, this is used to assess abnormal mucosal appearances (Figs 24.18 and 24.19).
- In the small intestine, it is performed to exclude coeliac disease, in the context of anaemia or malabsorption.

Complications are rare. The standard vital stain used is haematoxylin and eosin.

Duodenal aspirate is useful for the diagnosis of *Giardia lamblia* or to collect pancreatic juice for the estimation of enzyme activity.

Proctoscopy

Proctoscopy is undertaken with a translucent tube so that the walls of the anus can be inspected.

This technique is useful for anal fissures and haemorrhoids.

Sigmoidoscopy

Sigmoidoscopy is often undertaken in the clinic with a rigid tube and light source to inspect the anorectal margins and rectal mucosa. Biopsies can be taken for the diagnosis, or assessment of colitis/proctitis. Rectal biopsy is also indicated for the diagnosis of primary amyloidosis, where a Congo Red stain is used to produce green birefringence in polarized light.

Flexible sigmoidoscopy

Flexible sigmoidoscopy can also be undertaken to inspect the rectum and the lower sigmoid colon where up to two-thirds of colonic tumours are known to occur.

This is also useful as a prelude to barium enema for a complete examination of the colon.

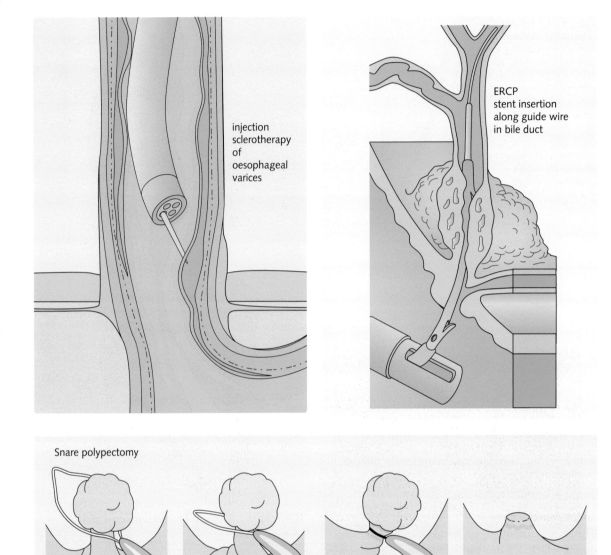

Fig. 24.18 Therapeutic procedures in endoscopy: examples of injection sclerotherapy to oesophageal varices, snare polypectomy with diathermy, and placement of an endoprosthesis across a tumour involving the lower bile duct at endoscopic retrograde cholangiopancreatography.

Full colonoscopy

Full colonoscopy is indicated when a lesion has been seen on barium enema which needs biopsy, or in the investigation of iron-deficiency anaemia or blood loss.

Enteroscopy

Enteroscopy is indicated when a lesion has been seen on barium meal that needs biopsy, or in the investigation of iron-deficiency anaemia or blood loss.

Endoscopic retrograde cholangiopancreatography

Endoscopic retrograde cholangiopancreatography (ERCP) is undertaken for the diagnosis and treatment of bile duct and pancreatic duct problems. Various interventions can be undertaken including sphincterotomy and removal of bile duct stones (choledocholithiasis). For obstructing lesions, an endoprosthesis can be inserted either into the bile duct or pancreas (Fig. 24.20). In the pancreas,

Fig. 24.19 Principle of ultrasound. A sound probe transmits an energy wave through the tissue. At the interface between layers of different density, some sound waves are reflected (echoed) back and can be translated into an image as shown in Fig. 24.20. Ultrasound probes can be used transcutaneously (transabdominal), endoscopically, or even endovascularly.

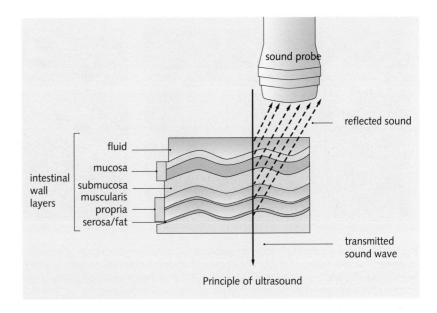

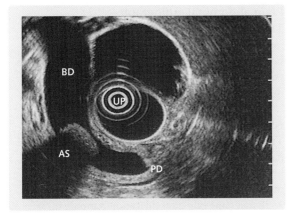

Fig. 24.20 Endoscopic ultrasound demonstrating a gallstone within the bile duct. An acoustic 'shadow' (AS) is cast behind the stone. Note the ultrasound probe (UP), bile duct (BD), and pancreatic duct (PD).

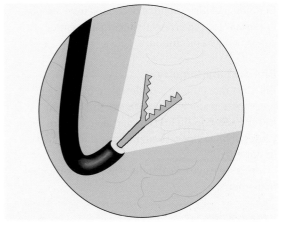

Fig. 24.21 Endoscopic biopsy—a grasping forceps can be used through the endoscope to obtain pinch biopsies of mucosa.

further intervention may involve removal of pancreatic duct concretions or passing a stent through the posterior stomach wall into a pancreatic pseudocyst (endoscopic cystgastrostomy). There is an increasing trend to reserve ERCP for therapeutic procedures; diagnosis of pancreatobiliary disorders can be achieved by endoscopic ultrasound or magnetic resonance cholangiopancreatography which have less procedure-related risks.

Endoscopic ultrasound

The principle of ultrasound is shown in Fig. 24.21.

Endoluminal ultrasound is an endoscopic examination of the oesophagus, stomach, duodenum, bile duct, pancreas, or rectum with an ultrasound probe on the end of the endoscope. It is useful for:

- Gaining more information on mucosal or submucosal lesions in these areas.
- For the staging of local spread of oesophageal tumours.
- For differentiating stones from malignant obstruction in the bile duct (Fig. 24.22).
- To assess ano-rectal damage (usually as a result of parturition or forceps delivery).

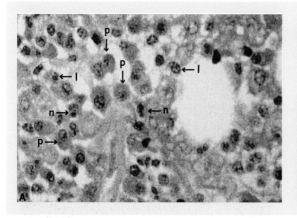
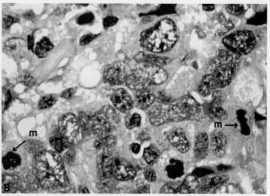

Fig. 24.22 Histological examination is important for identifying the cause of inflammation or for demonstrating malignant transformation in tissue. (A) Acute and chronic inflammation with neutrophils (n), plasma cells (p), lymphocytes (l), and the occasional eosinophil. (B) Large pleomorphic (bizarrely shaped) nuclei with little cytoplasm (increased nuclear:cytoplasmic ratio). Mitotic (m) figures can be seen.

Endoluminal ultrasound is becoming increasingly important for the investigation of pancreatic abnormalities and tumours.

Bile duct manometry

Bile duct manometry is undertaken by passing a pressure transducer on a catheter through an ERCP endoscope. This is undertaken for rare causes of biliary pain thought to be due to biliary dyskinesia.

Pressure waves are obtained as for oesophageal manometry.

Laparoscopy

Laparoscopy is now increasingly undertaken to perform surgical operations such as cholecystectomy. However, the original, and still very useful, indication is for inspection of intra-abdominal organs, including the liver. Ultrasound and biopsy can also be undertaken through the laparoscope.

Radiology
Chest radiograph

A chest X-ray is useful in the investigation of liver disorders to assess heart size and concomitant pulmonary disease. In the investigation of patients with an acute abdomen, it is essential to look for evidence of air under the diaphragm on an erect film, as this indicates a perforated intra-abdominal viscus (see Fig. 3.1). Conversely, absence of a gastric air bubble can be a feature of achalasia.

Plain abdominal radiograph

This is useful in suspected cases of obstruction to look for dilated bowel loops and fluid levels in the bowel (see Fig. 3.2). It is also useful in patients with colitis to assess mucosal oedema and colonic dilatation.

Abdominal ultrasound

This is undertaken in the investigation of abdominal pain, usually to exclude gallstones, or for the investigation of abnormal liver enzymes. It is useful:

- In assessing bile duct dilatation but only 60% sensitive in finding a cause.
- To screen for hepatic metastases or pancreatic tumours.
- To identify ascites.
- To look for occult gynaecological tumours.

Computed tomography (CT)

CT is an important investigative tool for gastroenterology. It is the main way of staging all intra-abdominal tumours. It is the most sensitive non-invasive technique for diagnosing chronic pancreatitis. It can be useful for CT-colography as an alternative to barium enema or colonoscopy in the elderly.

Magnetic resonance (MR)

Magnetic resonance can differentiate different tissue characteristics without using radiation. With

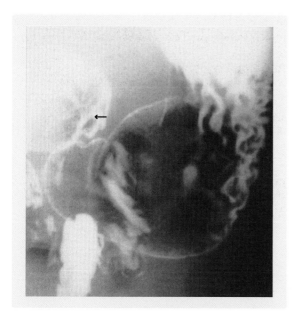

Fig. 24.23 Barium meal demonstration of a duodenal ulcer (long arrow) surrounded by oedema which appears as radiating folds (arrow).

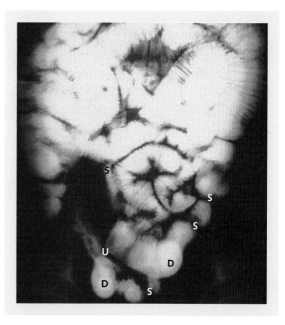

Fig. 24.24 Barium follow-through showing multiple areas of strictures (S), deep ulcers (U), and dilatation (D) resulting from Crohn's disease.

computer reconstruction it is a sensitive technique to examine the bile duct or pancreas as an alternative to ERCP (MRCP = magnetic resonance cholangiopancreatography).

Barium swallow

Barium swallow is frequently undertaken in the investigation or assessment of dysphagia. Compared with endoscopy:

- The additional advantage is that peristaltic pressure waves are observed and signs of gastro-oesophageal reflux can be sought.
- The disadvantage is that direct inspection of the mucosa cannot be undertaken and biopsies cannot be obtained.

Barium meal

This is an alternative to endoscopy for the investigation of dyspepsia or abdominal pain depending on local circumstances (Figs 24.23 and 24.24). Again, direct inspection of the mucosa cannot be undertaken and biopsies cannot be obtained.

Small bowel enema

The major indication for this study is for the investigation of malabsorption or abdominal pain, particularly if Crohn's disease is suspected.

Barium enema

Barium enema is frequently undertaken in the investigation or assessment of lower abdominal pain or altered bowel habit (Fig. 24.25). However, this method does not allow direct inspection of the mucosa and biopsies cannot be taken.

Nuclear medicine
White cell scan

The patient's leucocytes are removed and labelled with [111]indium. These are subsequently returned to the patient. The white cells accumulate in areas of inflammation or infection and can be detected by a gamma camera. It can be of particular clinical value in monitoring response to treatment in patients with colitis (particularly Crohn's disease).

Octreotide scan

Somatostatin (octreotide is a somatostain analogue) is taken up by neuroendocrine cells in certain tumours (e.g. carcinoid, gastrinoma) and can be detected by gamma camera.

MIBG scan

Metaiodobenzylguanidine (MIBG) is also taken up by neuroendocrine APUD cells and will accumulate

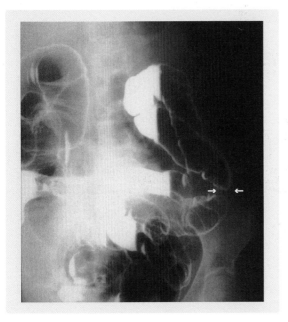

Fig. 24.25 Barium enema demonstrating an 'apple-core' lesion (carcinoma) in the ascending colon (arrows).

in areas of high content such as the pancreas, but also in liver tumours and carcinoid disease.

Red blood cell scan

An aliquot of patient's blood is labelled with ^{51}chromium and given back to the patient. In this situation, the leakage or a collection of isotope detected by a gamma camera and located to the lumen will indicate bleeding or red blood cell loss.

Sehcat scan is used to detect bile salt malabsorption.

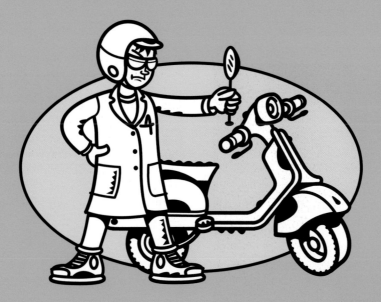

SELF-ASSESSMENT

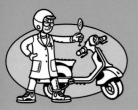

Multiple-choice Questions (MCQs)

Indicate whether each answer is true or false.

1. **The following are true of pain arising from the oesophagus:**

(a) It is often precipitated by exertion
(b) It can occur in the absence of heartburn
(c) It can mimic the pain of a myocardial infarction
(d) It is never relieved by glyceryl trinitrate
(e) It is associated with *Helicobacter pylori*

2. **The following are true of the investigation of indigestion:**

(a) A microcytic anaemia would be unconcerning
(b) Positive *H.pylori* serology indicates current infection
(c) The onset of melaena would prompt urgent investigation
(d) A chest x-ray is diagnostically unhelpful
(e) The presence of a hiatus hernia is diagnostic of acid reflux

3. **The following statements are true:**

(a) Elevated tone of the lower oesophageal sphincter (LOS) contributes to acid reflux
(b) Smoking increases LOS tone
(c) Normal endoscopy excludes reflux oesphagitis
(d) Pregnancy predisposes towards symptoms of reflux
(e) Conservative treatment is rarely effective in the management of acid reflux

4. **The following are true of Barrett's oesophagus:**

(a) Columnar epithelium is replaced by squamous epithelium
(b) It is a premalignant condition
(c) Endoscopic surveillance may be required
(d) The clinical features differ from reflux oesphagitis
(e) Severe dysplastic change is an ominous sign

5. **The following apply to a history of dysphagia:**

(a) Benign oesophageal stricture is often preceded by a history of heartburn
(b) If progressive suggests globus hystericus
(c) The patient can accurately assess the level at which it occurs
(d) Associated regurgitation of food suggests a benign stricture
(e) Significant weight loss is suggestive of carcinoma

6. **In the investigation of dysphagia:**

(a) Barium swallow is preferable to endoscopy if there is a history of regurgitation
(b) A chest X-ray may demonstrate evidence of prior pulmonary infection
(c) Endoscopic ultrasound best assesses local spread of oesophageal carcinoma
(d) If a stricture is suspected, endoscopy is the most appropriate investigation
(e) A full blood count is rarely necessary

7. **The following are true of achalasia:**

(a) Endoscopy is a sensitive diagnostic test
(b) A history of regurgitation is common
(c) It oftens presents in childhood
(d) Retrosternal chest pain is a frequent symptom
(e) Histology shows a reduction of Auerbach plexus ganglia cells in the oesophageal wall

8. **In the context of acute abdominal pain:**

(a) An elevated amylase is always indicative of acute pancreatitis
(b) An ECG is an important investigation
(c) The presence of ascites may suggest Budd–Chiari syndrome
(d) Respiratory rate is a useful parameter to assess
(e) A patient with peritonitis will be restless with the pain

9. **The following are bad prognostic factors in acute pancreatitis:**

(a) High white cell count
(b) High calcium levels
(c) High blood urea
(d) High amylase levels
(e) Hypoxia—pO_2 <8 kPa

10. **The following are true of the investigation of acute abdominal pain:**

(a) Microscopic haematuria would support a diagnosis of renal colic
(b) The absence of subdiaphragmatic gas on a chest X-ray excludes perforation
(c) A high CRP can be found in Crohn's disease
(d) Biliary colic is supported by high levels of liver enzymes
(e) An abdominal ultrasound is unhelpful

11. **The following clinical features can be associated with peptic ulcer disease:**

(a) A history of non-steroidal anti-inflammatory drug use
(b) Exacerbation of pain following eating
(c) The passage of fresh blood per rectum
(d) A palpable supraclavicular lymph node
(e) Radiation of pain to the back

12. **The following are true of the investigation of chronic abdominal pain:**

(a) A normal amylase excludes chronic pancreatitis
(b) A plain abdominal radiograph can be diagnostic
(c) Thrombocytosis can indicate a chronic inflammatory process
(d) Crohn's disease can present acutely with right iliac fossa pain
(e) A macrocytic anaemia is found with chronic blood loss

13. **The following are true of abdominal ascites:**

(a) Ascites with high protein content is found in the nephrotic syndrome
(b) Absence of malignant cells on cytological examination excludes cancer
(c) An echocardiogram may be indicated in its investigation
(d) Ultrasonography is sensitive diagnostic modality
(e) Assessment of jugular venous pressure is important

14. **For a patient with weight loss:**

(a) The patient's subjective assessment is usually accurate
(b) Malignancy can cause weight loss through anorexia
(c) Increased appetite may indicate hyperthyroidism
(d) Hypocalcaemia may suggest malabsorption
(e) Corticosteroid therapy may be a contributing factor

15. **The following drugs are known to commonly cause vomiting:**

(a) Corticosteroids
(b) Digoxin
(c) Antibiotics (e.g. metronidazole)
(d) Non-steroidal anti-inflammatory drugs
(e) Morphine

16. **The following metabolic conditions tend to produce vomiting:**

(a) Diabetic ketoacidosis
(b) Hypoglycaemia
(c) Hypercalcaemia
(d) Hypocalcaemia
(e) Uraemia

17. **The following are true of upper gastrointestinal bleeding:**

(a) Haematemesis and melaena rarely occur together
(b) The presence of a prosthetic heart valve influences management
(c) A postural drop in blood pressure may indicate a significant bleed
(d) The haemoglobin may be normal at the presentation of a large bleed
(e) A history of preceding vomiting suggests peptic ulcer disease

18. **In the investigation of upper gastrointestinal bleeding:**

(a) An elevated blood urea indicates chronic liver disease
(b) A coagulopathy can be expected with peptic ulcer disease
(c) A high leucocyte count can be seen in the context of a large bleed
(d) Thrombocytopenia can be associated with bleeding oesophageal varices
(e) Endoscopy is not always necessary

19. **The following features dictate that a gastrointestinal bleed is 'high risk':**

(a) Age over 65 years
(b) Non-steroidal anti-inflammatory drugs
(c) Coexisting cardiac failure
(d) Renal impairment
(e) A low haemoglobin at presentation

20. **The following drugs are well recognized to cause diarrhoea:**

(a) Codeine
(b) Amoxicillin
(c) Colchicine
(d) Corticosteroids
(e) Metronidazole

21. **Blood stained diarrhoea is associated with the following conditions:**

(a) Ulcerative colitis
(b) Giardiasis
(c) Radiation colitis
(d) Irritable bowel syndrome
(e) Thyrotoxicosis

22. The following are true of the investigation of diarrhoea:

(a) Macrocytic anaemia suggests underlying inflammatory bowel disease
(b) A 24-hour urine collection may be helpful
(c) Bacterial cultures are frequently positive in diarrhoea of infective origin
(d) Ferritin may be elevated in inflammatory bowel disease
(e) An abdominal radiograph is frequently of diagnostic value

23. Steatorrhoea is associated with the following conditions:

(a) Coeliac disease
(b) Bacterial overgrowth
(c) Chronic pancreatitis
(d) Ileal tuberculosis
(e) Whipple's disease

24. The following organisms are frequently implicated in infective diarrhoea:

(a) Rotavirus
(b) Cytomegalovirus
(c) *Salmonella* sp.
(d) *Staphylococcus aureus*
(e) Cryptosporidiosis

25. The following biochemical derangements can be associated with diarrhoea:

(a) Elevated blood urea
(b) Hyperkalaemia
(c) Hypomagnesaemia
(d) Hypercalcaemia
(e) Hyperglycaemia

26. In the context of rectal bleeding:

(a) Haemorrhoids produce dark red 'venous' bleeding
(b) Red blood mixed with stool is associated with low rectal lesions
(c) Pain on defecation is a feature of anal fissure
(d) Tenderness in the left iliac fossa suggests angiodysplasia
(e) Anaemia can usually be attributed to the blood loss

27. The following are true of the investigation of rectal bleeding:

(a) The majority of conditions can be diagnosed clinically with proctoscopy and sigmoidoscopy
(b) Angiography is only indicated if there is active bleeding at the time
(c) Rigid sigmoidoscopy can identify lesions up to 35 cm from the anal margin
(d) Anal fissure is frequently seen during proctoscopy
(e) The presence of haemorrhoids on proctoscopy makes more invasive investigation unnecessary

28. In the patient with anaemia:

(a) Conjunctival pallor is a sensitive correlate to the haemoglobin concentration
(b) Further tests are dependent on the full blood count parameters
(c) Gastroscopy should be undertaken in all cases of iron-deficient anaemia in the absence of an alternative explanation
(d) The presence of a duodenal ulcer is an adequate explanation for iron-deficiency anaemia
(e) Coeliac disease is an uncommon cause of malabsorption with anaemia in this country

29. The following are true of macrocytic anaemia:

(a) Methotrexate and anticonvulsant drugs can lead to B_{12} deficiency
(b) A reticulocytosis can result in a spurious macrocytosis
(c) Caecal carcinoma is a common cause in the elderly
(d) A Schilling test may be indicated if folate levels are low
(e) Hypothyroidism is a recognized cause

30. The following are true of iron deficiency:

(a) It is confirmed by a low serum iron *and* a low iron-binding capacity
(b) NSAIDs are commonly implicated
(c) It can result from heavy menstruation
(d) It can be a manifestation of coeliac disease
(e) Oval macrocytes are seen on a peripheral blood film

31. The following statements regarding jaundice are correct:

(a) It is only detectable clinically when the serum bilirubin level exceeds 80 mmol/L
(b) A rapid onset suggests autoimmune disease
(c) A palpable gallbladder suggests gallstones as the cause
(d) Abdominal ultrasound is the key investigation
(e) The level of bilirubin reflects hepatic synthetic function

32. The following drugs are *well recognized* to cause jaundice:

(a) Flucloxacillin
(b) Paracetamol
(c) Aspirin
(d) Gentamicin
(e) Antituberculous drugs

33. The following clinical findings can be associated with jaundice:

(a) Lymphadenopathy
(b) Ascites
(c) Features of Parkinsonism
(d) Palmar erythema
(e) Peripheral oedema

34. Regarding liver biochemistry:

(a) ALT is a good reflection of liver function
(b) Elevated GGT can also reflect bony metastases or Paget's disease
(c) GGT is an enzyme easily 'induced' by drugs or alcohol
(d) Elevated ALT and bilirubin suggests liver metastases
(e) T-cell lymphomas can derange liver enzymes

35. The following conditions cause clubbing of the nails:

(a) Coeliac disease
(b) Caecal carcinoma
(c) Crohn's disease
(d) Chronic pancreatitis
(e) Cirrhosis

36. The following clinical signs are correctly matched to the underlying condition:

(a) Grey–Turner's sign and acute pancreatitis
(b) Proximal myopathy and alcoholism
(c) Splenomegaly and cirrhosis
(d) Cullen's sign and Crohn's disease
(e) Pyoderma gangrenosum and ulcerative colitis

37. The following haematological findings are correctly matched to the disorder:

(a) Thrombocytosis and portal hypertension
(b) Neutrophilia and colonic inflammation
(c) Macrocytosis and iron deficiency
(d) Thrombocytosis and inflammatory disease
(e) Leucopenia and viral hepatitis

38. The following conditions typically cause pain in the right iliac fossa:

(a) Ectopic pregnancy
(b) Biliary colic
(c) Appendicitis
(d) Diverticulitis
(e) Crohn's disease

39. The following are recognized causes of a right iliac fossa mass:

(a) Ileocaecal tuberculosis
(b) Appendicitis
(c) Caecal carcinoma
(d) Coeliac disease
(e) Ectopic pregnancy

40. The following skin lesions can be associated with disease of the gastrointestinal tract:

(a) Dermatitis herpetiformis
(b) Psoriasis
(c) Eczema
(d) Spider naevi
(e) Xanthelasmata

41. The following investigations may be indicated following an acute upper gastrointestinal bleed:

(a) Endoscopy
(b) Endoscopic retrograde cholangiopancreatography
(c) Laparoscopy
(d) Labelled red blood cell scan
(e) Barium meal

42. The following statements regarding reflux oesophagitis are correct:

(a) It may manifest with nocturnal coughing
(b) Iron-deficiency anaemia can result
(c) The condition is more common in asthmatics
(d) Lying flat relieves symptoms
(e) It can mimic the pain of cardiac ischaemia

43. The following drugs may exacerbate symptoms of dyspepsia/reflux:

(a) Tricyclic antidepressants
(b) Domperidone
(c) NSAIDs
(d) Caffeine
(e) Proton pump inhibitors

44. The following are potential complications of reflux oesophagitis:

(a) Upper gastrointestinal bleeding
(b) Barrett's oesophagus
(c) Acute pancreatitis
(d) Benign oesophageal stricture
(e) Peptic ulceration

45. The following are true of Barrett's oesophagus:

(a) The majority of people with prolonged reflux will develop Barrett's
(b) Metaplastic change is from columnar to squamous epithelium
(c) Histological change correlates poorly with symptomatology
(d) Proton pump inhibitor therapy may allow return of normal epithelium
(e) Long-term endoscopic surveillance is often indicated

46. The following are true of benign oesophageal strictures:

(a) Weight loss can be marked
(b) Symptoms can mimic those of malignant strictures
(c) Symptoms of acid reflux often worsen as the condition progresses
(d) Endoscopic ultrasound may be necessary to exclude malignant infiltration
(e) A history of radiotherapy to the mediastinum may be pertinent

47. In the context of oesophageal carcinoma:

(a) Retrosternal chest pain is the commonest presenting feature
(b) Pernicious anaemia is associated
(c) The majority are squamous cell carcinomas
(d) Radiotherapy is often curative
(e) An elevated ALT and GGT may be seen

48. Regarding the stomach:

(a) The fundus extends to form the pylorus
(b) The antrum secretes gastrin from G-cells
(c) An acidic pH is required to activate enzymes
(d) It is a major site of absorption of glucose and amino acids
(e) Chief cells secrete pepsinogen

49. The following are true of H. pylori:

(a) It is noted for its ability to produce the enzyme urease
(b) Asymptomatic infection is uncommon
(c) Increasing prevalence is seen with advancing age
(d) It is a Gram-negative bacterium
(e) Peptic ulceration is the only manifestation of infection

50. Regarding diagnostic tests for H. pylori:

(a) Culture of the organism is a rapid and sensitive method of detection
(b) A serological antibody test indicates current infection
(c) Oesophagogastroduodenoscopy may demonstrate a blotchy mucosal appearance
(d) A normal full blood count makes infection unlikely
(e) The urease breath test involves inhalation of radiolabelled urea

51. The following are true of gastric ulcers:

(a) They occur more commonly in the elderly
(b) They occur more commonly than duodenal ulceration
(c) Retrosternal pain is common
(d) Eating may precipitate pain
(e) May be painless

52. Complications of gastric ulceration include:

(a) Gastric outflow obstruction
(b) Iron-deficiency anaemia
(c) Peritonitis
(d) Pancreatitis
(e) Dysphagia

53. In the context of duodenal ulceration:

(a) Iron-deficiency anaemia is common
(b) Association with H. pylori is unusual
(c) The patient's blood group may be relevant
(d) An acute gastrointestinal bleed may be the first manifestation
(e) Recurrent disease is typical

54. The following investigations are indicated in the presence of gastric carcinoma:

(a) Chest X-ray
(b) Abdominal X-ray
(c) Liver biochemistry
(d) Renal ultrasound
(e) Serum calcium

55. The following are recognized complications following gastrectomy:

(a) Vitamin D deficiency
(b) Bacterial overgrowth
(c) Constipation
(d) Diabetes mellitus
(e) Anaemia

56. The following may be manifestations of small intestinal disease:

(a) Steatorrhoea
(b) Constipation
(c) Weight loss
(d) Osteomalacia
(e) Abdominal pain

57. Regarding coeliac disease:

(a) It is commonly seen in Black Africans
(b) Hypersplenism is associated
(c) Intestinal lymphoma is associated
(d) There are documented HLA associations
(e) A dimorphic blood picture may be seen

58. The following are recognized complications of coeliac disease:

(a) T-cell lymphoma
(b) Peripheral oedema
(c) Macrocytic anaemia
(d) Microcytic anaemia
(e) Eczema

59. The following abnormalities can be seen in Crohn's disease:

(a) Normocytic anaemia
(b) Low albumin
(c) Low platelet count
(d) High CRP
(e) High serum calcium

60. The following are systemic manifestations of Crohn's disease:

(a) Uveitis
(b) Myocarditis
(c) Seropositive arthritis
(d) Osteopenia
(e) Pyoderma gangrenosum

61. The following statements are true of gastrointestinal manifestations of Crohn's disease:

(a) Oral ulceration is common.
(b) Transmural inflammation with non-caseating granulomas is seen
(c) The rectum is commonly involved
(d) Inflammation tends to be contiguous along the bowel
(e) Duodenal ulceration can occur

62. The following are true of Crohn's disease:

(a) Corticosteroids improve the overall prognosis of the condition
(b) Secondary amyloidosis can develop
(c) A small proportion of patients require surgical intervention
(d) Immunosuppression can be effective, even in severe disease
(e) Anaerobic infections are common in peri-anal disease

63. The following features are seen in the carcinoid syndrome:

(a) Abdominal pain
(b) Constipation
(c) Bronchoconstriction
(d) Pulmonary stenosis
(e) Peripheral neuropathy

64. The following are clinical features of bacterial overgrowth:

(a) Peptic ulceration
(b) Steatorrhoea
(c) B_{12} deficiency
(d) Gastrointestinal bleeding
(e) Weight loss

65. The following conditions are matched correctly to the type of organism responsible:

(a) Giardiasis—anaerobe
(b) Cholera—Gram-negative bacillus
(c) Tuberculosis—protozoan
(d) Yersinia—Gram-negative bacterium
(e) Tropical sprue—unknown

66. Regarding the large intestine:

(a) Its main role is the absorption of water and electrolytes
(b) Absorption takes place predominantly in the ascending colon
(c) The ascending colon is predominantly supplied by the inferior mesenteric artery
(d) The ileocaecal valve heralds the end of the large intestine
(e) The transverse colon is supplied solely by the superior mesenteric artery

67. The following statements regarding irritable bowel syndrome are true:

(a) Abdominal pain with weight loss are typical features
(b) LIF pain relieved by defecation is common
(c) Imaging of the large bowel is often diagnostically helpful
(d) Increased fibre intake is universally helpful in symptom control
(e) Psychological stress may be a precipitant

68. The following drugs commonly cause constipation:

(a) Tricyclic antidepressants
(b) SSRI antidepressants
(c) Iron sulphate
(d) Codeine phosphate
(e) Thyroxine

69. The following statements are true of colitis:

(a) Granulomas are present in collagenous colitis
(b) Rectal sparing is characteristic of Crohn's colitis
(c) Caseating granulomas in the terminal ileum are diagnostic of Crohn's disease
(d) Colitis in a smoker is more likely to be Crohn's than ulcerative colitis
(e) Pain is a characteristic feature of CMV colitis

70. The following are true of ulcerative colitis:

(a) It commonly presents with pain in the right iliac fossa
(b) It can be associated with ankylosing spondylitis
(c) It is a risk factor for toxic dilatation of the colon
(d) The appearance of abdominal tenderness is an ominous sign
(e) It often causes ischiorectal abscesses

71. The following are extra-intestinal features of ulcerative colitis:

(a) Pyoderma gangrenosum
(b) Renal calculi
(c) Sclerosing cholangitis
(d) Episcleritis
(e) Mononeuritis multiplex

72. The following are true of ulcerative colitis:

(a) Pseudopolyps can be seen macroscopically
(b) Crypt abscesses and goblet cell depletion are typical
(c) Longstanding colitis can lead to loss of haustra with fibrosis
(d) pANCA antibodies are often detected
(e) The small intestine is never affected

73. The following features are indicative of severity in ulcerative colitis:

(a) Fever
(b) Vomiting
(c) Tachycardia
(d) Hypoalbuminaemia
(e) Anaemia

74. The following are true of colon polyps and colon cancer:

(a) The larger the polyp, the greater the risk of cancer
(b) Malignant polyps can be successfully treated by colonoscopy and polypectomy alone
(c) Hyperplastic polyps have a higher malignant potential than villous polyps
(d) Polyps are common in the ascending colon
(e) Colonic polyps are often recurrent

75. The following statements are true of colonic carcinoma:

(a) Altered bowel habit is seen in greater than half of all patients
(b) Rectal bleeding is common with right-sided lesions
(c) Iron-deficiency anaemia is common with right-sided lesions
(d) Jaundice can occur
(e) It may present as an 'acute abdomen'

76. The following statements are true of bacterial infection of the colon:

(a) Is a common cause of diarrhoea
(b) Sigmoidoscopy is usually necessary
(c) Leucocytosis may be seen
(d) Anaemia is common
(e) Anti-diarrhoeal agents should be avoided

77. The following statements are true:

(a) Amoebiasis can result in bloody diarrhoea
(b) Cryptosporidiosis tends to be self-limiting in healthy individuals
(c) Schistosomiasis can cause a localized granulomatous reaction in the colon
(d) *Clostridium difficile* infection often follows treatment with narrow spectrum antibiotics
(e) Oral vancomycin can be used to treat *C. difficile*

78. The following are recognized functions of the liver:

(a) Synthesis of all the coagulation factors
(b) Iron storage
(c) Excretion of bilirubin
(d) Synthesis of insulin
(e) Synthesis of albumin

79. Of hepatitis A infection:

(a) Prodromal symptoms can mimic viral gastroenteritis
(b) Craving for nicotine is said to be enhanced in those who smoke
(c) Splenomegaly is common in the icteric phase
(d) Elevation of anti-HAV IgG implies acute infection
(e) Myocarditis is a potential complication

80. The following statements regarding hepatitis B are correct:

(a) Symptomless infected carrier rate can be up to 20% in some parts of the world
(b) The average incubation period is 14–21 days
(c) A polyarthritis can be a feature of acute infection
(d) Up to 90% of acute infections resolve without sequelae
(e) Carrier rate is much higher following vertical transmission

81. The following statements regarding hepatitis B are correct:

(a) HBsAg (surface antigen) is the first serological marker to appear
(b) HBeAg ('e') reflects viral replication and high infectivity
(c) Anti-HBe antibodies appear late (>3 months)
(d) Anti-HBs antibodies confer lifelong immunity
(e) Transaminase levels peak at around the same time as HBeAg levels

82. Regarding hepatitis C:

(a) Routine screening of blood products for the virus has been available since 1998
(b) Clinical jaundice appears in the majority of patients
(c) Synthetic function is usually preserved
(d) Viral RNA can be detected by PCR (polymerase chain reaction)
(e) Approximately two-thirds of patients will progress to cirrhosis

221

83. **The following statements are true of infections involving the liver:**

(a) Atypical lymphocytes can be seen in the blood with infectious mononucleosis
(b) Hepatitis due to EBV carries a poor prognosis
(c) CMV infection occurs predominantly in the immunocompromised
(d) Leptospirosis can be associated with renal failure
(e) Toxoplasmosis can cause a febrile illness with lymphadenopathy

84. **Haemachromatosis:**

(a) Is a genetic defect resulting in copper overload in the liver
(b) Is a risk factor for the development of hepatoma
(c) Has an equal sex incidence but presents earlier in males than females
(d) Can result in low blood glucose levels
(e) Can cause hypogonadism in the absence of cirrhosis

85. **Primary sclerosing cholangitis:**

(a) Occurs predominantly in middle-aged females
(b) Is a major risk factor for cholangiocarcinoma
(c) Occurs in 50% of patients with ulcerative colitis
(d) Ursodeoxycholic acid may be of some benefit
(e) May require insertion of an endoprosthesis for its treatment

86. **The following statements are true:**

(a) Kayser–Fleischer rings are seen in Wilson's disease
(b) Serum copper is grossly elevated (×10) in Wilson's disease
(c) Upper lobe emphysema is seen in homozygotes with Alpha-1-antitrypsin deficiency
(d) In Alpha-1-antitrypsin deficiency, prognosis depends on genotype
(e) Splenomegaly can be seen in cystic fibrosis

87. **The following are recognized extra-pulmonary features of cystic fibrosis:**

(a) Diabetes insipidus
(b) Impotence
(c) Malabsorption
(d) Small bowel obstruction
(e) Cirrhosis

88. **Primary biliary cirrhosis:**

(a) Predominantly affects women, with a ratio of 10 : 1
(b) Itching is a prominent feature, and often precedes jaundice
(c) Xanthomas are seen
(d) Vitamin D deficiency is common
(e) Membranous glomerulonephritis is associated

89. **The following statements regarding alcoholic liver disease are correct:**

(a) The majority of people dependent on alcohol will develop liver disease
(b) Fatty change is reversible with abstinence from alcohol
(c) Mallory bodies are characteristic of alcohol damage
(d) 75% of liver cirrhosis is due to alcohol
(e) Macrocytosis may be seen

90. **The following are recognized stigmata of chronic liver disease:**

(a) Leuconychia
(b) Kolionychia
(c) Jaundice
(d) Palmar erythema
(e) Cyanosis

91. **The following features are used to assess functional capacity of the liver:**

(a) Serum bilirubin levels
(b) Serum albumin
(c) Serum glucose
(d) Encephalopathy
(e) Spider naevi

92. **The following are true of tumours of the liver:**

(a) Metastases are the commonest tumours seen in the liver
(b) Cirrhosis is a risk for hepatocellular carcinoma, whatever the cause
(c) Hepatocellular carcinomas are particularly sensitive to chemotherapy
(d) Liver ultrasound will detect the majority of liver tumours
(e) Haemangiomas are the commonest benign liver tumour

93. **The following statements are true of paracetamol toxicity:**

(a) Glutathione depletion is a key biochemical feature
(b) Patients with pre-existing liver impairment are at greater risk of hepatic damage
(c) A prolonged prothrombin time correlates accurately with hepatic damage
(d) An elevated creatinine is a poor prognostic feature
(e) Metabolic alkalosis is seen

94. The following statements are true:

(a) Unconjugated bilirubin is water soluble
(b) Enterohepatic circulation of bilirubin occurs via the hepatic vein
(c) The majority of patients with gallstones will require a cholecystectomy at some stage
(d) The majority of gallstones are radio-opaque
(e) Patients with terminal ileal disease are at risk of developing gallstones

95. The following are potential complications of gallstone disease:

(a) Acute pancreatitis
(b) Pancreatic carcinoma
(c) Ascending cholangitis
(d) Primary biliary cirrhoisis
(e) Empyema of the gallbladder

96. The following are true of infections involving the biliary tract:

(a) Bile within the biliary tree is usually sterile
(b) Septicaemic shock with Gram-negative organisms can occur
(c) A 'cholestatic' picture may be seen biochemically
(d) Blood cultures are rarely positive
(e) Endoscopic retrograde cholangiopancreatography is a risk factor for cholangitis

97. The following are recognized clinical features of acute pancreatitis:

(a) Hypovolaemic shock
(b) Haematemesis
(c) Upper abdominal pain
(d) Vomiting
(e) Hypoxia

98. The following are recognized causes of acute pancreatitis:

(a) Hypocalcaemia
(b) Hyperglycaemia
(c) Corticosteroid therapy
(d) Alcohol excess
(e) Snake bite

99. The following are potential complications of acute pancreatitis:

(a) Septicaemia
(b) Hyperglycaemia
(c) Disseminated intravascular coagulation
(d) Ileus
(e) Acute renal failure

100. The following statements are true:

(a) Serum amylase is rarely normal in chronic pancreatitis
(b) Endoscopic retrograde cholangiopancreatography may be useful in the diagnosis of chronic pancreatitis
(c) Pseudocysts are an uncommon complication of acute pancreatitis
(d) Thrombophlebitis migrans is associated with pancreatic carcinoma
(e) Ascites occurs early in the course of pancreatic carcinoma

1. A 46-year-old woman presents with painless jaundice and pruritis. Alkaline phosphatase and GGT are three to five times the upper limit of normal. Transaminases are normal. What would your initial choice of investigations be? Why is a history of respiratory tract infection, for which she received treatment, of relevance?

2. A 22-year-old female presents with acute abdominal pain. She is tachycardic and hypotensive. She has marked tenderness in the right iliac fossa with signs of localized peritonitis. List five possible diagnoses and suggest one key investigation that could confirm each.

3. A man aged 55 years is found to have a microcytic hypochromic anaemia on a routine full blood count. How would you confirm iron-deficiency? An endoscopy reveals a duodenal ulcer. What would you do next?

4. A 38-year-old man presents with bloody diarrhoea with negative stool cultures and raised inflammatory markers. Describe five features that may help differentiate Crohn's disease from ulcerative colitis.

5. A 52-year-old man presents with severe upper abdominal pain and vomiting. Serum amylase is 3500. List the parameters that have prognostic significance and outline your initial management of the patient.

6. A 28-year-old man presents with diarrhoea. His brother is known to carry HLA-B27. What diagnostic possibilities should be considered for this patient and why?

7. A man aged 34 years presents with several weeks of diarrhoea and associated weight loss of 10 kg, despite a normal appetite. You suspect malabsorption. What biochemical and haematological tests would be relevant? List some causes of malabsorption and, given the history, name other conditions that could be easily excluded.

8. A 67-year-old man presented 3 months ago with obstructive jaundice. A diagnosis of carcinoma in the head of pancreas was made and the obstruction was relieved by endoscopic insertion of a biliary stent. He now presents with jaundice, rigors, pyrexia and pain in the right upper quadrant. What is the most likely explanation, and how would you investigate and treat him? What might you expect to find on blood cultures?

9. A 52-year-old woman presents with a history that is strongly suggestive of peptic ulcer disease. What diagnostic options do you have in establishing her *Helicobacter pylori* status? She is confirmed *H. pylori* positive. Give an example of an eradication regimen that may be used. Why might a patient be advised to avoid alcohol whilst taking this course?

10. A young woman attends A&E after taking 30 paracetamol tablets earlier that day. Which other pieces of information are particularly relevant? How would you decide whether or not to administer *N*-acetylcysteine? What are the three main parameters that have prognostic significance?

11. A 17-year-old male is referred with a bilirubin of 60, ALT normal, alkaline phosphatase slightly elevated and GGT normal. What is the most likely disgnosis and what is the mechanism of the hyperbilirubinaemia in this condition? Why is the alkaline phosphatase raised? List other situations in which an elevated alkaline phosphatase reflects a non-hepatological source.

12. A woman aged 70 years is found to have a macrocytic anaemia. Serum B_{12} levels are found to be low. She has a good diet. What tests could you perform to establish the aetiology of her B_{12} deficiency? What other causes of a macrocytic anaemia can you list?

13. A patient known to have hepatic cirrhosis is brought to A&E. He has become confused and disorientated over the last 2 days. He has a course flap with outstretched hands, sweet smelling breath and, shortly after admission, has a seizure lasting 1 minute. What is the diagnosis and what precipitants are commonly implicated in an acute onset such as this. Which four other parameters encompass the 'modified Child classification of cirrhosis'.

14. A man aged 32 years with recently diagnosed ulcerative colitis is admitted from clinic. He has been unwell for several days with profuse bloody diarrhoea, and feeling hot and shivery. List the clinical and laboratory features that would indicate severity in an exacerbation of ulcerative colitis such as this (up to eight). Which particular symptom would concern you? How would you explain the 'hot and shivery' symptoms? Outline your initial management of this patient.

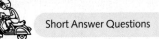

15. A man aged 46 years is found to have an elevated ALT and alk phosphatase and is subsequently investigated. Serum ferritin is found to be grossly elevated at 1200 and a presumptive diagnosis of haemachromatosis is made. How would you make a definitive diagnosis? Under what circumstances can an elevated ferritin be misleading? List the other manifestations of haemachromatosis according to site affected.

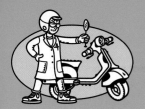
1.   THEME: Haematemesis and melaena

A.   Gastric ulceration
B.   Oesophageal varices
C.   Mallory–Weiss tear
D.   Gastric carcinoma
E.   NSAID-associated peptic ulcer
F.   Acute gastritis
G.   Severe haemophilia
H.   Atrophic gastritis
I.   Duodenal ulceration

The patients below have all presented with evidence of upper gastrointestinal bleeding. Select the most appropriate diagnosis from the above list.

1.   A 57-year-old lady presents to A&E with a 2-day history of tarry-black stools but no abdominal pain. She has a history of rheumatoid arthritis for 10 years but has not needed immunosuppressive therapy. She looks pale, has no signs of chronic liver disease, abdominal examination is unremarkable and melaena is confirmed on rectal examination. ☐

2.   A patient known to have alcoholic cirrhosis is brought in as an emergency after vomiting large amounts of fresh red blood and subsequently collapsing in the street. On examination, he is peripherally cold and clammy, hypotensive and tachycardic. There are signs of chronic liver disease evident. ☐

3.   A young man of 19 years presents to A&E after noticing blood in his vomit. He had consumed excess alcohol that night and was vomiting repeatedly. He says he noticed the streaks of red blood on the last two episodes of vomiting. There are no abnormal examination findings and FBC and U&E are normal. ☐

4.   A 70-year-old man presents to his GP with a 1-week history of tarry black stools. On questioning, he had been experiencing upper abdominal pain for some weeks. He was unsure how much weight he had lost, but his trousers had become very loose. FBC revealed a Hb 9.4g/dL, MCV 76, Plt 540, WCC 9.9. ☐

5.   A 45-year-old man visits his GP with an intermittent history of epigastric pain. This seems to be relieved by food or antacids. He points to a specific site in his epigastrium where the pain is experienced. *Helicobacter pylori* serology is positive. ☐

2.   THEME: Diarrhoea

A.   Crohn's disease
B.   Coeliac disease
C.   Pseudomembranous colitis
D.   Giardiasis
E.   Colonic carcinoma
F.   *Campylobacter* infection
G.   Ulcerative colitis
H.   Thyrotoxicosis
I.   Appendicitis

The following patients all give a history of diarrhoea. Select the most likely diagnosis from the above list.

1.   A 75-year-old Irish lady has had diarrhoea for a few months. This has been associated with 1 stone weight loss despite a normal appetite. On examination, she is pale and has a normal pulse rate. Iron deficiency anaemia is found on blood tests and lower gastrointestinal investigations are normal. ☐

2.   A 27-year-old man returns from a trip to Borneo. He has had watery diarrhoea for 10 days and has lost several kilograms in weight. Initial stool examination is negative but a repeat specimen is requested. There have been no previous episodes. ☐

3.   A young woman has had diarrhoea for a week. There is no abdominal pain or blood. Her weight is stable. Past history only comprises treatment for a skin infection 2 weeks ago. Standard stool culture is negative. ☐

4.   A man of 34 years presents to his GP with a 6-week history of diarrhoea associated with intermittent right iliac fossa pain. There is mucus but no blood on rectal examination. Blood tests demonstrate a normochromic normocytic anaemia with elevated CRP at 76. ☐

5.   A woman of 62 years has experienced diarrhoea for several weeks and has visibly lost weight, despite a healthy appetite. She is very anxious about her change in bowel habit. She tells you that her father died of 'a stomach tumour'. On examination, she has a normal blood pressure but her pulse is irregular. There are no palpable abdominal masses and she declines rectal examination. ☐

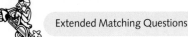

3. THEME: Acute abdominal pain

A. Peptic ulceration
B. Biliary colic
C. Acute cholecystitis
D. Bowel obstruction
E. Appendicitis
F. Acute pancreatitis
G. Acute hepatic vein thrombosis
H. Diabetic ketoacidosis
I. Ectopic pregnancy
J. Mesenteric thrombosis

The following patients all present with a short history of abdominal pain. Select the most appropriate diagnosis from the list above.

1. A man aged 74 years presents to A&E with central abdominal pain that had come on over the last few hours. He is known to be a smoker with atrial fibrillation but has no history of gastrointestinal disease. On examination, he is unwell with a tachycardia and low-grade pyrexia. Abdominal examination reveals diffuse tenderness, most marked in the umbilical region. Blood tests reveal a leucocytosis and a marked metabolic acidosis. Chest and abdominal radiographs are not diagnostically helpful.

2. A 52-year-old woman attends A&E with right upper quadrant pain. It had become gradually worse over the course of the day. Her liver enzymes are: alkaline phosphatase 600, GGT 205, bilirubin 56, ALT 57. *Escherichia coli* are grown in blood cultures.

3. A woman is brought to A&E by her husband with upper abdominal pain. She has been vomiting. On examination, she is in pain, tachycardic and hypotensive. Her upper abdomen is very tender. Her husband tells you a recent ultrasound scan showed gallstones. She beomes increasingly tachypnoeic in the few hours following admission.

4. A 19-year-old student attends A&E having experienced abdominal pain for 2 days. He has been vomiting but has had no diarrhoea. On examination, he is dehydrated and breathless at rest. His abdomen is soft with diffuse tenderness but no guarding. His chest sounds clear. Biochemistry: Na 135, K 6.2, urea 16, Cr 104, Bic 6.

5. A woman aged 24 years is brought to A&E with a history of right iliac fossa pain for a few hours. On examination she is pale, the pulse rate is 140bpm and she is noted to be peripherally cool. The right iliac fossa is very tender to palpation.

4. THEME: Chronic abdominal pain

A. Chronic pancreatitis
B. Mesenteric ischaemia
C. Peptic ulcer disease
D. Coeliac disease
E. Crohn's disease
F. Irritable bowel syndrome
G. Pancreatic carcinoma
H. Non-Hodgkin's lymphoma
I. Chronic cholecystitis
J. Gastric carcinoma

The following patients all give a history of persistent or recurrent abdominal pain. Select the most likely diagnosis from the list above.

1. A 59-year-old man gives a history of upper abdominal pain for several weeks. This has become progressively worse and recently has kept him awake at night, as the pain seems to radiate to his back. There has been no vomiting, change in bowel habit or melaena. He has been eating less and his wife thinks he has lost 2–3 stone in weight over a few months.

2. A 54-year-old lady attends her GP having experienced intermittent abdominal pain for some months. These episodes occur once or twice each week, and tend to be associated with nausea and vomiting. She indicates to her epigastric/right upper quadrant. Clinical examination is unremarkable. Blood tests reveal a CRP of 80 and a mild neutrophilia.

3. A 27-year-old nurse attends her GP surgery. She is worried about episodes of abdominal pain that have troubled her for several months. The pain tends to be intermittent in nature and usually in her lower abdomen, although a specific site could not be identified. Her bowel habit changes: often diarrhoea although she has been constipated recently. Her cousin has ulcerative colitis. Examination reveals an overweight women with no skin rashes, eye or joint abnormalities. Her abdomen is soft and she complains of tenderness across the central and lower regions. Inflammatory markers are normal.

4. A 64-year-old man has been troubled by central abdominal pain for many months. It tends to last for a few hours at a time with no identifiable relieving factors. It usually occurs in the evening, one or two hours before going to bed. He is currently under investigation by a neurologist for another problem and is awaiting carotid doppler scans. He sometimes has diarrhoea and thinks he has lost nearly a stone in weight, although he has deliberately been eating less. He has tar-stained fingers and abdominal examination is unrevealing.

5. A man aged 46 years has had central abdominal pain for several months. He describes the onset as insidious, and recently it has become quite uncomfortable. His wife complains that he has been sweating profusely at night, necessitating a change of bed clothes. He has been on a gluten free diet for many years and despite compliance, has lost 1 stone in weight over 2–3 months. On examination, his abdomen is slightly distended, but not particularly tender, and with no clinical evidence of ascites. A normocytic anaemia is found with normal U&E, LFT and LDH 720.

5. THEME: Anaemia

A. Pernicious anaemia
B. Coeliac disease
C. Metastatic carcinoma
D. Angiodyplasia
E. Caecal carcinoma
F. Bacterial overgrowth
G. Ileal tuberculosis
H. Crohn's disease
I. Barrett's oesophagus

The following patients are all found to be anaemic. Select the most likely diagnosis from the list above.

1. A routine FBC on a 74-year-old man declares him anaemic, with a MCV of 114. WCC and Plt counts are normal. On questioning, it is discovered that he has had loose motions for several months and his wife thinks he has lost some weight, although this could not be quantified. Past history is unremarkable aside from 'an operation for a stomach ulcer many years ago'. B_{12} levels are found to be low with an elevated folate level. Serum albumin, calcium and phosphate levels are all slightly low.

2. A 82-year-old man has been investigated for anaemia. Hb 8.7, WCC 9, Plt 510, MCV 73, MCH 26. Upper gastrointestinal endoscopy and duodenal biopsy are normal. Barium enema is reported as some colonic diverticulosis but nil else. He responds initially to oral iron supplementation but returns several times over the following months with further drops in his Haemoglobin, requiring red cell transfusion.

3. A women aged 48 years presents to her GP feeling tired. FBC: Hb 6, WCC 4, Plt 139, MCV 119. There are areas of skin depigmentation and she tells you that there is a family history of type 2 diabetes mellitus. Bilirubin is 45 and LDH 2900.

4. A man aged 32 years presents to his GP with weight loss and right iliac fossa pain. His symptoms have progressed over several weeks. He has been experiencing night sweats and is unsure whether he has lost weight. He has been taking corticosteroids intermittently for several years for 'brittle asthma'. He was fostered at the age of 14 years after arriving from Eastern Europe. He is found to be anaemic with a Hb 9, Plt 460, WCC 16 (differential: mild neutrophilia and monocytosis). MCV is 114 and B_{12} is low.

5. A 52-year-old man returns to surgical clinic for review. He had a gastrectomy a few months previously. He 'doesn't feel right'. Hb 8.2, WCC 2.4, Plt 89. Blood film comment: 'numerous nucleated red cells and myelocytes indicate a leucoerythroblastic picture'. His stools are dark but he is on iron supplementation. B_{12}, folate and iron all normal. Serum calcium 2.49 unadjusted. Albumin 25.

6. THEME: Dysphagia

A. Barrett's oesophagus
B. Oesophageal carcinoma
C. Achalasia
D. Benign oesophageal stricture
E. Pharyngeal pouch
F. Scleroderma
G. Oesophageal candidiasis
H. Oesophageal web
I. Antral carcinoma

The following patients all give a history of swallowing problems. Establish the most likely diagnosis from the selection provided.

1. A man in his fifties has been taking antacids for many years. He attends his GP complaining of difficulty swallowing solids which has progressed over several months. He has consequently changed his diet and his weight has remained steady. He is referred for an urgent oesophagogastroduodenoscopy.

2. A 42-year-old lady presents her GP with difficulty in swallowing over several months. She often coughs when swallowing liquids and food appears to stick retrosternally on occasions. She has also been experiencing exertional breathlessness for some time. Her blood pressure is 190/105 mmHg and there is proteinuria on dipstick examination. Oesophagogastroduodenoscopy demonstrates no mucosal lesion.

3. A man in his early sixties attends his GP with difficulty swallowing. He describes a sensation of food sticking behind his lower sternum and in the last 2 weeks has moved onto liquid or pureed food. He says he has lost 2 stone in weight and attributes this to the change in diet. He does not want an endoscopic examination.

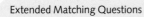
4. A man aged 45 years who has recently finished chemotherapy for lymphoma attends clinic complaining of painful swallowing that has got worse over the antecedent 10 days. He has lost some weight. He has just finished antibiotics for celluitis.

5. A women in her twenties attends her GP with an intermittent history of difficulty swallowing. This occurs with both liquids and solids and is associated with dyspeptic symptoms. She has attended A&E twice this year with episodes of central chest pain, following which she was reassured and discharged on both occasions.

7. THEME: Abnormal liver biochemistry

A. Hepatic metastases
B. Hepatitis C infection
C. Primary biliary cirrhosis
D. Drug induced hepatitis
E. Congestive cardiac failure
F. Primary amyloidosis
G. Haemachromatosis
H. Hepatitis A infection
I. Constrictive pericarditis

The following patients have all been found to have abnormal liver biochemistry. Attempt to identify the most likely diagnosis from the list provided.

1. A man aged 72 years is found to have an alkaline phosphatase of 980, a GGT of 645 and an ALT of 78. Bilirubin and albumin are normal. He has peripheral oedema but no ascites and there is a resting tachycardia with an audible third heart sound.

2. A man in his twenties presents to A&E with nausea and vomiting. He also has a dull headache and a temperature of 37.8 °C. On examination he has a 4-cm liver edge, a spleen tip is palpable and he is clearly jaundiced. Alkaline phosphatase 450, GGT 100, ALT 800, bilirubin 50. He is seen 4 weeks later and there has been complete clinical and biochemical resolution.

3. A man aged 65 years is referred by the cardiologists for investigation of abnormal liver biochemistry. Alkaline phosphatase 1200, GGT 550, ALT 89, bilirubin 39, albumin 21. He is being treated for cardiac failure of unknown aetiology (coronary angiography normal). He has peripheral oedema but a normal pulse rate, blood pressure, JVP and heart sounds. Proteinuria ++ is found on dipstick. There is evidence of hepatomegaly on clinical examination.

4. A woman aged 55 years is found to have abnormal liver biochemistry following investigation of a normocytic anaemia. Alkaline phosphatase 670, GGT 368, ALT and bilirubin normal. Albumin low at 29 and adjusted calcium 2.70. Clinical history is unrevealing. A week later, she fractures her right humerus following a fall in a shopping centre.

5. A man aged 47 years is referred for investigation of the following abnormalities. Alkaline phosphatase 400, GGT 90, ALT 107, bilirubin 20, albumin 30. He gives a history of joint stiffness and loss of libido. On examination, he has a healthy complexion, but evidence of hepatomegaly. There is no active joint inflammation and glucose is found on urine dipstick.

8. THEME: Jaundice

A. Haemolysis
B. Gilbert's syndrome
C. Carcinoma head of pancreas
D. Alcoholic liver disease
E. Sclerosing cholangitis
F. Intrahepatic cholestasis
G. α_1 antitrypsin deficiency
H. Epstein–Barr virus infection
I. Hepatic vein thrombosis
J. Gallstones

The following patients are all jaundiced. Select the most likely aetiology from the list above.

1. A 32-year-old man presents to his GP after his wife had noticed that he had become jaundiced. He was not sure of the exact timescale but had definitely got worse over the last 2 weeks. He had been experiencing some right upper quadrant pain intermittently for some weeks. His only medication was mesalazine for a history of well controlled ulcerative colitis. Bilirubin was 55 with elevated alkaline phosphatase of 980. The other liver enzymes are normal.

2. A woman aged 35 years presents to A&E. She has had abdominal pain since the previous morning and had subsequently become noticeably jaundiced. Her abdomen was distended but there were no signs of chronic liver disease. She was normally fit and well and had a history of DVT 2 years ago for which she completed 6 months of warfarin therapy. There was no family history of liver disease although her mother had died suddenly in her forties.

3. A medical student had not been feeling well for several days. His tutor had noticed jaundiced sclera and arranged hospital admission. On examination, he has a temperature of 37.8 °C, tender submandibular lymphadenopathy, tender hepatomegaly and was clearly jaundiced. The splenic tip is just palpable. He had consumed 45 units of alcohol over the previous weekend. Alkaline phosphatase 500, ALT 85, GGT 90, bilirubin 43. Atypical lymphocytes are reported on a blood film.

4. A man aged 64 years had become jaundiced over the preceding 2 weeks. This was not associated with pain or other gastrointestinal symptoms. On examination, he was thin without signs of chronic liver disease or hepatomegaly. Ultrasound demonstrated a dilated biliary tree and ERCP was suggested.

5. A young man in his twenties attends his GP after noticing 'yellow eyes' for 2 days. Alkaline phosphatase 95, GGT 35, bilirubin 46, ALT 26, albumin 37. He was usually fit and well although he was just recovering from a heavy cold. There were no abnormal examination findings.

9. THEME: Rectal bleeding

A. Diverticulosis
B. Haemorrhoids
C. Colonic carcinoma
D. Giardiasis
E. Diverticulitis
F. Angiodysplasia
G. Oesophageal variceal bleed
H. Ulcerative colitis
I. Amoebiasis
J. Cryptosporidiosis

The following patients all have a history of rectal bleeding. Select the most likely diagnosis from the list.

1. A 36-year-old man attends his GP as he is concerned about passing blood in his stools. This has occurred several times over the antecedent few weeks, with an associated history of 8–10 weeks of diarrhoea but no abdominal pain. He has no other significant medical history and is a non-smoker. There has been no recent travel abroad. Abdominal examination is interrupted by the patient having to rush to the toilet. FBC reveals a neutrophilia and a thrombocytosis.

2. A woman aged 56 years is brought to A&E as an emergency after collapsing in the street. She has cold peripheries, hypotension, tachycardia and is barely conscious. A large volume of red blood has been passed PR, but there is no melaena evident. She has numerous spider naevi over her upper chest and back and has bilateral parotid swelling.

3. A man aged 64 years presents to his GP with a history of several months of rectal bleeding. This has been intermittent, with small quantities of dark red blood sometimes mixed with the stool. His bowel habit has tended towards constipation. Abdominal examination reveals fullness in the left iliac fossa and rectal examination is normal. FBC and inflammatory markers are normal. He is referred for further investigation.

4. A 47-year-old man has had rectal bleeding associated with diarrhoea 3 days following a business trip to South East Asia. He has also been very nauseated and has vomited twice. There is some lower abdominal tenderness but no other helpful clinical signs. He responds to empiric treatment with metronidazole whilst stool samples are analysed.

5. A 54-year-old woman attends her GP with a history of dark red rectal bleeding. She has only noticed this over the last 10 days. The blood tends to be mixed with the stool. She has been opening her bowels twice a day for 2–3 months, whereas previously she was prone to constipation. She has lost 1 stone in weight over a 4-week period and attributes this to her thyroxine medication which started at this time. FBC demonstrates parameters consistent with iron deficiency.

10. THEME: Indigestion

A. Reflux oesophagitis
B. Achalasia
C. Gastric carcinoma
D. Oesophageal spasm
E. Gastric ulceration
F. Acute gastritis
G. Myocardial infarction
H. Oesophageal candidiasis
I. Non-ulcer dyspepsia
J. Duodenal ulcer

The following patients all present with symptoms that they attribute to "indigestion". Try and establish what the most likely underlying diagnosis is, given the following information.

1. A man aged 42 years complains of indigestion. On further questioning, this has occurred intermittently over several weeks and consists of epigastric pain and discomfort. There are no effects with change in posture but it is worse at night. His weight has been steady. FBC is normal.

2. A women aged 29 years attends her GP surgery complaining of persistent indigestion. She describes a sensation of epigastric fullness and early satiety. There have been no retrosternal symptoms or vomiting. Antacids are sometimes helpful. She does not take NSAIDS. Clinical examination is unrevealing. *Helicobacter pylori* serology is negative.

3. A woman aged 34 years asks her GP for 'a tablet for indigestion'. Her symptoms have become particularly worse over the last 6 weeks. She describes a feeling of retrosternal burning that is related to posture. Antacids provide temporary relief. There has been no vomiting or melaena. There are no urinary symptoms although her period is late. Examination reveals a slightly overweight women, but no other significant findings. ☐

4. A man aged 63 years attends his GP one evening. He has had 'indigestion' since 05.00 hours. He describes it as a retrosternal burning or heaviness. He is normally fit and well, his only medication is bendrofluazide for hypertension with no NSAID use. He takes occasional antacids for post-prandial dyspepsia but these have not helped today. On examination, he is sweating but there are no abnormal examination findings. ☐

5. A woman aged 44 years has had indigestion for several weeks. She describes epigastric discomfort and sometimes pain, precipitated by food. There are no retrosternal symptoms or a change in bowel habit. She is a smoker with no previous medical history. Routine FBC reveals Hb 10.8, WCC 9, Plt 440, MCV 74, MCH 22. ☐

11. THEME: Abdominal distension

A. Hypoproteinaemic ascites
B. Budd–Chiari syndrome
C. Pregnancy
D. Metastatic intra-abdominal malignancy
E. Cirrhotic ascites
F. Constrictive pericarditis
G. Acute bowel obstruction
H. Irritable bowel syndrome
I. Cardiac failure
J. Toxic megacolon

The following patients all present with a history of abdominal distension. Identify the most likely diagnosis.

1. A woman aged 63 years presents to A&E complaining of abdominal distension. This has occurred within the last 48 hours and is associated with pain. She has not opened her bowels for 3 days and had diarrhoea before this. On examination, she is clinically dehydrated, has a distended, tender, resonant abdomen with high-pitched, frequent, bowel sounds on auscultation. The rectum is empty with no discernible blood. ☐

2. A woman aged 26 years attends her GP. She has noticed increasing abdominal distension over several weeks at least. She is now unable to fit into her clothes. Bowel habit is normal and her only medication is the contraceptive pill. On examination: blood pressure, JVP and heart sounds are normal. There are no signs of chronic liver disease. Her abdomen is clearly distended with evidence of shifting dullness. Proteinuria is noted on urine testing. There is pitting oedema to the knees. ☐

3. A 31-year-old woman attends her GP as she is anxious about abdominal distension. This tends to occur intermittently and has bothered her for several months. Her last period ended 10 days ago. Her bowel habit is rather erratic: usually constipated but occasional diarrhoea. She has not lost weight. Her father died of bowel carcinoma at the age of 72 years. Examination reveals a slightly distended abdomen with active bowel sounds and no shifting dullness. PR is normal. ☐

4. A woman aged 64 years attends her GP because of abdominal distension. She has only noticed this over the past few weeks and has had no abdominal pain. Her bowels are unchanged although she has lost some weight. She drinks 20 units of alcohol each week and is a non-smoker on no regular medication. On examination, there is evidence of ascites clinically and a 4-cm liver edge. There were no signs of chronic liver disease and no splenomegaly. FBC: Hb 11, WCC 17 (neutrophilia), Plt 356, U&E normal. Alkaline phosphatase 540, GGT 165, Calcium 2.55, albumin 28, ALT and bilirubin normal. ☐

5. A man aged 48 years presents to A&E with abdominal distension. This had gradually progressed over several weeks and had become particularly uncomfortable on the day of presentation. On examination, it was noted that he had red palms but was not clinically jaundiced. His pulse was 100 bpm, JVP and heart sounds normal. The abdomen was distended and subsequently ascitic fluid was aspirated. This demonstrated a protein content of 19 g/L. LFTs were normal aside from a GGT of 90 and albumin 30. There was no peripheral oedema and ward-testing of urine was normal. ☐

12. THEME: Weight loss

A. Coeliac disease
B. Tuberculosis
C. Hyperthyroidism
D. Gastric carcinoma
E. Diabetes mellitus
F. Caecal carcinoma
G. Lymphoma
H. Bacterial overgrowth
I. Crohn's disease
J. Adrenal insufficiency

The following patients have all lost weight. Select the most likely cause on the basis of the information provided.

1. A women aged 27 years attends her GP after noticing 10 kg weight loss over 2 months. She was previously fit and well. There is an associated history of diarrhoea but no abdominal pain or excessive thirst. She has been feeling hot but has had no drenching sweats. On examination, she is anxious, there is no thyroid enlargement and abdominal examination is unremarkable.

2. A man aged 62 years has recently lost weight. He attributes the 1–2 stone weight loss to depression following a recent bereavement. He otherwise feels well although has had less energy recently. There has been no change in bowel habit. On examination, he is clinically euthyroid, with no palpable lymphadenopathy and only a fullness in the right lower abdomen. FBC: Hb 12 g/L, WCC 8, Plt 278, MCV 80, MCH 26. Serum iron 4, TIBC 55.

3. A woman aged 39 years attends her GP surgery concerned about weight loss. She thinks she has lost nearly 15 kg over several months. Her appetite has been reasonable. There has been some diarrhoea but no blood PR or abdominal pain. She has no medical history of note but her sister has diabetes mellitus. On examination, she is pale, pulse rate 70 bpm, evidence of vitiligo, no abdominal masses. She becomes dizzy on standing. FBC: normocytic anaemia, Na 129, K 5.3, urea 1.9, Cr 54. glucose 3.6, LFT normal.

4. A man aged 72 years is prompted to attend his GP by his wife, who is concerned about his weight loss. His trousers have become loose over the preceding 6 months. On questioning, he admits to diarrhoea over several months, but no blood PR or pain. FBC is consistent with iron deficiency and a colonoscopy is subsequently reported as normal. U&E normal, calcium 2.03, phosphate 0.6, prothrombin time 4 seconds prolonged.

5. A man aged 65 years is concerned about recent weight loss. There has been an 8 kg weight loss over 4–5 months. He has had no dyspepsic symptoms but his stools have become loose. He underwent a gastrectomy 10 years ago for gastric carcinoma. FBC macrocytic anaemia, B_{12} low, serum folate elevated. TSH and glucose normal.

13. **THEME: Vomiting**

A. Gastric outflow obstruction
B. Acute gastritis
C. *Staphylococcus enterotoxin*
D. *Salmonella* spp.
E. Digoxin toxicity
F. Autonomic neuropathy
G. Uraemia
H. Small bowel obstruction
I. Diabetic ketoacidosis
J. Hypercalcaemia
K. Gastric carcinoma

The following patients all present with vomiting. Select the most appropriate diagnosis on the basis of the details provided.

1. A man aged 37 years attends A&E with a history of repeated vomiting for the last few hours. He had attended a meal with friends several hours previously but had only consumed 4 units of alcohol. He feels dreadful and is retching as you examine him. There has been no diarrhoea or antecedent history of abdominal pain. He denies prescribed or illicit drug use.

2. A 56-year-old woman attends her GP with a history of vomiting that had gradually become worse over several months. This now occurred most days and she had become concerned. She was prone to constipation and had lost a few kg in weight. There was no dysphagia or abdominal pain. Aside from recent laser treatment for diabetic retinopathy, there was little else in the history. Examination of her abdomen was unrevealing.

3. A man is referred to a gastroenterology clinic on an urgent basis, with a 10-day history of persistent vomiting. He was now able to keep very little down and was becoming dehydrated. He is 50 years old and takes only ranitidine medication. Examination confirms dehydration and reveals a slightly distended, non-tender abdomen with an audible succussion splash. Blood glucose is normal and biochemistry tests reveal a metabolic (hypochloraemic) alkalosis.

4. A woman aged 42 years presents to A&E with a history of nausea and vomiting. She has not been feeling well for many weeks but had only recently started vomiting. She had lost her appetite, was lethargic, complained of headaches and had been in bed for several days. On examination, she looked pale and there were numerous excoriations on her arms and legs. Her blood pressure of 190/95mmHg. There was mild ankle oedema. Her only medication was low dose trimethoprim.

5. A man aged 70 years presents to A&E one evening. His wife tells you that he has been vomiting for 24 hours and she is concerned. He had been complaining of abdominal pain for the previous 2 days, but attributed it to constipation. He had undergone a laparotomy 10 years previously for a diverticular abscess but was otherwise fit and well. On examination, he was dehydrated and unwell. His abdomen was clearly distended, resonant and very tender. The rectum was empty. FBC: mild neutrophilia. Na 134, K 2.9, urea 16, Cr 98, amylase and glucose normal.

14. THEME: Infections of the gastrointestinal tract

A. Whipple's disease
B. Tuberculosis
C. Giardiasis
D. Yersinia
E. Pyogenic abscess
F. Hepatitis A
G. Cholera
H. Salmonella
I. Amoebic abscess
J. Cryptosporidiosis
K. Schistosomiasis

The following patients all have an infective illness involving the gastrointestinal tract. Identify the most likely pathogen from the list above

1. A man aged 43 years becomes unwell following a weekend on a livestock farm. He complains of watery (non-bloody) diarrhoea and cramping lower abdominal pain. This has been present for 2 days. On examination, he has a temp of 38 °C and some mild lower abdominal tenderness. An organism is identified on a modified Ziehl–Nielsen stain of faeces. The illness gradually subsides over the next few days without any specific antimicrobial treatment.

2. A man on holiday in Thailand develops profuse diarrhoea within a week of his arrival. He describes the diarrhoea as 'just water' with no visible blood and no abdominal pain. He feels dizzy on standing. Na 129, K 2.4, urea 26, Cr 204. He has a blood pressure of 110/70 mmHg and a pulse rate of 120 bpm. He is put on a drip and given tetracycline by the local hospital.

3. A woman has just returned from the East coast of Africa. She started to feel unwell on the plane journey home. She was initially just vomiting, but has now developed bloody diarrhoea. On examination, there are areas of urticaria visible on her arms and legs and she is febrile. Sigmoidoscopy reveals mucosal ulceration. A rectal biopsy is taken.

4. A man in his forties with known HIV infection has been feeling unwell for several weeks and attends his GP. He has lost weight and has been experiencing lower abdominal pain. His bowels are rather erratic and he attributes this to his medication. The right iliac fossa is tender and FBC demonstrates a macrocytic anaemia.

5. A middle-aged woman has been unwell for several days and she is brought to A&E by her husband. She has had a high temperature with sweats and has not been eating. Aside from a history of diabetes and diverticular disease, she has previously been well. There has been no foreign travel. On examination, a temperature of 38.4 °C is noted. She is tachycardic and the right lung base is dull to percussion. Alkaline phosphatase is 780 and bilirubin is 40. A Gram-negative organism is cultured in the blood.

15. THEME: Adverse drug effects and toxicity on the gastrointestinal tract

A. Digoxin
B. Amiodarone
C. Flucloxacillin
D. Diclofenac
E. Atenolol
F. Low-dose aspirin
G. Ciprofloxacin
H. Metformin
I. Ferrous sulphate
J. Prednisolone
K. Fluconazole

The following patients have gastrointestinal/hepatobiliary problems related to prescribed medication. Identify the most likely culprit.

1. A 55-year-old man attends his GP with symptoms of lethargy, and feeling dizzy on standing. His only history is that of hypertension and hypercholesteraemia. On examination, his pulse rate is 98 bpm, blood pressure 122/72 mmHg. Abdomen soft, non-tender. Rectal examination: tarry stool.

2. A 64-year-old woman is brought to A&E by her family. She is unwell, drowsy, dehydrated, and the only history is that of several days of diarrhoea. Na 135, K 6.3, urea 30, Cr 260 venous bicarbonate 10 (low), glucose 10.

3. A man aged 78 years attends A&E with a history of nausea and vomiting. Bowels are normal and no haematemesis. He has felt dizzy intermittently. He has a 10-year history of diabetes mellitus. On examination, he has an irregular pulse and there are no signs of chronic liver disease or adverse abdominal findings.

4. The boyfriend of a 27-year-old woman notices that her eyes look yellow and takes her to the GP. She is normally fit and well. She takes no regular medication but has recently been treated for a 'skin infection'. She also complains of vaginal thrush. She has a family history of hypercholesteraemia. On examination, she is jaundiced with no signs of chronic liver disease and no hepatomegaly.

5. A 66-year-old retired engineer gives a history of several weeks of progressively becoming jaundiced. He had noticed this in the mirror. Otherwise, he felt quite well. His only history was that of a coronary angioplasty last year and a previous history of atrial fibrillation. On examination, his pulse was regular and there was no hepatomegaly or signs of chronic liver disease.

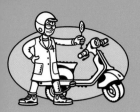
1. A 39-year-old male presents with a 3-month history of dysphagia for solids. He has lost 2 kg in weight, which he attributes to his recent avoidance of bread and meat. He has a long history of heartburn, but now that you ask, this has not troubled him recently. Discuss the differential diagnosis, and how features in the history would either support or discount these. Discuss the value of clinical examination in this setting. Outline your investigation strategy for this patient and how findings would influence your diagnosis.

2. A 15-year-old girl presents with acute onset lower abdominal pain. She has been vomiting for 24 hours. Examination reveals that she is pyrexial and tachycardic with guarding and tenderness in the right iliac fossa. What is your differential diagnosis? Outline your initial management strategy, including your choice of investigations.

3. A 35-year-old lady presents with a short history of gross abdominal distension and dyspnoea. She denies excessive alcohol ingestion. On examination, she is slightly icteric and has gross abdominal distension with shifting dullness evident. What is your differential diagnosis? Outline your investigation strategy, justifying your choices.

4. A 16-year-old male presents with loose pale stools, peripheral oedema and a vesicular rash. Outline your approach to diagnosis and management.

5. A 43-year-old man presents with central abdominal pain and diarrhoea. List the differential diagnoses and the investigations you would undertake to reach a final diagnosis.

6. A 26-year-old female presents with pain in the left iliac fossa and occasional spotting of blood on toilet paper following defecation. What additional features in the history would support a diagnosis of irritable bowel syndrome and how would this differ from inflammatory bowel disease? If you suspected inflammatory bowel disease, what would be your first choice of investigations?

7. A 48-year-old man presents with epigastric pain, weight loss and iron deficiency anaemia. Initial investigations include a gastroscopy which reveals a duodenal ulcer. Discuss your further management.

8. Discuss the problems associated with gastrectomy, and their management.

9. A 54-year-old female presents with weight loss, hot flushes and diarrhoea. An abdominal ultrasound reveals multiple metastatic deposits in her liver. What is the likely diagnosis? Explain the mechanism underlying the clinical symptoms and how you would confirm the diagnosis.

10. A 27-year-old man complains of occasional difficulty swallowing: 'food seems to stick half way down'. He has not lost any weight. He has found that he can resolve the problem by regurgitating food or by standing on his head! What is the likely diagnosis and what other clinical features are seen? A barium swallow demonstrates a 'bird's beak' appearance. Discuss your further management of this patient.

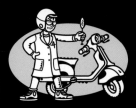

MCQ Answers

1. (a) F: Cardiac pain tends to be exertional, oesophageal pain can be positional
    (b) T: It can arise as a consequence of spasm
    (c) T: It can be difficult to differentiate the two and an ECG is often required
    (d) F: Oesophageal spasm can be relieved by GTN, which is often misleading
    (e) F: Oesophageal pain in itself is not associated with the bacterium

2. (a) F: This would raise concerns of either ulceration or neoplasia
    (b) F: The *H. pylori* IgG can indicate past infection, even following eradication
    (c) T: Evidence of upper gastrointestinal bleeding should be promptly investigated
    (d) F: It can be helpful if a hiatus hernia is demonstrable
    (e) F: It may be an incidental finding and not be the origin of the symptoms

3. (a) F: Reduction in LOS tone encourages acid reflux into the oesophagus
    (b) F: Smoking lowers LOS tone
    (c) F: Reflux can occur in the absence of macroscopic endoscopic findings
    (d) T: The LOS tone is lowered in pregnancy and intra-abdominal pressure increased
    (e) F: Lifestyle changes and simple antacids are frequently helpful

4. (a) F: Normal squamous epithelium is replaced by columnar epithelial cells
    (b) T: Dysplastic change does occur and can be pre-malignant
    (c) T: Repeated endoscopies may be required to monitor dysplastic change if present
    (d) F: The clinical features are the same for reflux oesophagitis
    (e) T: Severe dysplasia may herald malignant transformation

5. (a) T: Heartburn precedes the dysphagia, and the stricture often prevents further reflux
    (b) F: A progressive dysphagia suggests carcinoma, globus is a diagnosis of exclusion
    (c) F: The reported level of dysphagia by the patient is not a reliable clue
    (d) F: Regurgitation is not a feature of either benign or malignant strictures
    (e) T: Any significant weight loss is an ominous sign

6. (a) T: Barium swallow is useful in demonstrating anatomical problems such as pouches
    (b) T: Current or previous infective changes can be seen if there has been aspiration
    (c) T: This is best for local spread whereas CT is used for more gross metastatic spread
    (d) T: This allows biopsies to assess the histological nature of the stricture
    (e) F: A full blood count is important to look for anaemia

7. (a) F: Achalasia is often missed at endoscopy
    (b) T: Regurgitation is common and may result in aspiration if nocturnal
    (c) F: This would be rare—history is usually long and often intermittent
    (d) T: Common and can be severe due to uncoordinated contraction of oesophageal muscle
    (e) T: This is the typical histological finding

8. (a) F: There are other causes of a raised amylase, although acute pancreatitis gives the most marked rise
    (b) T: ECG is essential to exclude myocardial infarction
    (c) T: This is hepatic vein thrombosis causing acutely painful ascites
    (d) T: Tachypnoea may be a reflection of acidosis (e.g. diabetic ketoacidosis)
    (e) F: A patient with peritonitis will lie very still, as movement exacerbates the pain

9. (a) T: A leucocyte count $>15 \times 10^6$ is a poor prognostic marker
    (b) F: Hypocalcaemia is a bad sign (hypercalcaemia is a *cause* of pancreatitis)
    (c) T: A urea greater than 16 mmol/L is prognostically significant
    (d) F: High amylase levels support the diagnosis but are not of prognostic importance
    (e) T: Marked hypoxia (remember that ARDS is associated with acute pancreatitis)

10. (a) T: A ureteric stone often results in the detection of blood on urinalysis
    (b) F: Its presence would suggest this, but perforation cannot be excluded on its absence
    (c) T: Crohn's disease can present with acute abdominal pain and a high CRP
    (d) T: Alkaline phosphatase, gamma GT and bilirubin are commonly elevated
    (e) F: This can be helpful in assessing dilated bile ducts or detecting ovarian cysts

11. (a) T: This is often relevant (and may be painless)—do not forget low dose aspirin
    (b) T: Typically of gastric ulcers (may relieve pain of duodenal ulceration)
    (c) F: Altered blood, manifest as melaena, is sometimes a feature
    (d) F: This suggests a gastrointestinal malignancy and does not occur with peptic ulcers
    (e) T: This can be a feature—particularly of duodenal ulcers

12. (a) F: The amylase is frequently normal, in contradistinction to acute pancreatitis
    (b) F: Some features may be revealing but it is infrequently of diagnostic help
    (c) T: A high platelet count can also be seen with chronic blood loss
    (d) T: Particularly if the terminal ileum is involved
    (e) F: This occurs with B_{12} and folate deficiency—microcytosis is found in this context

13. (a) F: Nephrotic syndrome is a hypoalbuminaemic state leading to ascites with a low protein content
    (b) T: Cytological examination may reveal a neoplastic process, but this is not excluded by the absence of malignant cells
    (c) T: ECG changes of cardiac failure or constrictive pericarditis may be evident
    (d) T: This is the diagnostic modality of choice for the detection of ascites
    (e) T: The appearance may be suggestive of constrictive pericarditis or cardiac failure

14. (a) F: Patients often over- or underestimate the extent of their weight loss
    (b) T: A hypermetabolic state is thought to be the underlying mechanism although anorexia may contribute
    (c) T: This combination of symptoms would be typical for a hyperthyroid state
    (d) T: As would a low urea and low albumin
    (e) F: Corticosteroids tend to induce weight gain—hypoadrenalism can cause weight loss

15. (a) F: This would be unusual, although they can contribute toward peptic ulceration
    (b) T: Particularly if drug levels are in the toxic range
    (c) T: Many antibiotics are culprits. Metronidazole commonly does
    (d) F: NSAIDS tend to cause dyspepsia/reflux symptoms rather than vomiting *per se*
    (e) T: All opiates, including codeine, frequently cause vomiting

16. (a) T: Usually when the blood glucose gets very high
    (b) F: Different symptoms: sweating/hunger/tremor/altered consciousness/fits
    (c) T: Also constipation, abdominal pain, thirst and polyuria
    (d) F: Does not usually lead to vomiting
    (e) T: Particularly in chronic renal failure

17. (a) F: Melaena should always follow a true haematemesis
    (b) T: This indicates the patient is anticoagulated and subsequently at higher risk of a significant bleed
    (c) T: Suggests intravascular depletion and is often evident before systolic pressure falls
    (d) T: Until haemodilution of intravascular volume occurs
    (e) F: This history would more likely indicate a Mallory–Weiss tear

18. (a) F: A low urea can be seen with liver disease—a high urea indicates a significant bleed
    (b) F: Coagulopathy can indicate impairment of hepatic synthetic function
    (c) T: A reactive phenomenon of the bone marrow
    (d) T: Hypersplenism consequent upon portal hypertension is associated with varices
    (e) F: The national standard is that endoscopy should follow all gastrointestinal bleeds (although there is clearly a spectrum of urgency)

19. (a) T: Elderly patients have a poorer outcome from acute bleeding
    (b) F: Although aetiologically relevant, NSAIDs do not influence outcome
    (c) T: These patients are less able to cope with the haemodynamic stresses
    (d) T: Hypovolaemia results in 'pre-renal' deterioration in function
    (e) T: Can reflect preceding blood loss

20. (a) F: Constipation with opiates is the norm
    (b) T: Antibiotics such as the penicillins and cephalosporins are often culprits
    (c) T: (Used in gout) Is often dose-dependent
    (d) F: Not a well recognized side-effect of this drug class
    (e) F: This antibiotic is used to treat diarrhoea associated with pseudomembranous colitis (*Clostridium difficile* overgrowth)

21. (a) T: Reflects mucosal inflammation
    (b) F: Affects small intestine, watery, non-bloody diarrhoea
    (c) T: Can present a long time following radiotherapy
    (d) F: The presence of blood indicates more significant pathology
    (e) F: Causes diarrhoea, but not bloody

22. (a) F: A normocytic or microcytic picture is seen reflecting chronic disease or iron deficiency respectively
    (b) T: Urinary 5-HIAA, a serotonin metabolite is elevated in carcinoid syndrome
    (c) F: Aetiology is usually viral, although bacterial infection must be excluded
    (d) T: May occur despite iron deficiency—ferritin acts as an inflammatory protein
    (e) F: Not frequently—toxic dilatation/faecal impaction or pancreatic calcification may be seen

23. (a) T
     (b) T
     (c) T
     (d) F
     (e) T
     Steatorrhoea is seen with malabsorption, either due to (proximal) small intestinal disease or pancreatic insufficiency

24. (a) T: Commonly implicated
     (b) F: Although usually in the immunocompromised
     (c) T: Often as a consequence of poor food hygiene
     (d) F: Rarely causes diarrhoea
     (e) F: Often via contaminated water, severe in patients with AIDS

25. (a) T: Reflects dehydration; often disproportionately elevated to the serum creatinine
     (b) F: (Unless acute renal failure has resulted!) Hypokalaemia reflects excess gut loss
     (c) T: Often mirrors the potassium level
     (d) F: This tends to cause constipation
     (e) T: Poor diabetic control can lead to autonomic neuropathy

26. (a) F: Bright red blood is more typical of haemorrhoids
     (b) F: This pattern more often represents high rectal lesions such as carcinoma, angiodysplasia or inflamed diverticula
     (c) T: You would expect to find increased anal tone and pain on rectal examination
     (d) F: This would be a more characteristic feature of diverticulitis
     (e) F: Blood loss from 'simple' ano-rectal conditions is rarely severe enough to result in anaemia—carcinoma, inflammatory bowel disease or angiodysplasia is more likely

27. (a) T: Further investigation is only required in equivocal cases
     (b) T: And if there is a high level of clinical suspicion
     (c) F: Rigid sigmoidoscopy is limited to 15–20 cm range
     (d) F: Proctoscopy is rarely tolerated in patients with anal fissure
     (e) F: Haemorrhoids are common incidental findings and not always the culprit lesion

28. (a) F: Pale conjunctivae correlate very poorly with Hb concentration
     (b) T: Particularly the mean corpuscular volume, MCV
     (c) T: To exclude oesophagitis, gastric ulcer/erosions or carcinoma
     (d) F: In isolation, this finding is an insufficient explanation
     (e) F: This is a common cause in Britain and Ireland

29. (a) F: These drugs have an *anti-folate* action
     (b) T: Reticulocyte are large red cell precursors, seen in a marrow response to bleeding or haemolysis
     (c) F: Caecal carcinoma causes a microcytic, iron-deficient picture
     (d) F: This test helps differentiate between the different causes of B_{12} deficiency
     (e) T: On its own, or in association with pernicious anaemia

30. (a) F: This suggests anaemia of chronic disease. TIBC should be raised in Fe-deficiency
     (b) T: As a consequence of gastric erosions
     (c) T: Established from the context and history
     (d) T: Coeliac disease can lead to either iron or folate deficiency, or both
     (e) F: These are seen in B_{12}/folate deficiency

31. (a) F: Usually detectable in sclera at levels greater than 40 mmol/L
     (b) F: A rapid onset is more likely to be an infective cause
     (c) F: This contravenes Courvoisier's law
     (d) T: This differentiates obstructive jaundice from other causes
     (e) F: Prothrombin time is a better indicator of synthetic function

32. (a) T: Typically a cholestatic picture
     (b) T: In excess of therapeutic dose
     (c) F: Uncommon
     (d) F: Predominantly nephrotoxic
     (e) T: Such as isoniazid and rifampicin

33. (a) T: Infections such as CMV, EBV or Toxoplasmosis
     (b) T: Chronic liver disease/cirrhosis (Budd–Chiari if acute)
     (c) T: Wilson's disease also affects the basal ganglia
     (d) T: Another sign of chronic liver disease
     (e) T: Cardiac failure can lead to hepatic congestion

34. (a) F: Levels of ALT do not correlate well with liver *function*
     (b) F: Alk phos has non-hepatic sources: bone/placenta/small intestine
     (c) T: Raised GGT in isolation is very suggestive of this
     (d) F: A typical metastatic picture is elevated ALT and GGT
     (e) T: Enquire about night sweats, weight loss and skin rash

35. (a) T
     (b) F
     (c) T
     (d) F
     (e) T
     See Fig. 22.5 for a list of causes of clubbing.

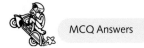

36. (a) T: Haematoma in the flank(s), seen in retroperitoneal haemorrhage
     (b) T: Also seen in corticosteroid use and Cushing's disease
     (c) T: As a consequence of portal hypertension
     (d) F: A sign of acute pancreatitis—bruising around the umbilicus
     (e) T: A characteristic ulcerating skin lesion, often on the lower leg

37. (a) F: Thrombocytopenia is seen, as a result of hypersplenism 2° splenomegaly
     (b) T: Particularly in an acute infective/inflammatory setting
     (c) F: Microcytosis with iron deficiency
     (d) T: For example inflammatory bowel disease
     (e) T: Viral illness can cause both neutropenia and lymphopenia

38. (a) T: This should always be excluded in pre-menopausal women
     (b) F: More typically in the RUQ or epigastrium
     (c) T: Classically starts centrally then localizes to RIF
     (d) F: Typically in the left iliac fossa
     (e) T: Terminal ileal inflammation is common in Crohn's disease

39. (a) T: Identify any risk factors for tuberculosis
     (b) F: An *appendix abscess* may present as a mass
     (c) T: Look for iron-deficiency anaemia
     (d) F: Abdominal masses only if progresses to lymphoma
     (e) T: Always consider in women of child-bearing age

40. (a) T: Associated with coeliac disease
     (b) T: Colitis (associated with HLA B27), and sometimes liver disease
     (c) F: Unrecognized
     (d) T: Dilated end-capillaries associated with liver disease
     (e) T: For example, eyelids—seen in primary biliary cirrhosis

41. (a) T: OGD should be undertaken following all upper gastrointestinal bleeds
     (b) F: Not indicated in this scenario
     (c) F: May be undertaken for the diagnosis of abdominal pain
     (d) T: At the time of active bleeding, may be useful if the site is not readily identifiable
     (e) F: Not in the acute setting

42. (a) T: As a result of reflux with microaspiration into the trachea
     (b) T: Insidious blood loss from chronic inflammation
     (c) T: A high prevalence of reflux in asthmatics is seen
     (d) F: This manoeuvre tends to exacerbate symptoms
     (e) T: Retrosternal chest pain is a common diagnostic problem

43. (a) T: Anticholinergic effects lower LOS tone
     (b) F: This is a *prokinetic* anti-emetic
     (c) T: Commonly implicated—interfere with prostaglandin synthesis
     (d) T: Lowers LOS tone
     (e) F: Potent therapeutic inhibitors of gastric acid production

44. (a) T: Oesophageal inflammation/ulceration
     (b) T: Well described
     (c) F: Unrelated
     (d) T: Prolonged reflux
     (e) F: Not a complication of reflux *per se*

45. (a) F: Approximately 15%
     (b) F: The converse is true, normal oesophageal epithelium is squamous
     (c) T: Severe reflux may be entirely asymptomatic
     (d) T: And prevent recurrence
     (e) T: Particularly if dysplastic change is present

46. (a) T: If caloric intake is not maintained
     (b) T: Progressive dysphagia from solids to liquids, with weight loss
     (c) F: Reflux symptoms often disappear as a fibrotic stricture forms
     (d) T: If endoscopic appearance is inconclusive
     (e) T: It may have been for oesophageal cancer or have resulted in fibrosis of the oesophagus.

47. (a) F: Dysphagia is much commoner
     (b) F: An iron deficiency picture is more likely
     (c) T: Just over 50% are squamous in origin
     (d) F: Predominantly to reduce tumour bulk and improve symptoms
     (e) T: Suggestive of liver metastases

48. (a) F: The antrum is distal, the fundus forms the upper portion
     (b) T: Which acts to stimulate H⁺ secretion
     (c) T: And act as a barrier to bacteria
     (d) F: This is of minor importance
     (e) T: In the upper two-thirds of the stomach

49. (a) T: This enzyme is utilized diagnostically in the urease breath test
     (b) F: Asymptomatic infection is very common
     (c) T: 50% of people aged over 50 years are infected
     (d) T: And a motile flagellate
     (e) F: Acute and chronic gastritis also occur

50. (a) F: Can be achieved in a special culture medium
     (b) F: IgG serology remains positive after eradication
     (c) T: A biopsy should be taken for histology or the urease test
     (d) F: FBC and biochemistry are frequently normal
     (e) F: This is ingested! CO_2 is produced by *H. pylori* which is then exhaled

51. (a) T: Peak incidence 50–60 years of age
    (b) F: Duodenal ulceration is commoner by a ratio of 4:1
    (c) F: Epigastric pain would be typical
    (d) T: cf. duodenal ulcer
    (e) T: Particularly if associated with NSAID use

52. (a) T: Pre-pyloric ulcers can cause pyloric stenosis—although commoner with duodenal ulcers
    (b) T: As a result of insidious blood loss
    (c) T: If acute perforation occurs
    (d) F: No causative association
    (e) F: Not a symptom of gastric ulcers

53. (a) F: An alternative source should be sought (e.g. caecal carcinoma)
    (b) F: Very common >90%
    (c) T: Blood group O have a 40% increased risk
    (d) T: There may be no antecedent history
    (e) T: If no maintenance or eradication therapy is given

54. (a) T: May identify pulmonary metastases
    (b) F: Usually diagnostically unhelpful
    (c) T: If deranged may suggest hepatic metastases (a liver ultrasound is often performed)
    (d) F: The renal tract is usually unaffected
    (e) T: May be elevated if bony metastases are present

55. (a) T: Osteomalacia can occur due to reduced absorption of vitamin D
    (b) T: Especially in Polya gastrectomy
    (c) F: Diarrhoea is much more common
    (d) F: Dumping syndrome can result in transient hyperglycaemia post prandially
    (e) T: May be iron deficient (less HCl to solubilize iron) or B_{12} deficient (less intrinsic factor)

56. (a) T: Common
    (b) F: Diarrhoea much more likely
    (c) T: As a consequence of malabsorption
    (d) T: Malabsorption of vitamin D
    (e) T: But usually associated with weight loss or diarrhoea

57. (a) F: Rarely seen in this group; commonest in the west of Ireland
    (b) F: Hyposplenism can be seen
    (c) T: Should be suspected if recurrence of symptoms or dramatic weight loss
    (d) T: HLA-A1, B8, DR3, DR7 and DQW2
    (e) T: If iron and folate deficiency coexist

58. (a) T: The risk may be reduced by compliance with a gluten-free diet
    (b) T: Hypoalbuminaemia as a result of malabsorption
    (c) T: As a result of folate malabsorption
    (d) T: Iron deficiency—malabsorption or bleeding
    (e) F: Dermatitis herpetiformis is the characteristic skin rash associated

59. (a) T: Reflecting anaemia of chronic disease
    (b) T: Correlates with the severity of the attack
    (c) F: A high platelet count reflects inflammatory activity
    (d) T: A very sensitive indicator of inflammation
    (e) F: Low calcium may be present if malabsorption is a feature

60. (a) T: Episcleritis and conjunctivitis can also occur
    (b) F: Pericarditis is associated
    (c) F: A seronegative inflammatory arthritis is seen
    (d) T: Exacerbated if steroid therapy has been necessary
    (e) T: A characteristic skin rash that is occasionally seen

61. (a) T: Aphthous mouth ulcers are commonly seen
    (b) T: A typical pathological appearance
    (c) F: Often spared; cf. ulcerative colitis
    (d) F: 'Skip lesions' are characteristic
    (e) T: Occurs in a small proportion of patients

62. (a) F: Are effective for acute exacerbations but don't significantly influence overall prognosis
    (b) T: Can occur with any chronic inflammatory condition
    (c) F: The majority (approximately 80%) will require surgery at some juncture
    (d) T: Drugs such as azathioprine can be very effective
    (e) T: And may require protracted courses of metronidazole

63. (a) T: A common feature
    (b) F: 'Secretory diarrhoea' is typically seen
    (c) T: Resulting in wheeze clinically—mediated by histamines
    (d) T: Tricuspid regurgitation can also occur
    (e) F: Not a feature

64. (a) F: Not directly associated
    (b) T: Reflecting malabsorption
    (c) T: As a result of bacterial metabolism (folate levels are often elevated)
    (d) F: Uncommon
    (e) T: Malabsorption

65. (a) F: *Giardia lamblia* is a protozoan
    (b) T: Faecal–oral spread
    (c) F: *Mycobacterium tuberculosis*!
    (d) T: Often self-limiting, sometimes treated with tetracyclines
    (e) T: Thought to be infective but exact aetiology unknown

66. (a) T: Glucose, amino acids etc are absorbed in the small intestine
    (b) T: Water + electrolytes are absorbed here
    (c) F: The superior mesenteric provides the ascending colon with blood
    (d) F: This is the *beginning* of the large intestine!
    (e) F: It has a dual blood supply from both inferior and superior vessels

241

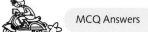

67. (a) F: Significant weight loss implies a more sinister pathology
     (b) T: A typical feature
     (c) F: Irritable bowel syndrome is a clinical diagnosis (imaging may exclude serious pathology though)
     (d) F: Can exacerbate symptoms but helpful in patients where constipation dominates
     (e) T: Often associated—depression is also a common feature

68. (a) T: Mediated via an anticholinergic effect
     (b) F: Not a common side effect
     (c) T: Also turns stools black, and may cause diarrhoea
     (d) T: All opiates can slow intestinal motility
     (e) F: More likely to cause diarrhoea in excess dose! (hypothyroidism can cause constipation)

69. (a) F: Not a pathological feature of this type of colitis
     (b) T: Compare with ulcerative colitis
     (c) F: *Non*-caseating granulomas are seen
     (d) T: Whereas ulcerative colitis is more common in non-smokers
     (e) T: Occurring predominantly in the immunosuppressed

70. (a) F: This is more typical of Crohn's
     (b) T: HLA-B27 associated
     (c) T: Which carries a significant mortality
     (d) T: Toxic dilatation or perforation should be considered
     (e) F: Typical of Crohn's disease

71. (a) T: A classical skin manifestation that can be difficult to treat
     (b) F: More commonly seen in Crohn's
     (c) T: Monitor liver biochemistry
     (d) T: Conjunctivitis and uveitis are also seen
     (e) F: Associated with e.g. diabetes, sarcoidosis, lymphoma

72. (a) T: Usually adjacent to areas of extensive ulceration
     (b) T: With an accumulation of inflammatory cells in the lamina propria
     (c) T: Fibrosis of mucosa and sub-mucosa, resulting in a 'lead-pipe colon'
     (d) T: In up to 60% of patients—although its significance is unclear
     (e) F: 'Backwash ileitis' can be seen in those with extensive disease

73. (a) T: >37.5°C, blood cultures must be performed
     (b) F: Not a usual feature and no reflection of severity
     (c) T: >100 bpm: reflecting dehydration +/− sepsis
     (d) T: <30 g/L—an 'acute phase' effect
     (e) T: Can be normocytic (chronic disease) or microcytic if bleeding is a significant feature

74. (a) T: Malignant potential correlates with size of polyp
     (b) T: Ensure the malignant area is fully resected with clear margins
     (c) F: The converse is true
     (d) F: More common in the distal colon
     (e) T: Colonoscopic screening may be indicated

75. (a) T: A common presenting feature
     (b) F: Left-sided lesions
     (c) T: Sometimes a RIF mass can be palpated
     (d) T: In the presence of liver metastases
     (e) T: Perforation and abscess formation is not uncommon

76. (a) T: Particularly in travellers outside their own country
     (b) F: Only if diarrhoea persistent or diagnosis in doubt
     (c) T: Usually a neutrophilia is seen
     (d) F: Not in uncomplicated acute bacterial infection
     (e) T: As they impair clearance of the pathogen from the bowel

77. (a) T: Ulceration of the colonic epithelium can occur
     (b) T: But can be protracted and debilitating in immunocompromised patients (e.g. AIDS)
     (c) T: Can be mistaken for colonic cancer
     (d) F: Broad spectrum antibiotics such clindamycin or cephalosporins
     (e) T: Metronidazole is also effective—the offending antibiotic should also be stopped where possible

78. (a) T: A coagulopathy can be seen in liver dysfunction
     (b) T: In addition to bone marrow iron stores
     (c) T: Via the bile duct
     (d) F: The pancreas is responsible (but glycogenolysis and gluconeogenesis do occur)
     (e) T: Half-life is 20 days under normal conditions

79. (a) T: Including nausea, vomiting, diarrhoea, headache, malaise
     (b) F: A distaste for cigarettes is said to be characteristic
     (c) F: Not common, but palpable in about 10%
     (d) F: Reflects prior exposure and lifelong immunity
     (e) T: Rare but recognized (along with arthritis, vasculitis and rarely hepatic failure)

80. (a) T: Particularly in parts of Asia and Africa
     (b) F: 90 days is typical (range 60–160 days)
     (c) T: Thought to be mediated via immune-complexes
     (d) T: 5–10% become carriers—5% develop chronic active hepatitis
     (e) T: Possibly due to immature immune response in the neonate

81. (a) T: Usually at 6 weeks to 3 months
    (b) T: And more severe disease, follows HBsAg
    (c) F: Approximately 8 weeks after infection, and imply low infectivity
    (d) T: Appear after 3 months
    (e) T: And tend to normalize as HBsAg disappears

82. (a) F: Since 1991
    (b) F: Less than a fifth of patients
    (c) T: Reflected by a normal prothrombin time, albumin and urea
    (d) T: Reverse transcription PCR method
    (e) F: 20% do—70% develop chronic indolent hepatitis of varying severity

83. (a) T: Although their presence is not specific for EBV infection
    (b) F: The prognosis is excellent, with the majority regaining normal liver function
    (c) T: Many patients are screened following organ transplantation
    (d) T: Weil's disease
    (e) T: Clinically similar to EBV infection

84. (a) F: *Iron* accumulation (autosomal recessive inheritance)
    (b) T: If cirrhosis ensues (almost inevitable if untreated)
    (c) T: Women are 'protected' by menstruation, and present later
    (d) F: Secondary diabetes can occur due to iron accumulation in the pancreas
    (e) T: Pituitary dysfunction may be the presenting manifestation

85. (a) F: More commonly presents in males 3:1
    (b) T: Up to 30% may develop this complication in the long tertm
    (c) F: Approximately 10% patients with ulcerative colitis have overt or subtle evidence of primary sclerosing cholangitis
    (d) T: Improves biochemical profile and has symptomatic benefits
    (e) T: Isolated stricture can be stented or balloon-dilated

86. (a) T: Seen in the cornea with a slit lamp
    (b) F: This is true of urinary copper, serum copper tends to be normal or low
    (c) F: Basal emphysema is classically seen
    (d) T: With MM being normal and ZZ being the severe type
    (e) T: If there is portal hypertension due to cirrhosis

87. (a) F: Diabetes mellitus can occur due to loss of pancreatic endocrine function
    (b) F: Infertility does occur in males
    (c) T: Due to pancreatic insufficiency
    (d) T: If meconium ileus occurs
    (e) T: Liver disease is a significant overall prognostic factor

88. (a) T: Presenting commonly between fourth and sixth decades
    (b) T: Often an early clinical feature
    (c) T: Cholesterol deposits may be seen in the cholesterol or skin
    (d) T: Malabsorption of fat-soluble vitamins
    (e) F: Renal tubular acidosis can also be a feature

89. (a) F: 20–30% will develop alcoholic liver disease
    (b) T: And is also seen in pregnancy, starvation, diabetes and obesity
    (c) F: Hyaline material that is also seen in chronic active hepatitis
    (d) F: Approximately 25% is thought to be due to alcohol
    (e) T: But microcytosis can also occur if there is bleeding from e.g. gastric erosions

90. (a) T: White nails, seen in liver disease
    (b) F: Spoon-shaped nails suggesting iron-deficiency
    (c) T: Check the sclera carefully
    (d) T: Also seen in pregnancy
    (e) F: Not a feature of chronic liver disease *per se*

91. (a) T: One parameter of the modified Child classification
    (b) T: Although low albumin is often seen in the 'sick' patient (e.g. sepsis)
    (c) T: Does not reflect hepatic function
    (d) T: May be subtle: irritability or constructional apraxia
    (e) F: A sign of chronic liver disease but does not reflect function

92. (a) T: Commonly from the gastrointestinal tract, but most tumours can metastasize here
    (b) T: And is more common in males than females with cirrhosis
    (c) F: There is little response to radiotherapy or chemotherapy
    (d) T: CT may be required if there is diagnostic uncertainty
    (e) T: And should be recognized so as to avoid biopsy! (bleeding risk)

93. (a) T: With a resultant build-up of toxic metabolite
    (b) T: Or those on enzyme-inducing drugs
    (c) T: A sensitive indicator of damage in this context
    (d) T: Acute (renal) tubular necrosis can occur
    (e) F: Metabolic acidosis occurs and is a bad prognostic sign

94. (a) F: This is bound to albumin—*conjugated* bilirubin is water soluble
    (b) F: Via the *portal* vein
    (c) F: About 15% have a cholecystectomy for symptoms attributable to gallstones
    (d) F: Only approximately 10% are seen on plain X-ray
    (e) T: Cholesterol stones (reduced bile salts in the liver)

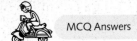
95. (a) T: Obstruction/swelling of the ampulla of Vater caused by gallstones
    (b) F: Not causally associated
    (c) T: Infection spreading into intra-hepatic ducts
    (d) F: An entirely distinct pathology
    (e) T: Can present with swinging fever and septicaemia

96. (a) T: Sphincter of Oddi and gastric acid help maintain this
    (b) T: *E. coli* being the commonest organism implicated
    (c) T: With elevation of alkaline phosphatase and bilirubin—transaminase elevation usually mild
    (d) F: Frequently positive—90% if repeated cultures are taken
    (e) T: Especially if a stent is inserted

97. (a) T: Massive pooling of intravascular fluid around the pancreas—'third space losses'
    (b) F: Not a typical presentation
    (c) T: Very common, severe and often radiates to the back
    (d) T: Almost invariable
    (e) T: Particularly in severe cases and if ARDS is a complication

98. (a) F: A potential complication (*hyper*calcaemia is a cause)
    (b) F: A potential complication due to loss of endocrine function
    (c) T: Particularly at high doses
    (d) T: A common cause
    (e) F: Scorpion bite!

99. (a) T: Blood cultures should always be performed at presentation
    (b) T: Oral hypoglycaemics/insulin may be required, short or long-term
    (c) T: Can be life threatening, perform a coagulation screen, fibrinogen and d-dimers
    (d) T: Paralytic ileus is commonly seen
    (e) T: Usually as a result of hypovolaemia +/– sepsis +/– DIC

100. (a) F: Usually normal in chronic pancreatitis
     (b) T: Pancreatic duct dilatation/distortion may be seen
     (c) F: Can be seen in up to 50% of moderate to severe cases
     (d) T: A paraneoplastic skin manifestation
     (e) F: Late—often with hepatomegaly and liver metastases

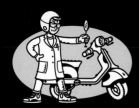

1. The pattern of enzyme abnormality (and the history of itching) suggests a cholestatic process. The single most useful investigation is a hepatobiliary ultrasound to assess the biliary tree. If the bile ducts are not dilated, all hepatic causes (especially those causing intrahepatic cholestasis) should be considered. In a middle-aged woman, primary biliary cirrhosis is a distinct possibility [check anti-mitochondrial (M_2) antibodies]. She may have been given co-amoxiclav for a respiratory infection, which would be a prime suspect as an aetiological agent in cholestatic jaundice.

2. There is clinical evidence of shock. This could be as a result of sepsis, intravascular volume loss, or both. You should consider acute appendicitis with perforation or abscess, Crohn's disease, ectopic pregnancy, ruptured ovarian cyst and acute pyelonephritis. Investigations should include a pregnancy test, ultrasound scan, mid-stream urine for culture, and possibly further imaging with a small bowel enema.

3. A low ferritin would confirm iron-deficiency, although a normal or high ferritin should be interpreted with caution, as it is an acute phase (inflammatory) protein. Low serum iron and high iron-binding capacity are also supportive of iron deficiency. The finding of a duodenal ulcer should prompt acid-suppression and *Helicobacter pylori* eradication if appropriate, but should not necessarily be accepted as the cause of the iron-deficiency. The lower gastrointestinal tract should be investigated with colonoscopy or barium enema. Check whether duodenal biopsies were taken at the time of the initial endoscopy (exclude coeliac disease).

4. Ulcerative colitis (UC) is more likely to present with bloody diarrhoea than Crohn's disease. Mouth ulcers are common in Crohn's as the entire length of the gastrointestinal tract can be affected. It characteristically affects the terminal ileum or small intestine which are usually unaffected by UC. The rectum is almost always inflamed in UC and usually spared in Crohn's. UC causes superficial ulceration, whereas Crohn's is a transmural disease causing deep ulcers. Histology may demonstrate crypt abscesses in UC and granulomata in Crohn's. Crohn's is more common in smokers. Perianal disease, with abscesses or fistulae, are more common in Crohn's disease.

5. Low pO_2, high LDH, high WCC, high glucose, low calcium, high urea, low albumin and high AST are poor prognostic signs in acute pancreatitis. Initial management should include: oxygen if hypoxic (and perform a chest X-ray), adequate venous access and fluid resuscitation, a urinary catheter is often required, consider a central venous line (particularly if there is existing cardiac impairment), adequate analgesia and antiemetics, blood cultures and broad spectrum antibiotics if there is evidence of sepsis. A coagulation screen should be performed to look for evidence of disseminated intravascular coagulation. Always get senior help.

6. The human leucocyte antigen B_{27} is associated with a group of inflammatory conditions known as the spondylarthritides because a prominent feature is an inflammatory arthritis, usually of the spine. They include ankylosing spondylitis, psoriatic arthropathy and Reiter's disease (an asymmetrical arthritis with urethritis, uveitis and occasionally colitis). All of these conditions are associated with ulcerative colitis. It is postulated to be an immune phenomenon related to Salmonella or Chlamydial infection.

7. Characteristically, a low albumin, low calcium and phosphate (vitamin D deficiency) are seen. Urea may also be low, although does not correlate well with nutritional state. Prothrombin time may be prolonged if vitamin K deficiency has occurred. Anaemia may be seen: microcytic if iron-deficient, macrocytic if B_{12}/folate deficient, or normocytic if combined haematinic deficiency exists. Normocytic anaemia may also reflect a 'chronic disease/inflammatory process'. Abnormal LFTs may give aetiological clues. Inflammatory markers such as CRP may also help in his respect. Causes of malabsorption in a man this age include Coeliac disease, Crohn's disease, chronic pancreatitis, bacterial overgrowth and infections such as giardiasis. Hyperthyroidism and diabetes mellitus should be excluded.

8. This man presents with features suggestive of cholangitis. It is likely that the endoprosthesis has become occluded and the bilary tree has ascending infection. Blood cultures may reveal the causative organism, most commonly *Escherichia coli*. Broad spectrum antibiotics to cover Gram-negative and anaerobic organisms should be used in the first instance. LFTs will suggest cholestais, a neutrophilia may be seen with elevated inflammatory markers. He should undergo an urgent biliary ultrasound and the stent should subsequently be removed and replaced.

9. Endoscopy with biopsy for histology, culture or a 'clo (urease) test' can be employed at the time of biopsy. Alternative, non-invasive approaches would include a serological (IgG) test that indicates past infection, but will remain positive following eradication. A urease

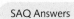

breath test can also be employed (see Chapters 15 and 24). Triple therapy may include amoxicillin, metronidazole and a proton pump inhibitor such as lansoprazole. Alcohol should be avoided in combination with metronidazole, as extremely unpleasant reactions would occur (nausea, vomiting and flushing). This occurs because metronidazole inhibits the enzyme acetaldehyde dehydrogenase, resulting in accumulation of the offending metabolite.

10. You need to establish the exact timing of the overdose and whether or not any other prescription or illicit drugs were consumed. A history of alcohol excess or underlying liver or renal impairment is also relevant. A psychiatric history should also be taken to assess suicidal intent. Serum paracetamol levels are plotted on a Prescott nomogram and correlated to time post-ingestion to establish the need for treatment, but the timing may be difficult if the history is unreliable. It is usually safer to treat if any doubt remains. A low pH, high creatinine and prolonged prothrombin time have been shown to adversely affect outcome.

11. This is a common age for Gilbert's syndrome to present, and is the most likely explanation for the isolated hyperbilirubinaemia in this context. The normal GGT implies that the alkaline phosphatase may be from a non-hepatic source (isoenzymes of alkaline phosphatase can be measured to determine the organ of origin). In this case, the elevated alkaline phosphatase reflects actively growing bones. Red cell haemolysis should be considered, and a reticulocyte count performed. The mechanism of the hyperbilirubinaemia involves a reduction in enzyme activity (glucuronosyl transferase or UGT-1), and thus a reduction in conjugation of bilirubin.

12. Pernicious anaemia should be considered. Autoantibodies to parietal cells are found in 90%, there may also be antibodies to intrinsic factor. A Schilling test (see Chapter 24) may be appropriate to differentiate between lack of intrinsic factor and terminal ileal disease (e.g. Crohn's or tuberculosis). Malabsorption due to small intestinal disease should be considered, particularly in younger patients with B_{12} deficiency. Other causes of a macrocytosis include alcohol excess, folate deficiency, hypothyroidism,

myelodysplasia, hyperlipidaemia, chronic hypoxia. A reticulocytosis can also manifest as a 'spurious' macrocytosis.

13. This patient has clear evidence of hepatic encephalopathy. Convulsions and coma are seen in severe cases, or signs may be as subtle as constructional apraxia or mild irritability. Acute onset usually has a precipitating factor which can be potentially reversible; for example, bleeding, infection (bacterial or fungal) or drugs. Grade of encephalopathy is one parameter used to assess the functional capacity of the liver. The others are raised bilirubin, lowered albumin, ascites and coagulopathy (prolonged PT).

14. Features indicating severity in ulcerative colitis include; stool frequency >8 times/day with blood, abdominal pain and tenderness, fever >37.5, tachycardia >100 bpm, CRP >20, ESR >35, Hb<10, albumin <30. Abdominal pain is often an ominous sign and an abdominal radiograph should be performed to look for evidence of toxic megacolon. The history of 'shivers' may indicate superimposed sepsis (bacteraemia resulting from damaged colonic mucosa). Blood and stool cultures should be performed and broad spectrum antibiotics initiated if suspicion exists. Aggressive fluid resuscitation is often required. A stool chart, strict fluid balance charting and a daily weight are imperative. Corticosteroids are usually given during an acute attack to induce remission. Further immunosuppression and surgical intervention may be required.

15. Liver biopsy is the definitive test for diagnosis and at the same time assesses the extent of liver damage. The hepatic iron index is of particular value (see Chapter 18). Ferritin is an 'acute phase' protein and can be (misleadingly) elevated in infections or inflammatory states. Other manifestations of haemachromatosis include: hypogonadotrophic hypogonadism (pituitary), pigmentation of skin, porphyria cutanea tarda (skin photosensitivity), arthritis of the small joints of the hand, chondrocalcinosis (knees), cardiomyopathy, diabetes mellitus (pancreatic damage). The patient is also at risk of hepatoma and the other complications of cirrhosis.

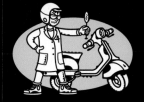

EMQ Answers

Haematemesis and melaena

1. E: This lady is taking NSAIDs for her arthritis, these ulcers are often painless and may present with acute bleeds.

2. B: Large variceal bleed in a patient with known cirrhosis and consequent portal hypertension. These patients sometimes have thrombocytopenia because of liver disease/splenomegaly/alcohol toxicity, thus increasing the bleeding risk.

3. C: A typical history of Mallory–Weiss. Of note, the streaks of blood only appeared in later episodes of vomiting.

4. D: Significant weight loss has occurred and the indices are those of iron-deficiency. Gastric carcinoma is commoner with advancing age. Note the high platelet count, consistent with chronic bleeding.

5. I: Pain from duodenal ulceration is classically worse with hunger and relieved with food. 95% of duodenal ulcers are associated with *Helicobacter pylori* infection.

Diarrhoea

1. B: Coeliac disease is particularly common in the West of Ireland and has a second peak of incidence in this age group. It commonly causes an iron-deficiency picture through malabsorption.

2. D: Giardiasis is common in the tropics and can cause malabsorption. Repeat stool culture is often necessary to identify cysts. Campylobacter is less likely because of the significant weight loss and no blood in the stool.

3. C: *Clostridium difficile* toxin-associated diarrhoea often occurs following recent antibiotic treatment (e.g. penicillins, cephalosporins, clindamycin).

4. A: Terminal ileum involvement is common in Crohn's, producing RIF pain. 'Anaemia of chronic disease' with elevated inflammatory markers can occur.

5. H: The clues to thyrotoxicosis here are: weight loss with a good appetite, anxiety, irregular pulse atrial fibrillation).

Acute abdominal pain

1. J: Acute bowel infarction caused by mesenteric thrombosis. He has 'vascular' risk factors of smoking and notably atrial fibrillation. A lactic (metabolic) acidosis is very common. The mortality is high.

2. C: A jaundiced middle-aged woman with RUQ pain. The diagnosis is supported by the pattern of liver enzymes and *Escherichia coli* septicaemia.

3. F: Gallstones are a common cause of acute pancreatitis in the UK. She has evidence of shock and is likely to be

tachypnoeic as a result of a metabolic acidosis, or may be developing acute respiratory distress syndrome.

4. H: He is dehydrated (polyuria) clinically and biochemically and has a very low venous bicarbonate (metabolic acidosis). The hyperkalaemia and breathlessness are as a result of the acidosis. Never forget glucose!

5. I: The differential, of course, includes appendicitis. However, the history is short and she has evidence of significant intravascular volume loss.

Chronic abdominal pain

1. G: Pancreatic carcinoma is often associated with significant weight loss and the pain is persistent and often severe. The NSAID history is a red herring.

2. I: There is evidence of inflammation and the site of pain suggests a biliary origin. Ultrasound may demonstrate a shrunken gall bladder with evidence of chronic inflammation.

3. F: A typical history for irritable bowel syndrome, alternating bowel habit with a rather vague history of abdominal pain. The negative findings mentioned and normal inflammatory markers lead one away from an inflammatory aetiology.

4. B: This man has probably been seeing neurology for transient ischaemic attacks. The timing of the pain coincides with a few hours after the evening meal. A degree of malabsorption can occur with mesenteric ischaemia.

5. H: This man probably has a history of coeliac disease although the recent story of soaking night sweats, abdominal pain, weight loss and elevated LDH are suggestive of Non-Hodgkin's lymphoma. This may well be an Enteropathy Associated T-Lymphoma (EATL).

Anaemia

1. F: The operation was likely to be a partial gastrectomy and the resulting anatomy has encouraged bacterial overgrowth. Clinical and biochemical features of malabsorption are typical and a high folate is the consequence of bacterial metabolism.

2. D: The indices indicate iron deficiency with the slightly high platelet count suggestive of chronic bleeding. No lesion was identified at upper or lower gastrointestinal investigation but the bleeding evidently was recurrent. A radioisotope labelled red cell scan is sometimes helpful if bleeding is active.

3. A: Pernicious anaemia is often associated with a personal or family history of autoimmune disease. The high

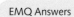
bilirubin and LDH are typical and indicate ineffective erythropoesis.

4. G: This man was probably never vaccinated against tuberculosis. The corticosteroid therapy is immunosuppressive and puts him at higher risk of tuberculosis. A monocytosis is often seen in occult infection and the mild thrombocytosis indicates chronic inflammation. Ileal disease has resulted in malabsorption of B_{12}. The differential includes Crohn's, although less likely in this case.

5. C: The gastrectomy was a curative attempt for gastric carcinoma. The pancytopenia and blood film appearances are suggestive of bone marrow infiltration by metastatic disease. Although not the commonest site for metastases, it is well recognized. Adjusted (for albumin) calcium is high.

Dysphagia

1. D: A long history of dyspepsia with more recent dysphagia without weight loss. However, weight loss can occur with benign strictures if caloric intake is unable to be maintained.

2. F: This lady has a multisystem disorder, with dysphagia, hypertension, symptoms of respiratory disease (pulmonary fibrosis) and proteinuria suggestive of renal disease. Patients with scleroderma often have recurrent episodes of aspiration pneumonia due to the dysphagia.

3. B: Progressive dysphagia and significant weight loss. Barium swallow is an alternative investigation although a biopsy for histology cannot be performed.

4. G: This patient is immunosuppressed and has had antibacterial agents putting him at risk for mucosal candidiasis. Swallowing tends to be painful. Always ask yourself why a patient has developed extensive candidiasis – think of HIV/AIDS.

5. C: A classic history of this rare condition. The episodes of chest pain are as a result of oesophageal spasm.

Abnormal liver biochemistry

1. E: Signs of cardiac failure with a characteristic enzyme pattern.

2. H: Clinical features of hepatitis A infection (palpable splenomegaly is seen in approximately 10%). ALT is moderately raised and the condition is self limiting, usually within 4 weeks.

3. F: This is a multisystem disorder with deposition of amyloid fibrils resulting in organ dysfunction. Oedema and proteinuria suggests nephrotic syndrome. Biopsy is often risky as there is an associated bleeding tendency.

4. A: The enzyme pattern, the high calcium and anaemia are suspicious of malignancy. The fracture is likely to be pathological.

5. G: Chondrocalcinosis, secondary diabetes mellitus, testicular atrophy and a 'tanned' complexion are indicative of this condition.

Jaundice

1. E: 10% of patients with ulcerative colitis have overt or subtle evidence of primary sclerosing cholangitis. It more commonly presents in males. Patients may have no bowel symptoms.

2. I: There is a personal history of thrombosis and a suggestion of a family history. This patient should have a full thrombophilia screen.

3. H: Characteristic clinical findings of infectious mononucleosis. Atypical ('viral') lymphocytes are common. The alcohol history is a red herring in this case.

4. C: Painless, progressive jaundice with extrahepatic viliary obstruction is very suspicious. Weight loss is almost universal.

5. B: Isolated hyperbilirubinaemia, more common in males, often precipitated by fasting, viral illness or dehydration.

Rectal bleeding

1. H: Bloody diarrhoea with an FBC suggestive of underlying inflammation in a young non-smoker with no recent travel history. Ulcerative colitis is most likely from the list given.

2. G: This lady has signs of chronic liver disease and has clearly had a massive bleed. Upper gastrointestinal bleeding can present with red blood PR if it is large enough due to 'intestinal hurry'.

3. A: Diverticulosis is the most likely diagnosis given the information supplied. The fullness in the LIF is the sigmoid colon loaded with faeces. Normal inflammatory markers (and the absence of diarrhoea) make active diverticulitis less likely. Carcinoma should, of course, be considered and excluded.

4. I: Amoebiasis is seen in the tropics and presents with this type of history. Cryptosporidiosis causes watery, non-bloody, diarrhoea and is self-limiting. Giardiasis causes malabsorption and not rectal bleeding.

5. C: Weight loss, PR bleeding, iron deficiency and a change in bowel habit. Note the change in bowel habit precedes the thyroxine – this is a red herring.

Indigestion

1. J: Classically worse at night or when hungry, usually localized to the epigastrium. Iron-deficiency is not usually attributable to a duodenal ulcer.

2. I: A young woman with no features of peptic ulceration or weight loss and no serological evidence of *Helicobacter pylori*.

3. A: This woman is pregnant and gives a history consistent with acid reflux.

4. G: Pain from myocardial infarction is often attributed to indigestion. The clues here are the history of hypertension and the observation of sweating (vagal mediated).

5. C: New onset dyspepsia associated with iron deficiency. She warrants an urgent endoscopy.

Abdominal distension

1. G: An acute presentation with clinical signs of bowel obstruction. She needs fluid resuscitation and urgent surgical attention.

2. A: She is likely to have nephrotic syndrome with hypoproteinaemic ascites as a consequence. A 24-hour urine collection for protein, U&Es, albumin and serum cholesterol should be performed in the first instance.

3. H: A typical history of irritable bowel syndrome. Further investigation not warranted at this stage.

4. D: Hepatomegaly, ascites, weight loss and elevated calcium (adjust for albumin). A neutrophilia can be seen in disseminated malignancy.

5. E: LFTs can be surprisingly normal in cirrhosis. He has palmar erythema, a transudative ascites and a slightly low albumin. He should be investigated for the cause of the chronic liver disease.

Weight loss

1. C: Anxiety, heat intolerance and diarrhoea in a young woman. Also ask about menstruation, examine her eyes carefully and perform an ECG.

2. F: Weight loss, iron deficiency and a possible mass in the RIF. Urgent lower gastrointestinal investigation is necessary.

3. J: The dizziness is postural hypotension, there is associated autoimmune disease (vitiligo and sister's diabetes mellitus) and the biochemical derangement is typical of steroid deficiency. Perform an early morning cortisol and seek help!

4. A: Coeliac disease has two peaks of incidence at extremes of age. The prolonged prothrombin time is due to malabsorption of vitamin K (required for synthesis of II, VII, IX, X). Malabsorption of iron and vitamin D also occurs.

5. H: Recurrence of gastric carcinoma is possible but unlikely in this case. The B_{12} deficiency and high folate are typical for bacterial overgrowth. Establish exactly what surgical procedure was performed.

Vomiting

1. C: *Staphylococcus aureus* enterotoxin is heat-stable and, classically, results in vomiting 1–4 hours after a meal.

2. I: You are told of existing end-organ damage, with reference to retinal photocoagulation. Diabetic gastroparesis can be difficult to treat effectively.

3. A: He was taking rantidine empirically for symptoms of duodenal ulceration. Outflow obstruction has now occurred, with a characteristic biochemical derangement.

4. G: Chronic renal failure often presents in a 'non-specific' way. She has been itchy and is hypertensive with oedema. The aetiology is chronic pyelonephritis (prophylactic antibiotics for recurrent urinary infection).

5. H: The aetiology of the small bowel obstruction is adhesions, as a consequence of previous intra-abdominal surgery. Also remember to check the hernial orifices. U&Es reflect vomiting and dehydration.

Infections of the gastrointestinal tract

1. J: The parasite has its major reservoir in cattle and usually spread via contaminated water. Unless immunocompromised (e.g. HIV), the disease is usually self-limiting.

2. G: Significant intravascular volume loss with resultant renal failure and electrolyte loss. Tetracycline can shorten the duration of the illness.

3. K: Specific antibodies can be detected in the serum and sigmoidoscopy reveals mucosal inflammation (not in itself diagnostic). Urticaria is a clue to diagnosis here.

4. B: Tuberculosis of terminal ileum with resultant B_{12} malabsorption. Resistant organisms can be a problem in those with HIV.

5. E: Sepsis, abnormal LFTs, the effusion at the right base is reactive. Pyogenic favoured over amoebic as diverticulitis a potential source (bacteraemia via the portal circulation).

Adverse drug effects and toxicity on the gastrointestinal tract

1. F: There are signs of intravascular volume loss (dizzy on standing and tachycardia). He is taking aspirin 75 mg as primary prevention of coronary or cerebral vascular events.

2. H: Not easy! Metformin often causes diarrhoea and should be used with particular care in those with renal (and liver) impairment. The diarrhoea has caused dehydration, renal impairment, metformin toxicity and a lactic acidosis.

3. A: Early signs of digoxin toxicity. The dizziness could be cardiac dysrhythmia. (Ventricular arrhythmias can be fatal).

4. C: A bacterial infection such as folliculitis is often treated with flucloxacillin to cover skin staphylococci. Both the thrush and jaundice are consequences of this treatment. The liver enzyme abnormalities may take many weeks to resolve after cessation of the offending drug.

5. B: A clue is the **previous** history of atrial fibrillation. The anti-arrhythmic drug is clearly maintaining sinus rhythm. Jaundice and hepatitis can be seen. Dose reduction or withdrawal may be necessary.

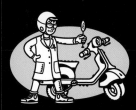
1. The history suggests a benign, fibrotic, oesophageal stricture on a background of long-standing reflux oesophagitis. However, you should include carcinoma and achalasia in your differential. Consider the duration and progression of dysphagia and seek to quantity the weight loss. Clinical examination is often unrewarding in this setting but should always be performed, as a positive finding may clinch the diagnosis. See Chapter 14 for a comprehensive investigation strategy, but endoscopy is clearly indicated here and a histological diagnosis should be sought.

2. Acute right iliac fossa pain is a common clinical scenario with which you should be familiar. The points to note here are that she has systemic upset evidenced by fever and tachycardia. The important diagnoses to consider in a young female are acute appendicitis, ectopic pregnancy, Crohn's disease, tubo-ovarian abscess and salpingitis. There is evidence of localized peritonitis. Investigations should be performed as for any acute abdomen (see Chapter 3), but should include a pregnancy test, an urgent abdominal ultrasound, blood and urine cultures. Intravenous fluid resuscitation and broad spectrum antibiotics are indicated. Do not forget pain relief!

3. Recent onset ascites and jaundice. The history of dyspnoea may lead you to think of a primary cardiac cause: constrictive pericarditis is a possibility (history of rheumatic fever or tuberculosis?) or congestive cardiac failure (unlikely in a woman of this age). Hepatic vein thrombosis can cause 'acute' ascites but is usually associated with pain and would not necessarily explain the dyspnoea (unless pulmonary emboli had resulted). Obviously, a primary liver problem should not be discounted, although the history is short and the dyspnoea is not readily explained. Investigation should include haematological and biochemical indices, an ECG and echocardiogram. Ascitic fluid for protein content may be helpful. A liver ultrasound with colour Doppler to assess vein patency is also indicated. These investigations should, of course, be anteceded by a thorough clinical examination!

4. You should immediately think of coeliac disease. The history is suggestive of steatorrhoea, hypoalbuminaemic oedema and dermatitis herpetiformis. See Chapter 16 for details, but specific investigations should include anti-endomyseal antibody and a duodenal biopsy as the 'gold standard' diagnostic test. Haematological and biochemical evidence of malabsorption should be sought. Management should comprise a gluten-free diet and vitamin replacement where necessary. If the rash does not respond well to dietary restrictions, dapsone can be used.

5. The history is suggestive of small intestinal pathology. Inflammatory bowel disease, coeliac disease and infective aetiologies should be considered. Chronic pancreatitis is also a possibility. Small intestinal malignancies, including lymphoma, are rare causes. Look for evidence of malabsorption, check FBC, biochemistry and inflammatory markers, consider upper gastrointestinal endoscopy (with biopsy) and small bowel imaging such as a barium follow-through. Abdominal X-ray may show pancreatic calcification. Do not forget to send stool for microscopy and culture.

6. A history of alternating diarrhoea and constipation, abdominal pain that is relieved by defecation, abdominal distension and bloating. These features would support a diagnosis of irritable bowel syndrome. Features of depression may also be present. However, a history of protracted diarrhoea, rectal bleeding (may be mixed with the stool), weight loss, cramping abdominal pain and fever would prompt further investigation for inflammatory bowel disease. Examination may reveal extra-intestinal manifestations of inflammatory bowel disease or positive abdominal findings, such as a right iliac fossa mass (Crohn's). FBC, biochemistry and inflammatory markers are often helpful in the first instance. Lower gastrointestinal endoscopy or barium studies may then be performed. The former allows opportunity for biopsy.

7. In the context of a history of chronic blood loss and weight loss, the finding of a duodenal ulcer should not be accepted as the aetiological culprit. Duodenal ulcers rarely cause significant iron-deficiency. The duodenum should be biopsied to exclude coeliac disease. The lower gastrointestinal tract should also be investigated to include the caecum (colonoscopy or barium enema). As an additional point, the patient's *Helicobacter pylori* status should be established and triple therapy eradication instituted if positive.

8. You should discuss common symptomatic problems such as diarrhoea, proposed mechanisms, and how to address them (bile salt diarrhoea and bacterial overgrowth). Anaemia is a late, common complication usually resulting from haematinic deficiency (B_{12} +/− iron). Describe the features of each. Malabsorption is often seen and may manifest in numerous guises (see Chapter 15). 'Mechanical'

problems such as afferent loop syndrome (rare) can be mentioned, as should the increased risk of carcinoma that is observed.

9. Carcinoid syndrome fits with the clinical picture and ultrasound findings. Clinical features can also include bronchospasm and cardiac lesions (seen in 50%). The tumour originates from APUD (amine precursor uptake and decarboxylation) cells. Common primary sites include the appendix, terminal ileum and rectum. The hormones most commonly secreted are serotonin (5-HT), bradykinin and histamines. The syndrome is only seen in those with liver metastases (see Hints and Tips 20.5). Diagnosis can be supported by detecting the major metabolite of serotonin in the urine or by radioisotope techniques. See Chapter 16 for further details.

10. The history is strongly suggestive of achalasia. Presentation in childhood is unusual. This rare condition also commonly presents with chest pain as a result of oesophageal spasm. Dysphagia can also be overcome by drinking large quantities of fluid (with the risk of aspiration). Endoscopy can be useful to obtain biopsy, although can sometimes miss the oesophageal narrowing. An endoscopic ultrasound is helpful in excluding malignant infiltration, should this be suspected. Specific treatment can include balloon dilatation or surgical division of muscle fibres. Calcium channel-blockers can reduce oesophageal spasm and can be useful in elderly patients who may not be suitable for invasive procedures. The risk of carcinoma is significantly higher and reflux oesophagitis is common following treatment.